Atlas of Laparoscopic Gynecological Anatomy

Helizabet Salomão Ayroza • Paulo Ayroza Ribeiro
Editors

Atlas of Laparoscopic Gynecological Anatomy

Springer

Editors
Helizabet Salomão Ayroza
Obstetrics and Gynecology Department
Faculdade de Ciências Médicas da Santa
São Paulo, Brazil

Paulo Ayroza Ribeiro
Obstetrics and Gynecology Department
Faculdade de Ciências Médicas da Santa
São Paulo, Brazil

ISBN 978-3-031-63522-9 ISBN 978-3-031-63520-5 (eBook)
https://doi.org/10.1007/978-3-031-63520-5

This Springer imprint is published by the registered company Springer Nature Switzerland AG
The registered company address is: Gewerbestrasse 11, 6330 Cham, Switzerland

Foreword

It is an honor for me to write the foreword of a book written by Prof. Dr. Paulo Ayroza Ribeiro and Prof. Dr. Helizabeth Salomao Abdalha Ayroza Ribeiro and their collaborators.

With them, I am united by the bonds of teacher, student, friend, and partner, with total complicity in the development of knowledge and conception of life; we are even compadres. This has been a long time ago.

Since the beginning of laparoscopic surgery, a time we had the privilege of seeing, the priority was the specific instruments, then the indications for the use of this approach, and the surgical training of the team.

With the passing of time, the instrumental development and the use of technological advances have been splendid, the indications were and are already well defined, and much progress has been made in the teaching of the surgical technique and the training of those who are initiated in the laparoscopic surgical technique.

We have always wished to have an anatomy book with a laparoscopic view, with all that this means, very necessary, current, and very useful.

This is a great opportunity, the presentation of an absolutely necessary book, which goes to the most essential part of surgery, which is the anatomical knowledge, to be able to recognize it in each surgical act, with the identification of the anatomical repairs, the spaces they delimit, and the structures they contain.

The "Atlas of Gynecological Laparoscopic Surgical Anatomy" is an excellent work, with its nine chapters: Abdominal and Pelvic Wall, Abdominopelvic Organs, Fascia and Ligaments, Pelvic Floor, Pelvic Spaces, Pelvic Irrigation, Pelvic Innervation, Retroperitoneum: Digestive System, and Retroperitoneum: Urinary System.

It is a characteristic and an objective of our teaching group to transmit our knowledge with the best possible quality, with generosity and humility. In this "Atlas of Gynecologic Laparoscopic Surgical Anatomy," I consider that this objective has been achieved.

I recommend consulting it systematically before each surgery. My most sincere congratulations.

Instituto Callao
Buenos Ayres, Argentina

Leopoldo Carlos Videla Rivero

Message from the Editors

> I will praise you, because I have been formed in such an admirable way; wonderful are your works, and my soul knows it very well.
>
> (Psalms 139:14, Almeida Atualizada)

Through the body, we come into contact with the world, and also through it, the world invades the soul. Alongside science goes art, and, through art, the beauty of transformation. Human anatomy has been portrayed and revered by masters of art with a doctor's soul, such as Leonardo da Vinci, Raffaello Sanzio, Michelangelo Buonarroti, Titian, and Rembrandt, who, with their brush, quill, or chisel, have exalted the human form and made it easier to study and understand human anatomy.

From Vitruvian Man, through Leonardo da Vinci's Last Supper, to David, a masterpiece by Michelangelo, where the structure of a leg is dissected to perfection, we come to the ceiling of the Sistine Chapel, with biblical passages in large proportions and anatomically correct characters.

The forms are camouflaged, shown by gestures, by angels, and perfection is made.

It is fascinating! I was mesmerized the first time I saw it. Michelangelo considered himself essentially a sculptor, dissatisfied with having to use brushes. He was given a few dues to paint the ceiling of the chapel, but he tried to perform his function with primacy.

Artists sought the proportion of beauty that would bring the world of men and the universe of the gods closer together.

Michelangelo had the theory that the real thing cannot be seen. He spent 20 years engaged in anatomical dissections—largely performed in the Basilica of the Holy Spirit in Florence, Italy—in search of knowledge. And if the real thing could not be seen, he tried and succeeded to portray the real thing through his noble art. He incredibly portrayed various human forms in his paintings.

> Nowhere does God show Himself more to me in His grace than in some beautiful human form. And that alone I love, for in that He mirrors Himself.
>
> Michelangelo

To heal surgically, based on anatomical knowledge, to warm the heart torn by pain, and to reassure the soul restless by the certainty of good-bye is to love the other as yourself. This atlas shows the beautiful human form and its anatomical landmarks and also brings the way and the strategy to treat the disease, preserving such a beautiful form, the human body.

Helizabet Salomão Ayroza
Paulo Ayroza Ribeiro

Acknowledgments

To God, who has granted us, by his infinite goodness, the gifts of teaching and pain relief.

To the co-authors for their friendship and for making their knowledge available for this work.

To the NAVEG group, which allowed us to transmit our knowledge, forming this group of friends who are involved, dedicated, and accomplices in the art of teaching.

"One swallow alone does not make summer!" Together we are a team, a strong current!

Contents

Contributors

Mauricio Simões Abrão Hospital Beneficência Portuguesa of São Paulo (HBPSP), São Paulo, Brazil

Department of Obstetrics and Gynecology, School of Medicine, University of São Paulo (FMUSP), São Paulo, Brazil

Fernanda de Almeida Asencio Santa Casa de Misericórdia de São Paulo (SCMSP), São Paulo, Brazil

FEBRASGO (Brazilian Society of Obstetri s and Gynecology), São Paulo, Brazil

Albert Einstein Hospital, São Paulo, Brazil

Priscila de Almeida Barbosa Faculty of Medicine, University of São Paulo (FMUSP), São Paulo, Brazil

Invasive Gynecologic Surgery Program, Hospital Beneficência Portuguesa of São Paulo (HBPSP), São Paulo, Brazil

Ricardo de Almeida Quintairos Brazilian Federation of Gynecology and Obstetrics Associations (FEBRASGO), São Paulo, Brazil

Helizabet Salomão Ayroza Obstetrics and Gynecology Department, Faculdade de Ciências Médicas da Santa Casa de Misericórdia de São Paulo (SCMSP), São Paulo, Brazil

Gynecological Endoscopy and Endometriosis Division, Santa Casa de São Paulo Hospital, São Paulo, Brazil

Paulo Ayroza Ribeiro Brazilian Federation of Gynecology and Obstetrics Associations (FEBRASGO), São Paulo, Brazil

Department of Obstetrics and Gynecology, School of Medical Sciences, Santa Casa de Misericórida São Paulo (SCMSP), São Paulo, Brazil

Department of Obstetrics and Gynecology, Santa Casa de São Paulo School of Medical Sciences, São Paulo, Brazil

Camila Veckhaouser Calegari FEBRASGO (Brazilian Society of Obstetri s and Gynecology), São Paulo, Brazil

Daniel Bier Caraça Hospital Israelita Albert Einstein (HIAE), São Paulo, Brazil

Faculty of Medicine, University of São Paulo (FMUSP), São Paulo, Brazil

Hospital das Clínicas of the Medical School of the University of São Paulo (HCF-MUSP), São Paulo, Brazil

Graziele Vidoto Cervantes Ob/Gyn Department, Santa Casa de São Paulo School of Medical Sciences, São Paulo, Brazil

Brazilian Federation of Gynecology and Obstetrics Associations (FEBRASGO), São Paulo, Brazil

Beatriz Taliberti da Costa Porto Santa Casa São Paulo School of Medical Sciences (SCMSP), São Paulo, Brazil

Brazilian Federation of Gynecology and Obstetrics Associations (FEBRASGO), São Paulo, Brazil

Raquel Silveira da Cunha Araújo Federal University of Paraíba (UFPB), João Pessoa, Brazil

Brazilian Federation of Gynecology and Obstetrics Associations (FEBRASGO), São Paulo, Brazil

Faculty of Medical Sciences, Santa Casa de Misericórdia de São Paulo (SCMSP), São Paulo, Brazil

Adriano Silva Farah Santa Casa de Misericórdia de São Paulo (SCMSP), São Paulo, Brazil

Brazilian Federation of Gynecology and Obstetrics Associations (FEBRASGO), São Paulo, Brazil

Gustavo Leme Fernandes Faculty of Medical Sciences, Santa Casa de Misericórdia de São Paulo (SCMSP), São Paulo, Brazil

Santa Casa de São Paulo School of Medical Sciences, São Paulo, Brazil

Department of Obstetrics and Gynaecology, Faculty of Medicine, University of Toronto, Toronto, ON, Canada

Department of Gynecology, Paulista School of Medicine, Federal University of São Paulo (EPM/UNIFESP), São Paulo, Brazil

Rodrigo Fernandes Cancer Institute of the State of São Paulo - University of São Paulo Medical School (FMUSP), São Paulo, Brazil

Luciano Gibran FEBRASGO (Brazilian Society of Obstetri s and Gynecology), São Paulo, Brazil

Faculty of Medicine, University of São Paulo (FMUSP), São Paulo, Brazil

Anna Luiza Lobão Gonçalves Gynecological Endoscopy and Endometriosis Division, Faculty of Medical Sciences, Santa Casa de Misericórdia de São Paulo (SCMSP), São Paulo, Brazil

Santa Casa de Sao Paulo School of Medical Sciences, São Paulo, Brazil

Brazilian Federation of Gynecological and Obstetrical Associations (FEBRAS-GO), São Paulo, Brazil

Gil Kamergorodsky Santa Casa de Sao Paulo School of Medical Sciences (FCMSCSP), São Paulo, Brazil

Brazilian Federation of Gynecology and Obstetrics Associations (FEBRASGO), São Paulo, Brazil

Fábio Sakae Kuteken Brazilian Federation of Gynecology and Obstetrics Associations (FEBRASGO), São Paulo, Brazil

Faculty of Medical Sciences, Santa Casa São Paulo School of Medical Sciences (SCMSP), São Paulo, Brazil

Guilherme Karam Corrêa Leite Brazilian Federation of Associations of Gynecology and Obstetrics (FEBRASGO), Santos, Brazil

Faculdade de Ciências Médicas da Universidade Metropolitana de Santos (UNIMES), Santos, Brazil

Faculty of Medical Sciences, Santa Casa de Misericórdia de São Paulo (SCMSP), São Paulo, Brazil

Hospital Ana Costa de Santos/United Health Group (UHG), Santos, Brazil

Nucélio Barros Moreira Lemos Department of Obstetrics and Gynaecology, Faculty of Medicine, University of Toronto, Toronto, ON, Canada

Department of Gynecology, Paulista School of Medicine, Federal University of São Paulo (EPM/UNIFESP), São Paulo, Brazil

Raquel Ferreira Lima Brazilian Federation of Gynecological and Obstetrical Associations (FEBRAS-GO), São Paulo, Brazil

Faculty of Medical Sciences, Santa Casa de Misericórdia de São Paulo (SCMSP), São Paulo, Brazil

Marina Miyuki Maekawa Santa Casa São Paulo School of Medical Sciences (SCMSP), São Paulo, Brazil

Brazilian Federation of Gynecology and Obstetrics Associations (FEBRASGO), São Paulo, Brazil

Augusta Morgado Brazilian Federation of Associations of Gynecology and Obstetrics (FEBRASGO), São Paulo, Brazil

Pelvic Neuropsychiatric Outpatient Clinic of the Urogynecology Section of the Gynecology Department of the Federal University of São Paulo, São Paulo, Brazil

Fabio Ohara Santa Casa de Misericórdia de São Paulo (SCMSP), São Paulo, Brazil

Brazilian Federation of Gynecology and Obstetrics Associations (FEBRASGO), São Paulo, Brazil

Andresa Maria Felipe de Paiva Ob/Gyn Department, Santa Casa de São Paulo School of Medical Sciences, São Paulo, Brazil

Brazilian Federation of Gynecology and Obstetrics Associations (FEBRASGO), São Paulo, Brazil

Marina de Paula Andres Endometriosis Department, University of São Paulo School of Medicine Hospital das Clínicas (HC-FMUSP), São Paulo, Brazil

Hospital Beneficência Portuguesa of São Paulo (HBPSP), São Paulo, Brazil

Sérgio Podgaec Department of Gynecology and Obstetrics, School of Medicine, University of São Paulo (FMUSP), São Paulo, Brazil

Albert Einstein Hospital and School of Medicine Education, São Paulo, Brazil

Francisco Cesar Rodrigues Ob/Gyn Department, Santa Casa de Sao Paulo School of Medical Sciences, São Paulo, Brazil

Mariana Rossette Federal University of São Paulo (UNIFESP), Albert Einstein Hospital, São Paulo, Brazil

Rômulo Müller dos Santos Melo Brazilian Federation of Gynecology and Obstetrics Associations (FEBRASGO), São Paulo, Brazil

Fundação Santa Casa de Misericórdia do Pará (FSCMPA), Belém, Brazil

Eduardo Schor Gynecology Department, Escola Paulista de Medicina of the Universidade Federal de São Paulo (EPM-UNIFESP), São Paulo, Brazil

Deusdedit Cortez Vieira da Silva Neto Rede D'Or Sao Luiz, São Paulo, Brazil

Mariano Tamura Federal University of São Paulo (UNIFESP), Albert Einstein Hospital, São Paulo, Brazil

Uterine Myoma Outpatient Clinic, Escola Pau-list de Medicina da Universidade Federal de São Paulo (EPM/UNIFESP), São Paulo, Brazil

Ludimila Neris Teles Tatsu Santa Casa de Sao Paulo School of Medical Sciences (FCMSCSP), São Paulo, Brazil

Brazilian Federation of Gynecology and Obstetrics Associations (FEBRASGO), São Paulo, Brazil

Mariana Carpenedo Tomasi Santa Casa de Misericórdia de São Paulo (SCMSP), São Paulo, Brazil

Brazilian Federation of Gynecology and Obstetrics Associations (FEBRASGO), São Paulo, Brazil

Aline Estefanes Eras Yonamine Department of Obstetrics and Gynecology, Santa Casa de Misericórdia de São Paulo (ISCMSP), São Paulo, Brazil

Santa Casa de Sao Paulo School of Medical Sciences (FCMSCSP), São Paulo, Brazil

Brazilian Federation of Gynecology and Obstetrics Associations (FEBRASGO), São Paulo, Brazil

Chapter 1
Abdominal and Pelvic Wall

Aline Estefanes Eras Yonamine, Eduardo Schor, Gil Kamergorodsky, Ludimila Neris Teles Tatsu, Mariana Rossette, and Mariano Tamura

Quick Tips

The anterior abdominal wall is the first barrier to be crossed for surgical access, and the mastery of this anatomy is fundamental to reduce risks. Puncture accidents

Supplementary Information The online version contains supplementary material available at https://doi.org/10.1007/978-3-031-63520-5_1.

A. E. E. Yonamine (✉)
Department of Obstetrics and Gynecology, Santa Casa de Misericórdia de São Paulo (ISCMSP), São Paulo, Brazil

Santa Casa de Sao Paulo School of Medical Sciences (FCMSCSP), São Paulo, Brazil

Brazilian Federation of Gynecology and Obstetrics Associations (FEBRASGO), São Paulo, Brazil

E. Schor · L. N. T. Tatsu
Gynecology Department, Escola Paulista de Medicina of the Universidade Federal de São Paulo (EPM-UNIFESP), São Paulo, Brazil

G. Kamergorodsky
Santa Casa de Sao Paulo School of Medical Sciences (FCMSCSP), São Paulo, Brazil

Brazilian Federation of Gynecology and Obstetrics Associations (FEBRASGO), São Paulo, Brazil

M. Rossette
Federal University of Minas Gerais (UFMG), Belo Horizonte, Brazil

Federal University of São Paulo (UNIFESP), Albert Einstein Hospital, São Paulo, Brazil

M. Tamura
Federal University of São Paulo (UNIFESP), Albert Einstein Hospital, São Paulo, Brazil

Uterine Myoma Outpatient Clinic, Escola Pau-list de Medicina da Universidade Federal de São Paulo (EPM/UNIFESP), São Paulo, Brazil

H. Salomão Ayroza, P. Ayroza Ribeiro (eds.), *Atlas of Laparoscopic Gynecological Anatomy*, https://doi.org/10.1007/978-3-031-63520-5_1

account for over 50% of complications in laparoscopy (1) and may cause delays, sequelae, or change in the procedure. The preferred positioning for the main trocar is the umbilical scar, where there is complete fusion of the skin with the peritoneum and with a shorter distance to be covered by the trocar. The distance from the umbilical scar to the great vessels may vary according to the BMI and the patient's positioning, important criteria for the adoption of the most appropriate technique. The lateral punctures should take into account the path of the vessels that compose the superficial and deep irrigation networks, especially the inferior epigastric artery, a branch of the external iliac artery, and the main blood supply of the anterior wall. This vessel ascends medially to the internal inguinal canal and travels below the transverse fascia, composing the lateral peritoneal fold, toward the umbilical scar. As it crosses the lateral border of the rectus abdominis muscle, at the arcuate line, it is susceptible to injury during insertion of the lateral trocars. At this site, there may also be nerve injury, especially to the iliohypogastric and ilioinguinal nerves, which pass medially to the anterosuperior iliac crest.

General Vision

The abdominal wall protects the abdominopelvic organs from the outside environment. It is the first barrier to be overcome for successful surgery. An entry accident early in the videolaparoscopy represents a delay in surgical time and stress to surgeons and, in extreme cases, can determine the end of the surgery, without the proposed procedure having been performed.

Although every procedure carries inherent risk, full mastery of the structures that make up the abdominal wall can minimize the risk of first puncture accidents, one of the main complications in laparoscopic procedures.

Anatomic Limits and Landmarks

The limits of the abdomen are superiorly, the inferior border of the ribs and the xiphoid process; inferiorly, the iliac crests, the inguinal line, and the pubic bone; and posterolaterally, the lumbar spine and adjacent muscles.

The midline, located between the xiphoid process of the sternum and the pubic symphysis, indicates the position of the linea alba, a dense tensile stripe that divides the anterior abdominal wall into right and left halves. The semilunar lines, two curved grooves observed about 5–8 cm either side of the midline, demarcate the lateral border of the rectus abdominis muscle (Fig. 1.1).

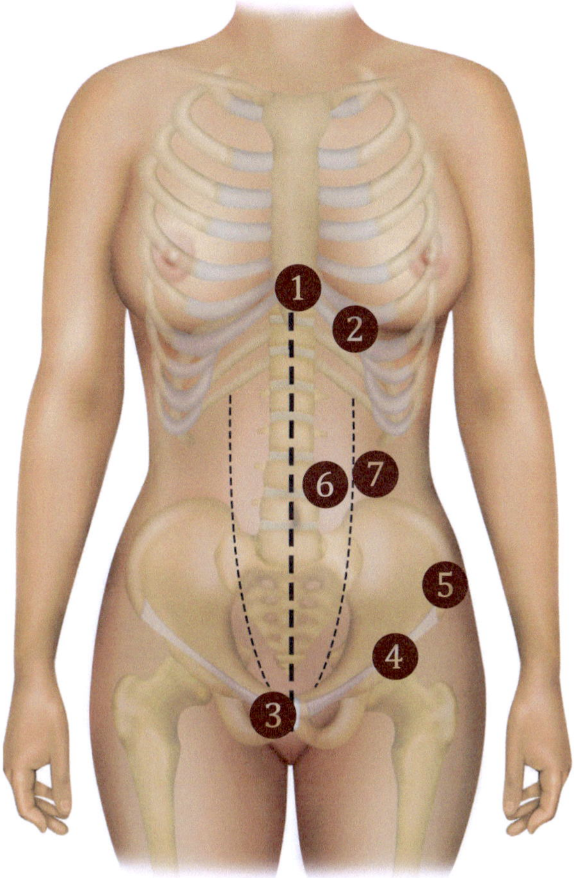

Fig. 1.1 Anatomical boundaries and landmarks of the abdomen. (1) Xiphoid process of the sternum, (2) inferior edge of the ribs, (3) pubis, (4) inguinal ligament, (5) iliac crest, (6) linea alba, (7) semilunar lines

Umbilical Scar

Generally, the most evident structure of the lower abdominal wall, the umbilicus, represents a defect in the linea alba, which, during gestation, allows the passage of blood vessels toward the placenta. Its location may vary, with a tendency to be lower in children and the elderly, but, in general, it is located at the level of the intervertebral disc, between the L3 and L4 vertebrae, midway between the xiphoid process and the pubic symphysis (Fig. 1.2).

For laparoscopic surgeons, a complete understanding of this structure is especially important, as it is the preferred site for positioning the main trocar, and, in the closed technique of first puncture, the entry of the laparoscopic trocar will occur without direct vision.

The umbilicus is the only place where there is complete fusion of the skin with the peritoneum and therefore the place with the shortest distance to be covered by the trocar, which facilitates the technique. With the patient in horizontal dorsal

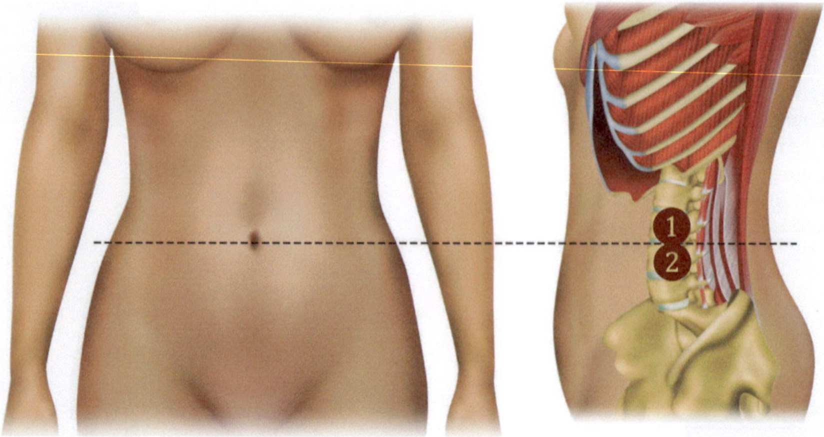

Fig. 1.2 The umbilical scar is located between the L3 and L4 vertebrae. (1) L3 vertebra, (2) L4 vertebra

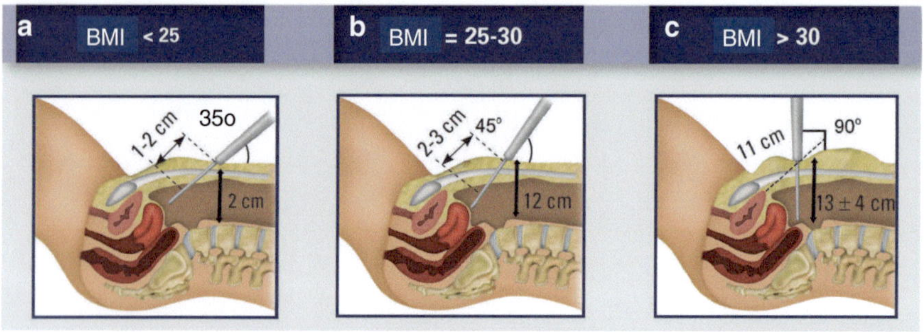

Fig. 1.3 Relationship between BMI and distance from the umbilicus to the great vessels; (a) distance from the wall to the vessels (2 cm, 12 cm, and 13 ± 4 cm); (b) the distance the trocar needs to travel to enter the cavity 1–2, 2–3, and 11 cm; (c) angulation of the trocar (35°, 45°, and 90°)

decubitus, the distance from the umbilicus to the great vessels is variable and can be estimated according to the body mass index (BMI). This distance can vary from only 2 cm in thin patients to about 13 cm in obese patients (Figs. 1.3 and 1.4).

Tips and Tricks 1 and 2

1. In thin or overweight patients, the infraumbilical abdominal wall should be well elevated, and the needle should form a 45° angle with the horizontal plane (Fig. 1.4). In obese patients, it is recommended to maintain an angle of about 90° with the horizontal plane, because with a smaller angle, there is a higher risk of failure due to the thickness of the skin, which can be up to 11 cm (Fig. 1.3).
2. To minimize the risk of injury to large vessels, the first puncture should always be performed with the patient in horizontal dorsal decubitus and always respecting the most appropriate angulation for her physical size. Only after

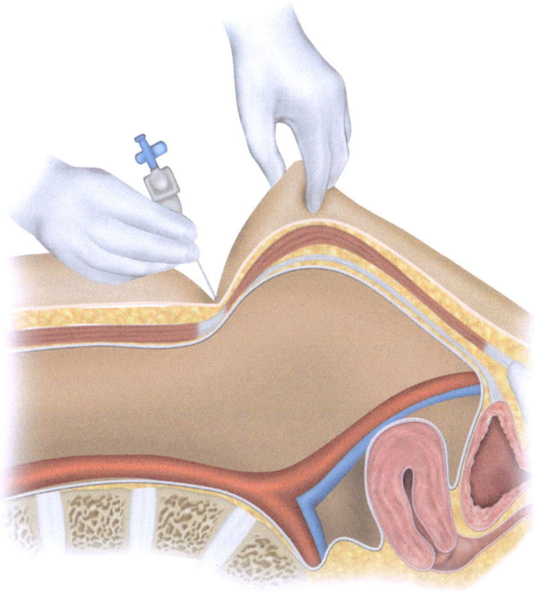

Fig. 1.4 In nonobese patients, the infraumbilical abdominal wall should be elevated well, and the needle should form a 45° angle with the horizontal plane

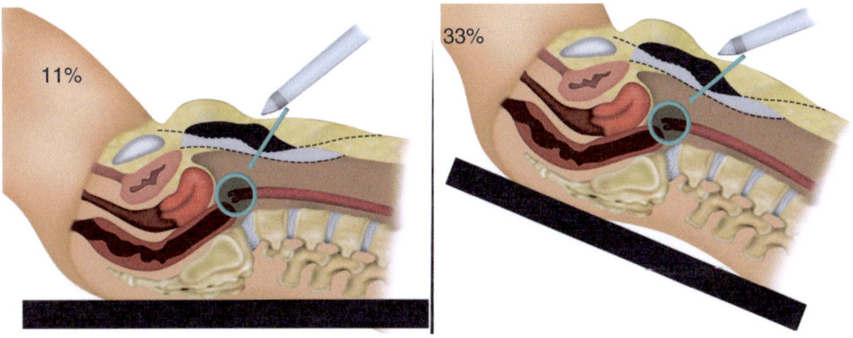

Fig. 1.5 Relation between umbilicus and bifurcation of the aorta according to the angulation of the operating table. The great vessels are located caudal to the umbilicus in 11% of the patients in DDH and in 33% of the patients in reverse Trendelenburg

entering and reviewing the puncture site should the patient be placed in reverse Trendelenburg position.

Another factor to be observed during the first puncture is the positioning of the patient. It has been shown that the location of the aortic bifurcation varies greatly according to the angulation of the table. In the supine position, the bifurcation is caudal to the umbilicus in 11% of the cases; in reverse Trendelenburg position, this occurs in 33% of the cases. This difference was statistically significant and unrelated to BMI (Fig. 1.5).

Abdominal Wall Layers

Skin: The skin fibers in the abdominal region are predominantly transverse in direction, with a slight upward curvature laterally, which results in greater tendency to put the skin under tension in vertical incisions, which can lead to wider scars.

Subcutaneous cellular tissue: Just below the skin, the subcutaneous tissue is identified, composed of adipose tissue and supported by several thin fibrous septa. In its most superficial portion, called Camper's fascia (or adipose panicle of the abdomen), there is a predominance of fat tissue.

In its deeper portion, Scarpa's fascia (or subcutaneous membranous stratum), the fibrous tissue predominates over the fatty tissue, and inexperienced surgeons should be careful not to confuse it with the aponeurosis of the rectus abdominis muscle, especially laterally, where this layer is more developed.

Musculoaponeurotic layer: Below the subcutaneous tissue lies a layer of fibrous tissue and muscles that not only protects the intra-abdominal organs but also allows movement of the back.

The anterolateral wall of the abdomen has five pairs of muscles: two vertical muscles and three flat muscles. Laterally to the rectus abdominis muscle are the three flank muscles, whose fascia joins to form an aponeurosis that covers the rectus abdominis (Fig. 1.6).

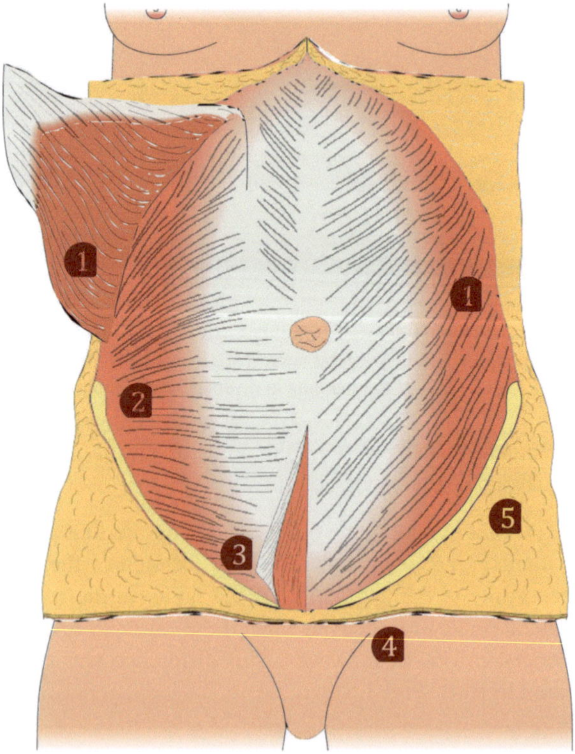

Fig. 1.6 Muscle for the abdominal wall: (1) external oblique muscle; (2) internal oblique muscle; (3) pyramidal muscle; (4) inguinal ligament; (5) anterosuperior iliac crest

The most superficial of the flat muscles is the external oblique, whose oblique fibers run inferomedially. It originates in the last costal cartilages (V–XII) and attaches to the linea alba, the pubic tubercle, and the anterior half of the iliac crest.

Below the external oblique muscle, another flat muscle is located, the internal oblique muscle, whose fibers, also oblique, are connected to the external oblique. Its fibers, also oblique, originate in the thoracolumbar fascia and iliac crest and run superior medially toward the last costal cartilages (X–XII), the linea alba, and the pubic pectineal line.

For the most part, the fibers of these two muscles are arranged perpendicular to each other, although they run, in the lower region, almost in the same direction.

The transverse abdominis, also a flat muscle, is the deepest of the anterior wall muscles, and its transversely oriented fibers originate in the thoracolumbar fascia, the last costal cartilages, and the iliac crest, inserting in the linea alba and the pubic crest.

The most caudal part of the internal oblique fuses with the transverse abdominis, which is why in transverse incisions, only two muscle layers are distinguished in the lateral regions.

It is between the internal oblique and transverse muscles that the nerves and blood vessels of the flanks are located, which is called the **neurovascular plane** of the anterolateral wall. In the anterior portion of the abdominopelvic wall, however, these nerves and vessels leave the neurovascular plane and are located mainly in the subcutaneous tissue (Fig. 1.7).

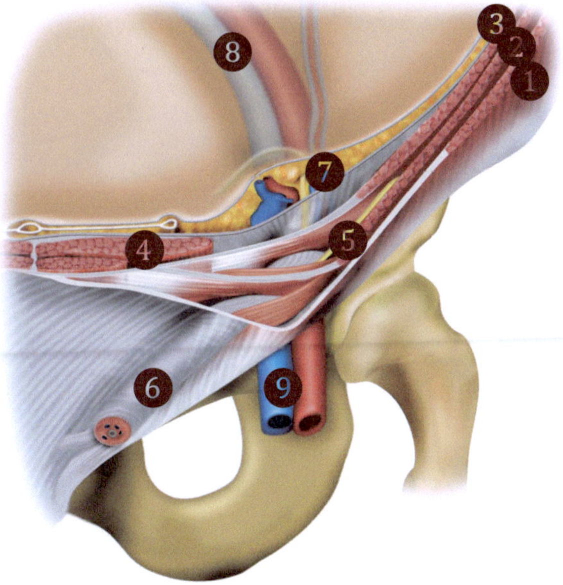

Fig. 1.7 Between the internal oblique and transverse muscles is located the neurovascular plane of the anterolateral wall. (1) External oblique muscle; (2) internal oblique muscle; (3) transverse abdominis muscle; (4) rectus abdominis muscle; (5) ilioinguinal nerve; (6) inguinal canal; (7) inferior epigastric vessels; (8) external iliac vessels; (9) femoral vessels

Medially, the muscle fibers of these three muscles become aponeurotic, forming sheets of tendinous fibers that cross and interlace at the midline, forming the linea alba.

It is interesting to understand that most of the fibers on one side of the linea alba continue with fibers that follow the same direction on the other side. Thus, the contralateral internal and external oblique muscles together form a "digastric muscle," with two bellies and a common tendon, which act as a unit to allow the main movements of the trunk (Fig. 1.8).

The rectus abdominis is a muscle with vertically directed fibers, positioned laterally to the midline and covered by the sheath formed by the aponeuroses of the flat muscles (external oblique, internal oblique, and transverse abdominis). This muscle

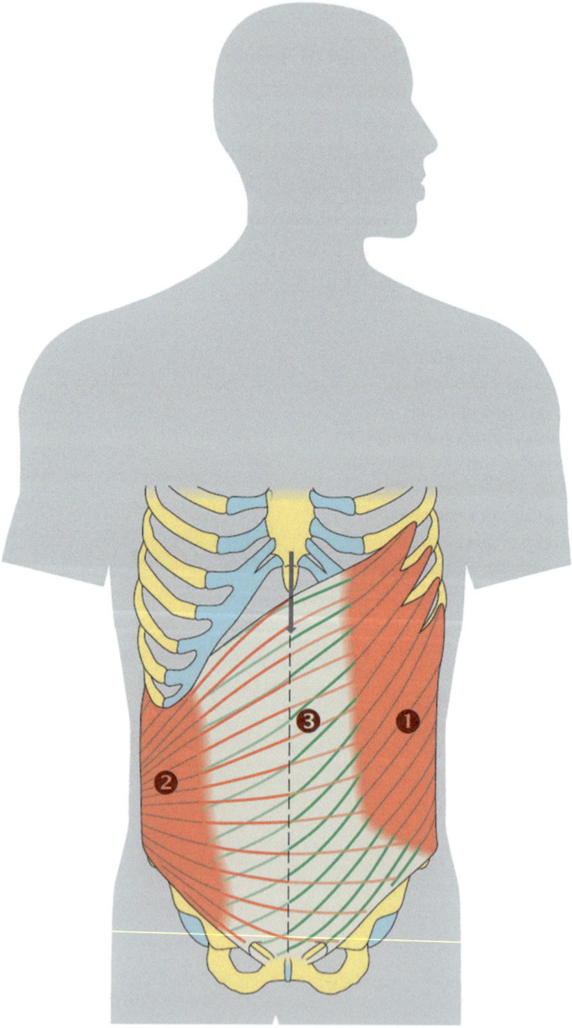

Fig. 1.8 The contralateral internal and external oblique muscles work as a "digastric muscle," with two ventricles and one common tendon: (1) external oblique muscle; (2) internal oblique muscle; (3) linea alba

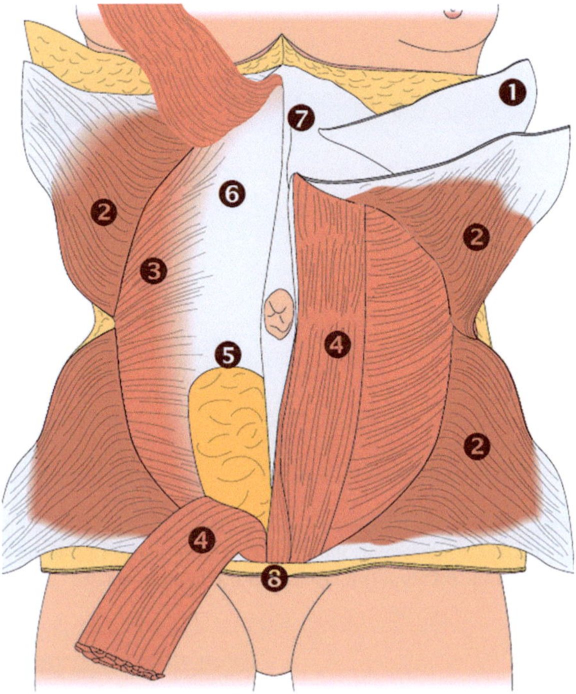

Fig. 1.9 Muscles of the abdominal wall and dorsal sheath. (1) External oblique muscle; (2) internal oblique muscle; (3) transversus abdominis muscle; (4) rectus abdominis muscle; (5) arched line; (6) posterior leaflet of the rectus abdominis sheath; (7) anterior leaflet of the rectus abdominis sheath; (8) pyramidal muscle

has three tendinous insertions that ensure its attachment to this sheath, usually located above the navel. These sheaths should not be cut, as they are crossed by cutaneous nerves and by branches of the superior epigastric artery.

The second muscle of vertical direction, the pyramidal muscle, originates in the pubis and inserts in the linea alba, a few centimeters above the pubic symphysis. These are small, triangular shaped muscles of little importance, absent in 20% of people (Fig. 1.9).

The aponeuroses of the flat muscles stretch anteriorly and fuse together to form the rectus abdominis sheath. The conformation of the rectus abdominis sheath varies in different regions. This variation is limited by the arched line, a crescentic border, not visible under the skin, located midway between the umbilicus and the pubic bone.

Below the arched line, all aponeuroses of the three muscles (external oblique, internal oblique, and transverse oblique) pass anteriorly to the rectus abdominis muscle, so that its posterior surface is in direct contact with the transversalis fascia.

Above the arched line, the aponeurosis of the internal oblique muscle divides into two: its anterior leaflet fuses with the aponeurosis of the external oblique to pass anteriorly to the rectus abdominis muscle. Its posterior leaflet fuses with the aponeurosis of the transverse and passes posteriorly to the rectus muscle, which is therefore completely covered (anteriorly and posteriorly) by its sheath (Figs. 1.10 and 1.11).

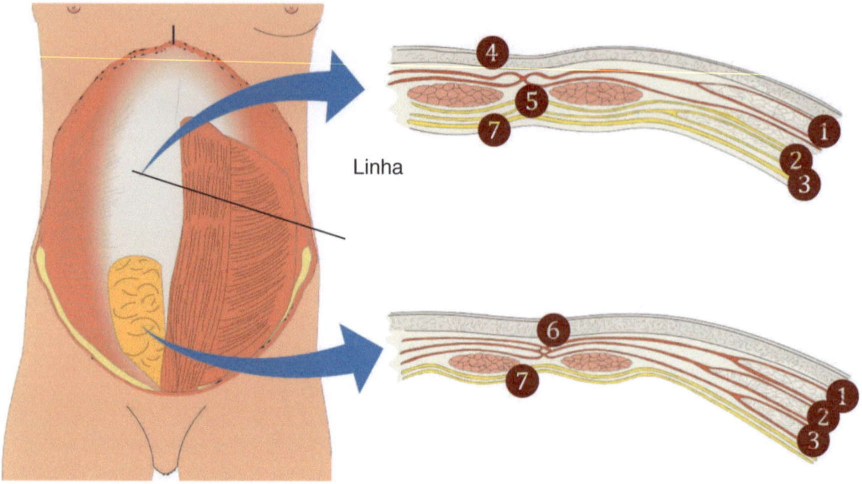

Fig. 1.10 Sheath of the rectus abdominis muscle. (1) Oblique muscle; (2) internal oblique muscle; (3) transverse abdominis muscle; (4) anterior leaflet of the sheath; (5) posterior leaflet; (6) single leaflet of the sheath; (7) transversalis fascia/peritoneum

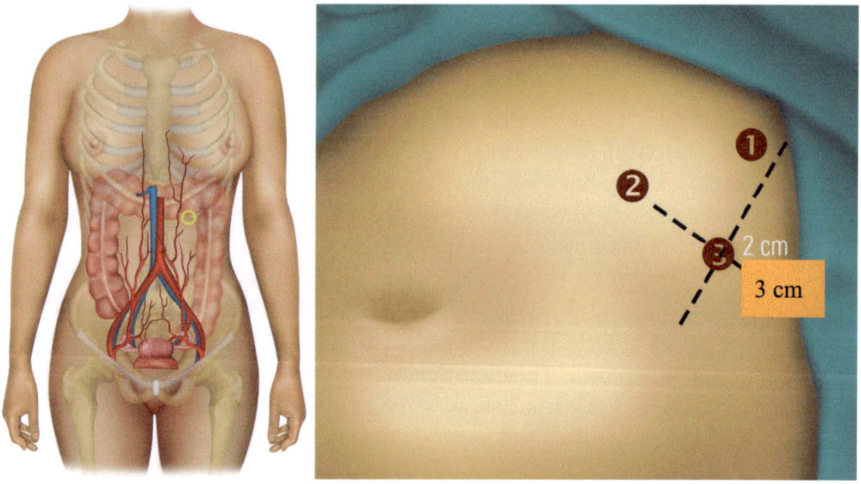

Fig. 1.11 Palmer's point is located on the left hemiclavicular line, 3 cm below the costal arch (yellow circle). (1) Hemiclavicular line; (2) costal arch; (3) Palmer's point

The internal surface of the abdominal wall is clothed by membranous and areal laminae of variable thickness. The part of the fascia that lines both the transverse abdominal muscle and its aponeurosis posteriorly is called the transversalis fascia, which is separated from the parietal peritoneum by a variable amount of extraperitoneal fat (Fig. 1.12).

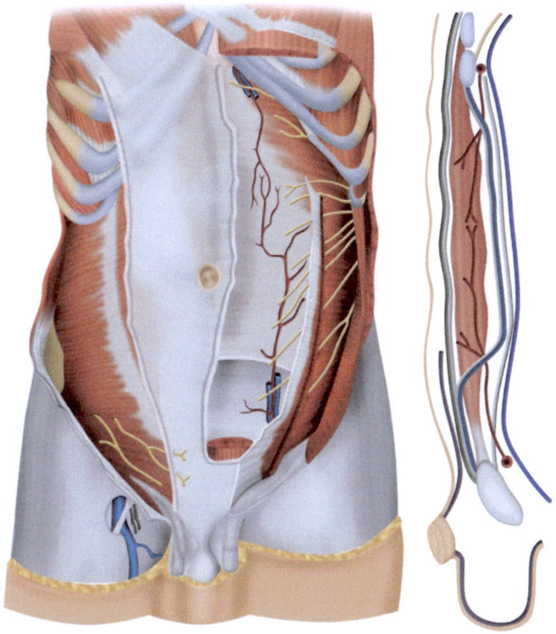

Fig. 1.12 Layers of the abdominal wall
Origin of the rectus abdominis muscle on the costal cartilages (there is no posterior sheath to the muscle at this site)
Posterior wall of the sheath of the rectus abdominis muscle formed by:
Posterior lamina of the aponeurosis of the internal oblique muscle of the abdomen
Aponeurosis of transverse abdominis muscle
Posterior wall of the sheath of the rectus abdominis muscle formed by:
Aponeurosis of the external oblique muscle
Anterior lamina of the aponeurosis of the internal oblique muscle
Arched line posterior wall of the sheath of the lower part of the rectus abdominis muscle; only transverse fascia
Diaphragm
Extremity of thoracic artery
Peritoneum
Transverse fascia
Body of pubis

Tips and Tricks 3

Understanding these different conformations is important when performing the first puncture. If the Veress needle is introduced in the umbilicus or below the arcuate line, there will be a tactile sensation that the needle overcomes two resistances, that of the rectus sheath and that of the peritoneum. However, in situations where there is great risk in umbilical puncture (suspected intestinal adhesions, failed umbilical puncture attempts, large umbilical hernia, and very thin patients) and the Palmer's point puncture is indicated, there will be the sensation that the needle overcomes three resistances (anterior leaflet of the sheath, posterior leaflet, and transversalis fascia/peritoneum).

Internal Aspect of the Anterolateral Abdominal Wall

Some structures cross the abdominal wall, forming five peritoneal folds visible on the posterior aspect of the anterior wall, which serve as anatomical landmarks, helping in surgical steps.

The median peritoneal fold runs from the apex of the bladder to the umbilicus and covers the urachus (median umbilical ligament). Lateral to it, there are the medial peritoneal folds that cover the occluded portions of the umbilical arteries. More laterally then, we can find the lateral umbilical folds, which cover the inferior epigastric vessels and therefore bleed if they are cut. The latter are the only ones that do not reach the umbilicus (Fig. 1.13).

Tips and Tricks 4

Easily identifiable, the obliterated umbilical arteries are important anatomical landmarks in surgeries that require occlusion of the uterine artery at its origin, such as myomectomy, because the mobilization of the obliterated umbilical artery allows the precise identification of the uterine artery, located medially to it (Fig. 1.14). This structure also delimits medially the paravesical space, whose dissection is essential in surgeries such as hysterectomy and pelvic lymphadenectomy (Figs. 1.15 and 1.16).

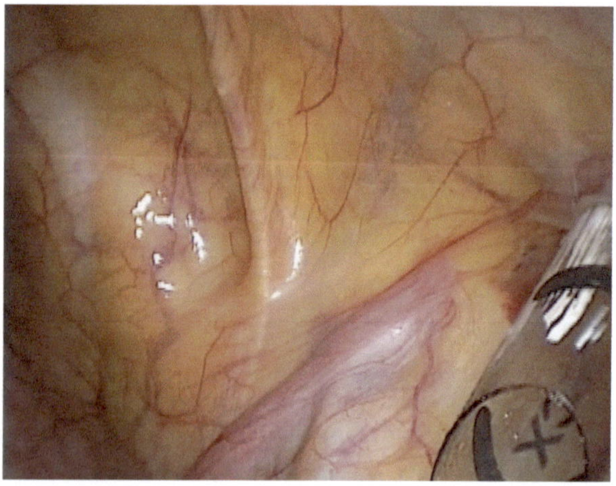

Fig. 1.13 Laparoscopic view of the lateral peritoneal fold [1]

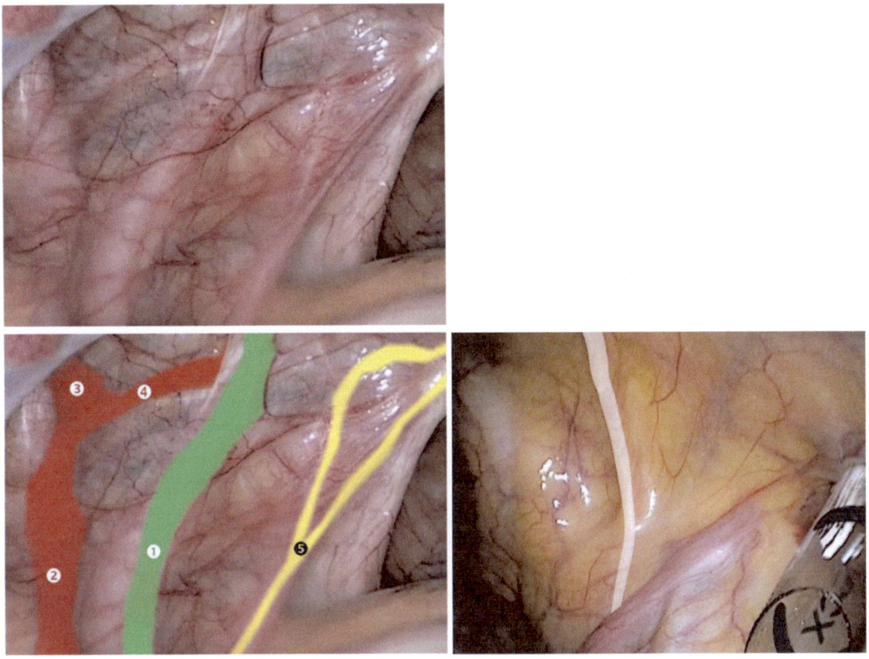

Fig. 1.14 The uterine artery in its origin, found from the mobilization of the obliterated umbilical artery. (1) Ureter, (2) iliac-internal artery, (3) umbilical artery, (4) uterine artery, (5) hypogastric nerve

Vascularization

Knowing the course of the vessels that supply the abdominal wall allows the surgeon to anticipate their location, thus preventing vascular accidents during incision and trocar insertion.

The anterior abdominal wall has a superficial and deep blood supply. The deep system is formed by the superior epigastric artery, the inferior epigastric artery, and the deep circumflex arteries, as well as their corresponding veins.

The deep inferior epigastric artery is the main blood supply of the abdominal wall. It originates from the external iliac artery approximately 1 cm above the inguinal ligament and ascends medially into the internal inguinal canal (Fig. 1.17a and b). It proceeds toward the umbilical scar, crossing the lateral border of the rectus abdominis muscle at the arcuate line, where it perforates the transversalis fascia and enters the space between the rectus abdominis muscle and its posterior sheath (Figs. 1.18, 1.19, and 1.20).

After reaching the sheath of the rectus abdominis muscle, the inferior epigastric vessels branch extensively and ascend until they anastomose with the superior epigastric artery between the umbilicus and the xiphoid process. The main

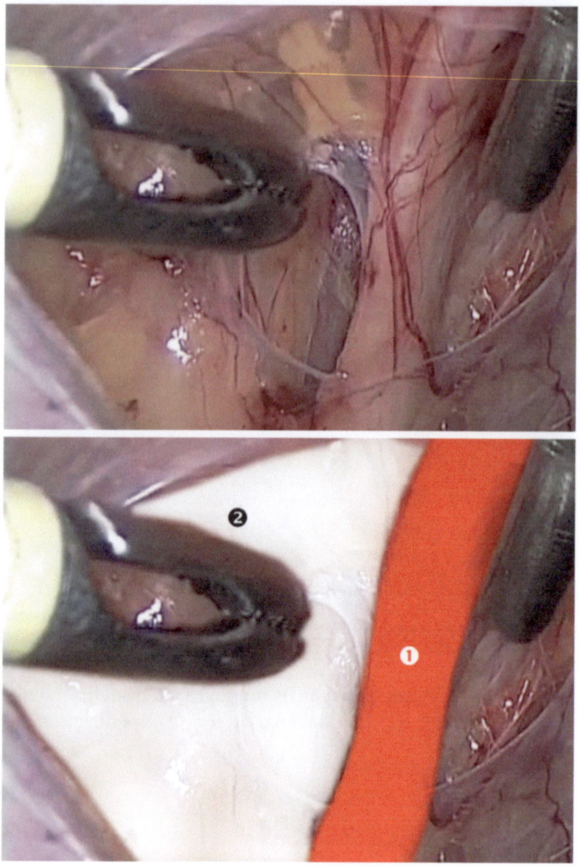

Fig. 1.15 Surgical photo of the obliterated umbilical artery delimiting the paravesical space. (1) Umbilical obliterated artery, (2) left paravesical space

skin-piercing branches are located in the periumbilical region and are derived exclusively from the inferior deep epigastric artery (Fig. 1.18).

The superior deep epigastric artery originates from the internal thoracic artery, a branch of the subclavian artery. It passes behind the seventh costal cartilage and perforates the posterior sheath of the rectus abdominis muscle, sending muscle branches that give rise to myocutaneous perforating branches, before anastomosing with the inferior deep epigastric artery (Figs. 1.18, 1.19, and 1.20).

The superficial network is composed of the superficial epigastric and circumflex arteries and their corresponding veins. The superficial epigastric artery originates from the femoral artery, is located in the subcutaneous tissue, and runs medially toward the rectus abdominis muscle, forming a diagonal path toward the umbilicus. It starts as a single vessel and starts issuing numerous branches as it approaches the umbilical scar. The superficial circumflex artery also originates from the femoral artery and runs laterally toward the flank (Figs. 1.18, 1.19, and 1.20).

The epigastric arteries are usually located between 4 and 8 cm from the midline in the abdominal region, but anatomic variations may occur. Joy et al. identified, by

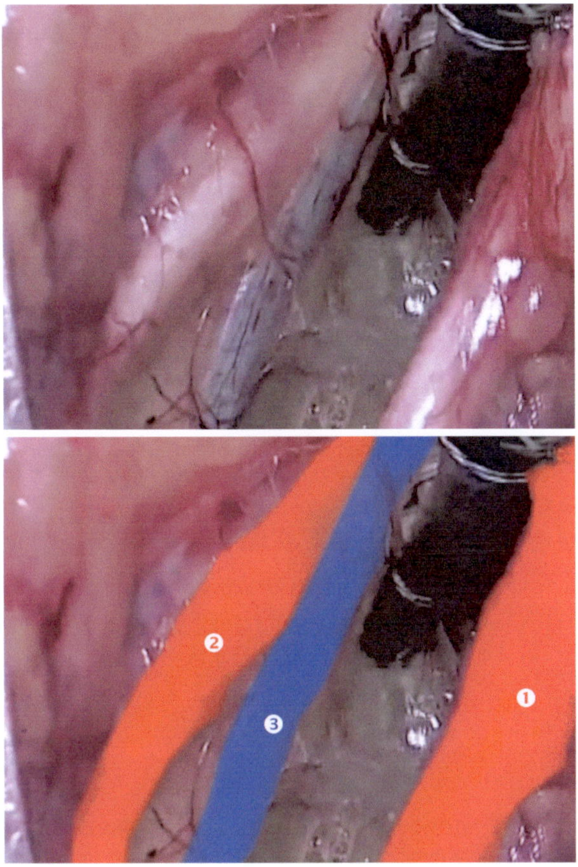

Fig. 1.16 Structures of the lateral paravesical space. (1) Umbilical obliterated artery, (2) obturator artery, (3) obturator vein

means of cadaver dissection, that the mean distance of the inferior epigastric arteries from the midline was 4.45 ± 1.42 cm at the internal inguinal ring and 4.10 ± 1.15 cm at the anterior superior iliac spine (Fig. 1.21).

Tips and Tricks 5
Some anatomical variations of the inferior epigastric artery were described: it may emerge from the external iliac artery up to 6.2 cm above the inguinal ligament; it may originate from the femoral artery or be like a common trunk to the circumflex artery; it may originate from the obturator artery; and it may also be found duplicated. At the level of the upper branch of the pubis, the inferior epigastric artery passes through anastomosis with branches of the obturator artery, forming the corona mortis. Knowledge of this anatomical variant is of surgical interest, as it is susceptible to injury during gynecological surgery and hernia repair, and its hemostasis may be difficult to perform (Figs. 1.17a–c and 1.22).

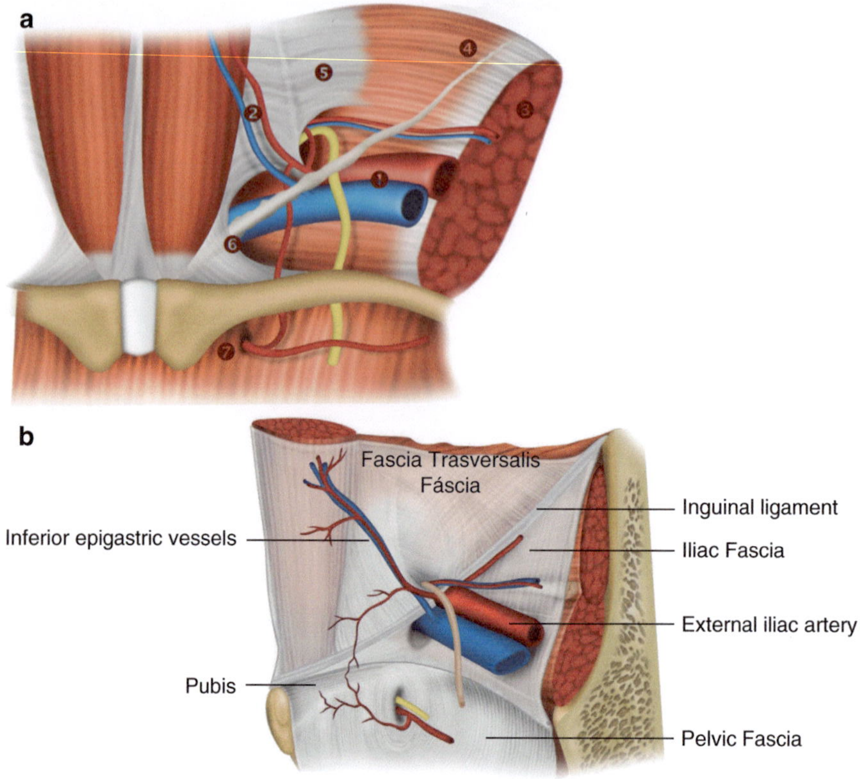

Fig. 1.17 (**a**) Lower deep epigastric vessels. (1) External iliac vessels; (2) inferior epigastric vessels; (3) psoas muscle; (4) inguinal ligament; (5) deep inguinal ring; (6) femoral ring; (7) obturator ring. (**b**) Lower deep epigastric vessels and fascia

Tips and Tricks 6

The anatomical location of the inferior and superficial epigastric arteries makes them susceptible to injury during abdominal procedures, such as insertion of laparoscopic trocars, drains, dialysis catheters, and paracentesis. It is estimated that in laparoscopy, injury occurs in about 0.3–2.5% of cases, leading to difficult-to-control bleeding that may result in the need for blood transfusion, management of abdominal hematomas, or even conversion to laparotomy.

A number of measures can be taken to avoid injury to the epigastric arteries. During laparoscopy, for example, it is possible to identify the inferior epigastric arteries by direct vision as they pass along the peritoneal fold, lateral to the obliterated umbilical artery (medial peritoneal ligament) (Fig. 1.23).

The superficial epigastric arteries, in turn, can be identified by transillumination. The success of this technique, however, is reduced with increasing weight of the patients, and the arteries can be identified in 80% of normal-weight patients and only in 63% of obese patients (Fig. 1.24).

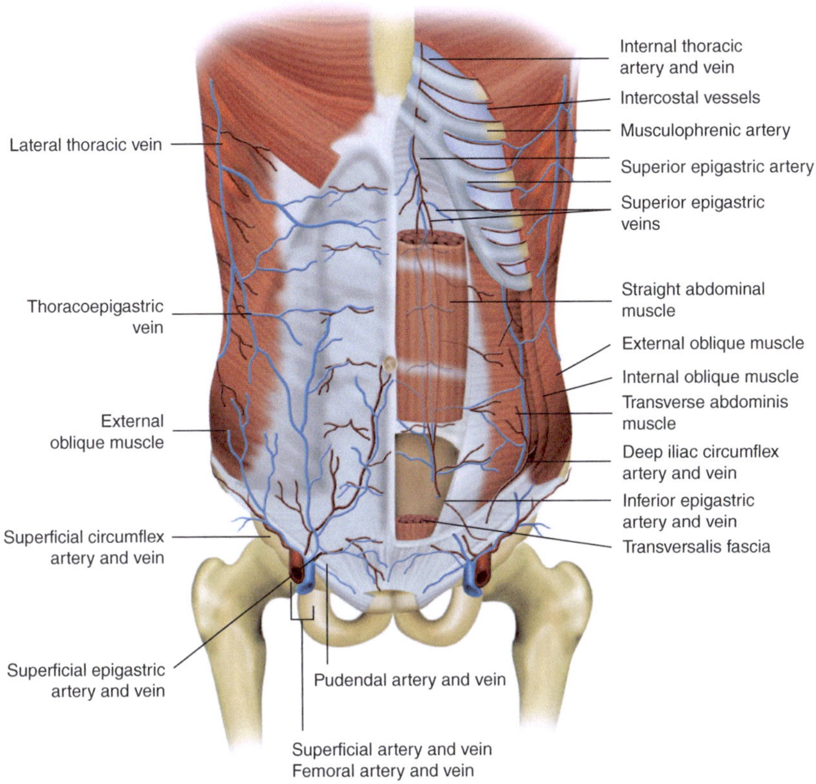

Fig. 1.18 Irrigation of the abdominal wall with emphasis on the epigastric vessels
The superficial network is seen on the left of the illustration, and the deep network on the right.
Captions on the left side of the figure:
Lateral thoracic vein
Thoracoepigastric vein
External oblique muscle
Superficial circumflex artery and vein
Superficial epigastric artery and vein
Captions on the inferior part of the figure
Pudendal artery and vein
Superficial artery and vein
Femoral artery and vein
Captions on the right side of the figure:
Internal thoracic artery and vein
Intercostal vessels
Musculophrenic artery
Superior epigastric artery
Superior epigastric veins
Straight abdominal muscle
External oblique muscle
Internal oblique muscle
Transverse abdominis muscle
Deep iliac circumflex artery and vein
Inferior epigastric artery and vein
Transversalis fascia

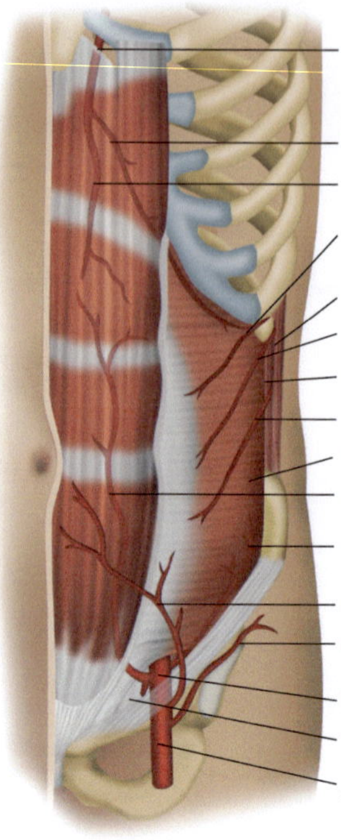

Fig. 1.19 Detailed illustration of the upper and lower epigastric vessels
Internal thoracic artery
Musculophrenic artery
Superior epigastric artery
10th superior intercostal artery
External oblique muscle of the abdomen
11th posterior intercostal artery
Internal oblique muscle of the abdomen
Subcostal artery
Transverse abdominal muscle
Inferior epigastric artery
Superficial circumflex iliac artery
Deep circumflex iliac artery
External iliac artery
Femoral artery
Transverse fascia

Tinelli et al. selected an area called "yellow island" for trocar insertion. This is an avascular area of subperitoneal adipose tissue accumulation located in the lateral third of a line between the anterosuperior iliac spine and the umbilical scar. This is also an effective strategy to avoid vascular injuries in obese patients in whom identification of the epigastric arteries is not possible by laparoscopic vision. Based on measurements obtained by computed tomography, it has been suggested as the safest points for lateral trocar insertion (Figs. 1.25, 1.26, and 1.27).

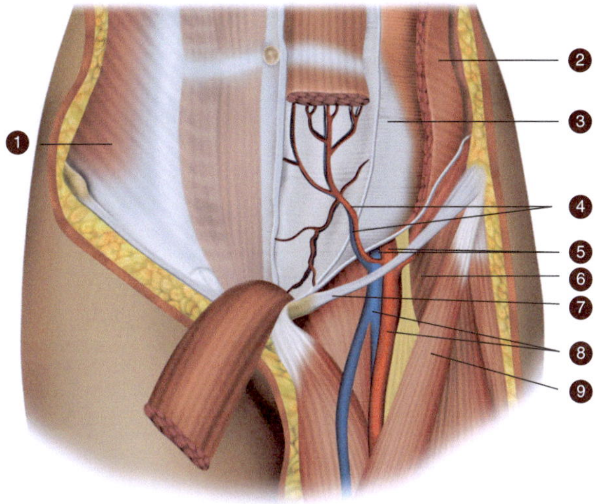

Fig. 1.20 Superficial net on the left and deep net on the right. (1) Internal oblique muscle, (2) external oblique muscle, (3) transverse abdominal fascia, (4) inferior hypogastric artery, (5) external iliac artery, (6) iliopsoas muscle, (7) inguinal ligament, (8) femoral artery and vein, (9) sartorius muscle

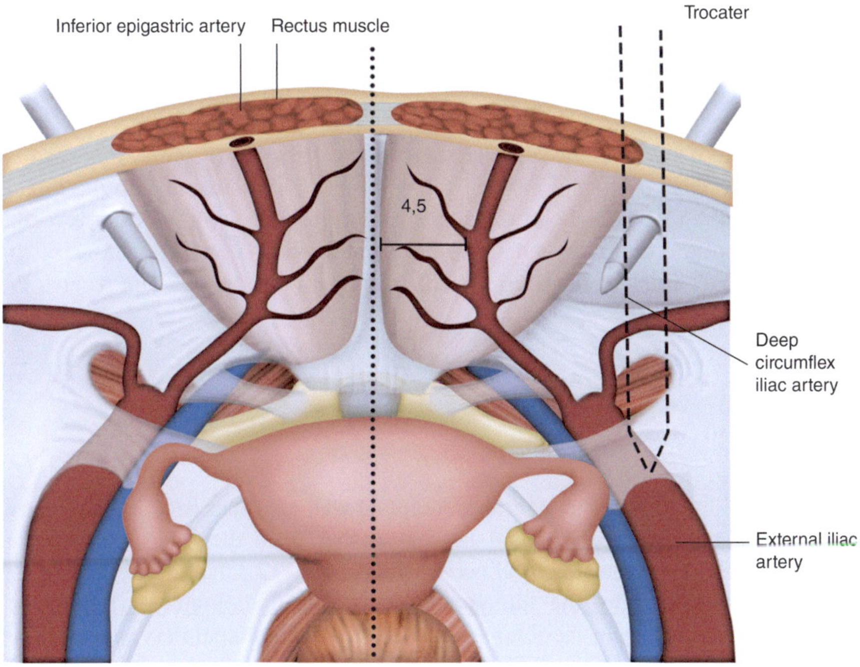

Fig. 1.21 Inferior epigastric artery and anatomic boundaries
Inferior epigastric artery
Rectus muscle
Trocar
Deep circumflex iliac artery
External iliac artery

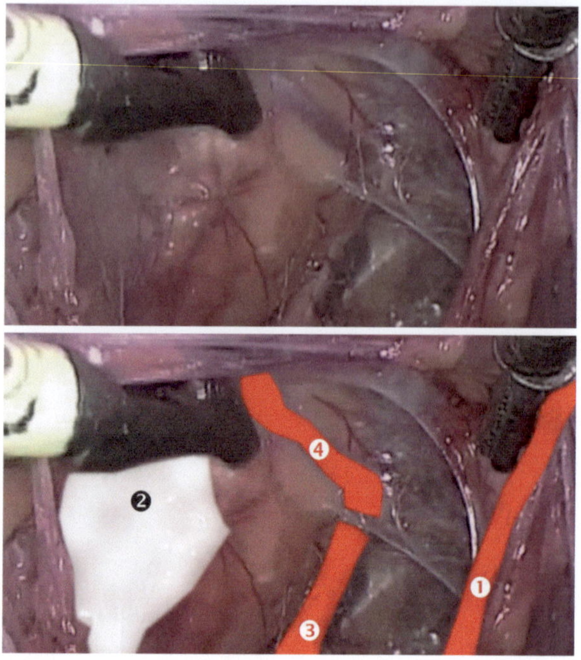

Fig. 1.22 Corona mortis. (1) Umbilical obliterated artery, (2) left paravesical space, (3) obturator artery, (4) corona mortis

The venous network of the superficial system is formed by a complex plexus that drains superomedially to the internal thoracic vein, superolaterally to the lateral thoracic vein, and inferiorly to the superficial epigastric vein, and, close to the umbilical scar, the drainage is done to the paraumbilical veins, tributaries of the portal vein. The veins of the deep system accompany the arteries and receive the same name.

Innervation

The skin and muscles of the anterior abdominal wall are innervated by the ventral branches of the thoracoabdominal nerves, arising from the inferior intercostal nerves (T7–T11) and the subcostal nerves (branch of T12); the inferior part of the abdomen is supplied by the iliohypogastric (L1) and ilioinguinal (L1) nerves (Fig. 1.28). Starting from the intercostal spaces, the abdominal nerves descend in the neurovascular plane toward the anterior aspect of the abdomen. In the anterior axillary line, the thoracoabdominal muscles emit their lateral cutaneous branches, which pierce the muscles of the anterolateral wall and enter the subcutaneous tissue.

After reaching the lateral border of the rectus sheath, they then issue their anterior cutaneous branches, which, in turn, perforate the abdominal musculature and its sheath, near the linea alba, to innervate the skin and subcutaneous tissue (Fig. 1.29).

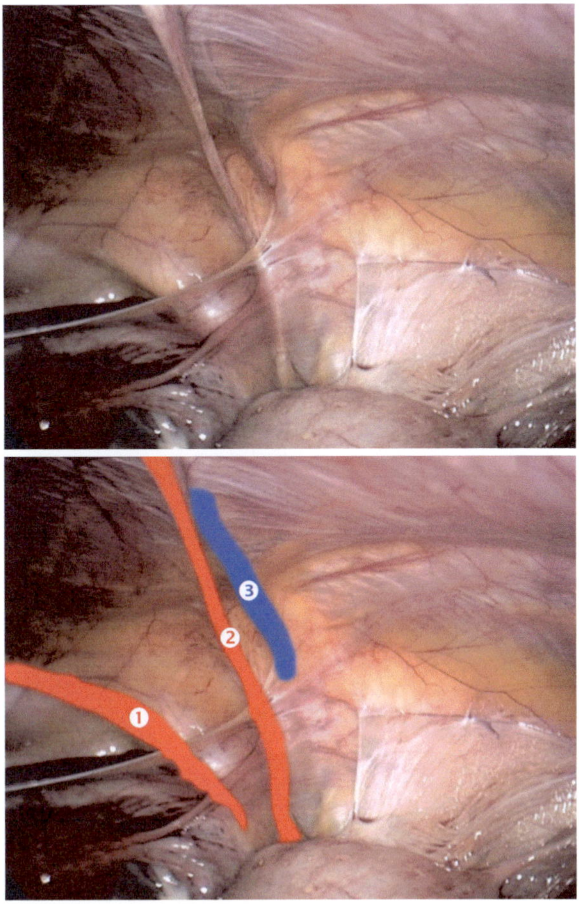

Fig. 1.23 Laparoscopic view of the deep epigastric vessels. (1) Obliterated umbilical artery, (2) deep epigastric artery, (3) deep epigastric vein

Tips and Tricks 7

The lesion of these nerves has been documented in about 3.7% of gynecological procedures, either through Pfannenstiel incisions or during the insertion of a lateral trocar during laparoscopy. The most common clinical manifestations of these lesions include severe chronic pain or burning pain in the inguinal region with vulvar irradiation that may manifest in the immediate postoperative period or later.

Incisions on the lateral border of the rectus abdominis may lead to muscle denervation, with atrophy and loss of strength. Similarly, when detaching the muscle from its sheath and performing hemostasis, as performed in the Pfannenstiel incision, there may be distension of the perforating nerves, causing localized cutaneous anesthesia.

The iliohypogastric and ilioinguinal nerves pass medially through the anterosuperior iliac crest. The former innervates the skin of the suprapubic area and groin; the latter innervates the lower abdominal wall, the labia majora, and the anterosuperior thigh (through branches that follow the inguinal canal) (Figs. 1.29 and 1.30).

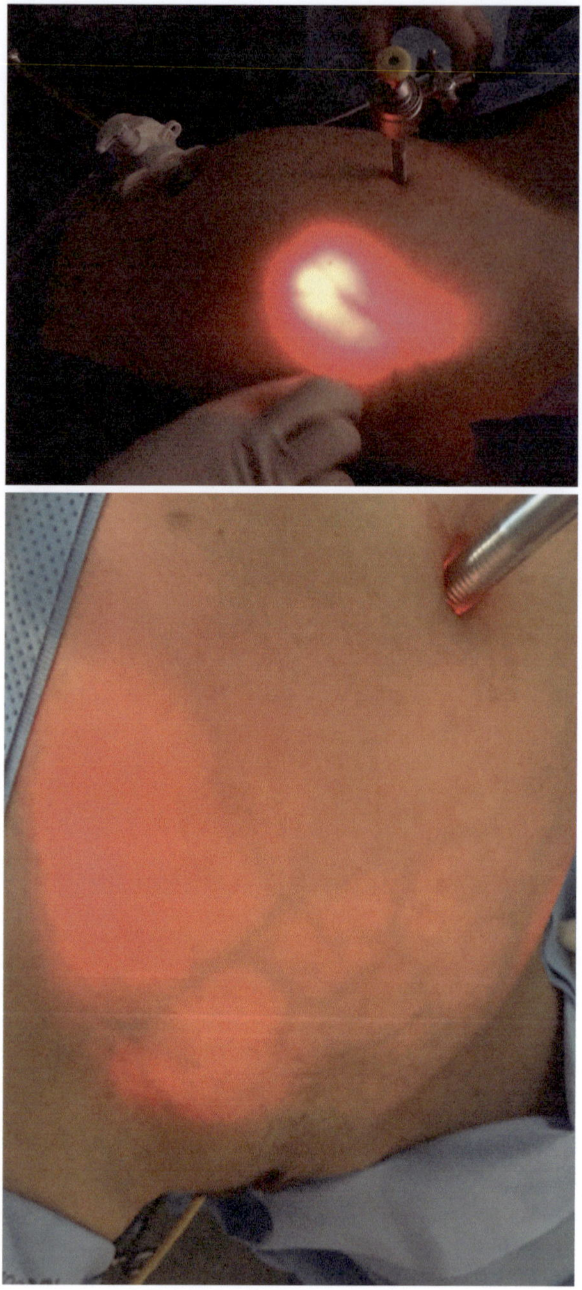

Fig. 1.24 Identification of the superficial epigastric arteries by transillumination

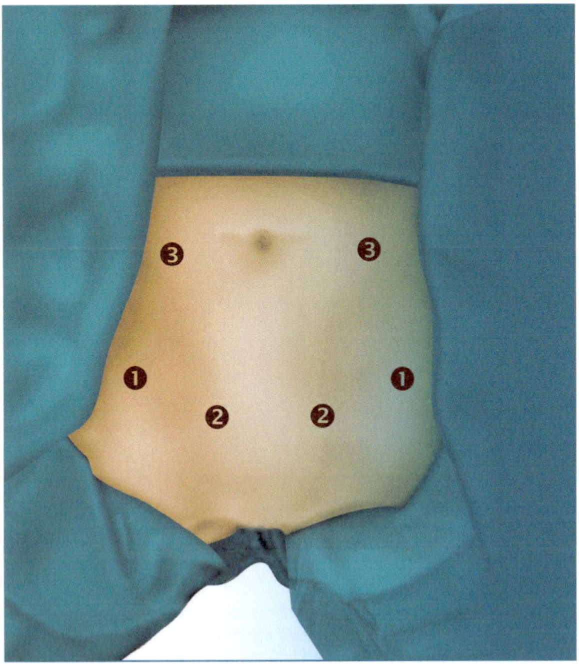

Fig. 1.25 Landmarks for accessory punctures to minimize vascular injury. (1) Ideal location for the lateral trocar 5 cm above the symphysis pubis and 8 cm lateral to the midline, (2) alternative location for the lateral trocar 3 cm above the symphysis and 4 cm from the midline, (3) trocar location near umbilicus 8 cm from midline

The genitofemoral (L1 and L2) and cutaneofemoral (L2 and L3) nerves can also be injured during gynecological surgery. The genitofemoral runs above the psoas muscle in the posterior abdominal wall, where the use of retractor may result in anesthesia of the labia majora and the medial thigh.

The cutaneofemoral nerve can be compressed either by the use of retractor or by excessive flexion of the thigh during lithotomy positioning, causing anesthesia of the anterior thigh (Fig. 1.31).

Careful planning of the position of the lateral trocar is essential for a safe puncture. When placed inferiorly to the anterosuperior iliac spine, there is a higher risk of nerve damage. Its placement above the anterosuperior iliac spine and 8 cm from the midline minimizes the risk of vascular and nerve injury (Fig. 1.32).

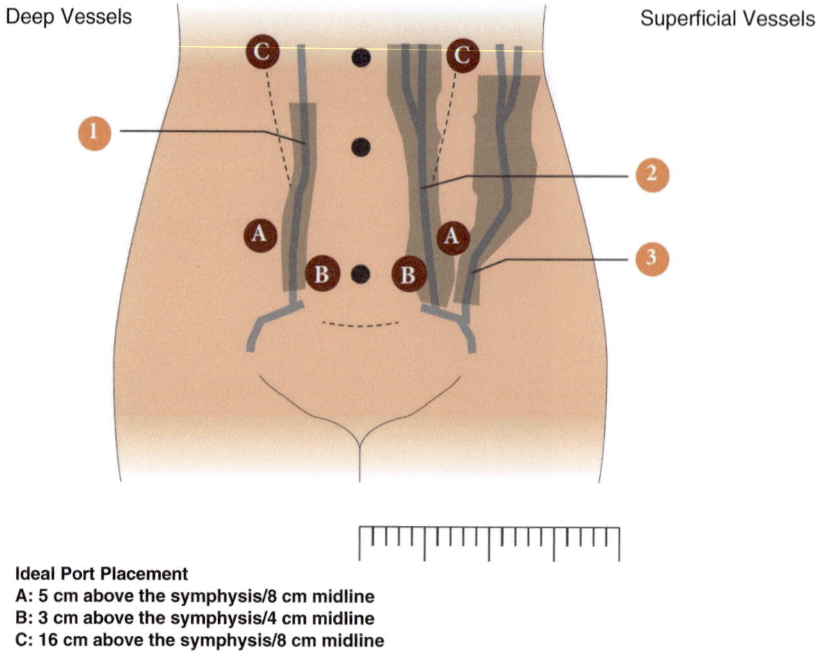

Fig. 1.26 Trocar positioning to reduce the risk of vascular injury. (1) Inferior epigastric vessels, (2) superficial epigastric vessels, (3) circumflex superficial iliac artery
Ideal Port Placement
A: 5 cm above the symphysis/8 cm midline
B: 3 cm above the symphysis/4 cm midline
C: 16 cm above the symphysis/8 cm midline

Fig. 1.27 Insertion of the side trocar in the "yellow island"

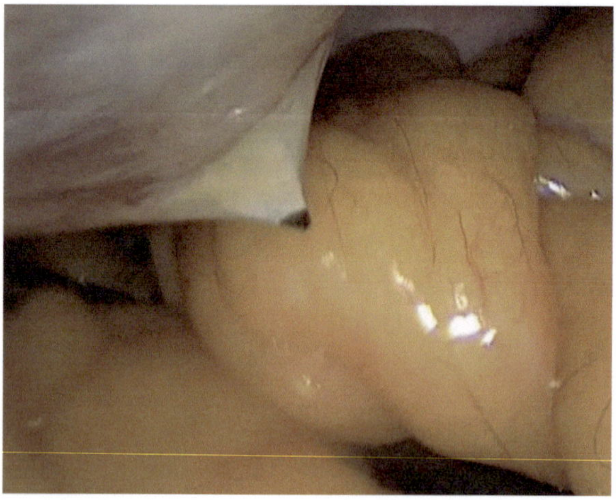

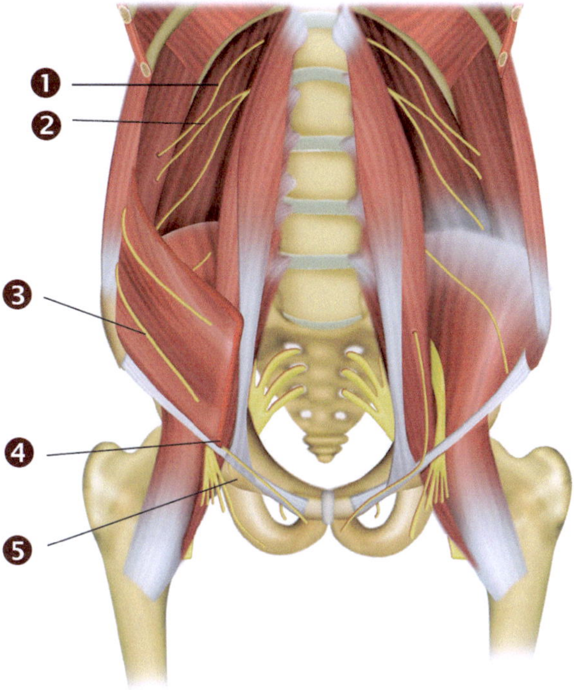

Fig. 1.28 Abdominal wall innervation. (1) Subcostal nerve, (2) hypogastric iliac nerve, (3) inguinal nerve, (4) genital branch of the genitofemoral nerve, (5) femoral branch of the genitofemoral nerve

a

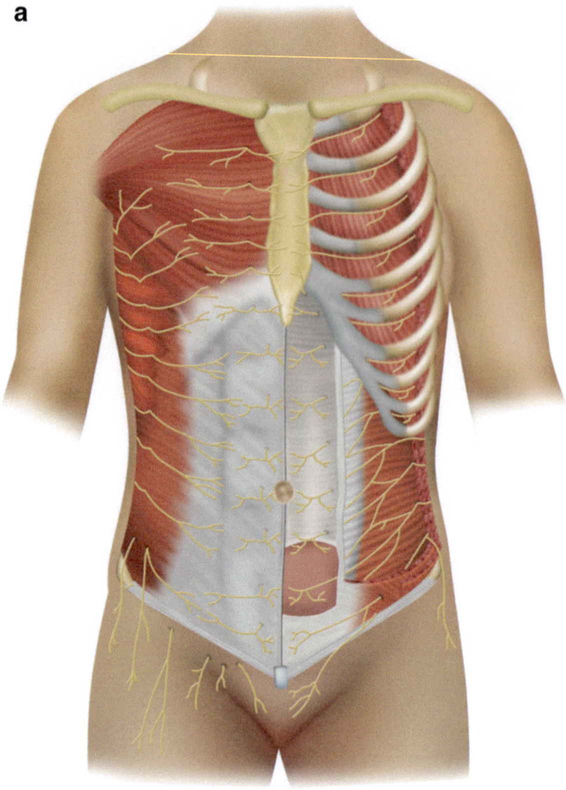

Fig. 1.29 Abdominal wall innervation
Left side of the picture
Anterior cutaneous branches of the intercostal nerves (T1–T11)
Thoracic intercostal nerves (T1–T6)
Lateral cutaneous branches of the intercostal nerves (T3–T11)
Anterior cutaneous branches of the subcostal nerves (T12)
Lateral cutaneous branches of the subcostal nerve (T12)
Lateral cutaneous branch of the iliohypogastric nerves
Femorolateral cutaneous nerves
Right side of the picture
Thoracic intercostal nerves (T1–T6)
Intercostal abdominal nerves (T7–T11)
Anterior cutaneous branch of the subcostal nerves (T12)
Ilioinguinal nerve
Anterior branch of the iliohypogastric nerve
Inguinal canal
Ilioinguinal nerve

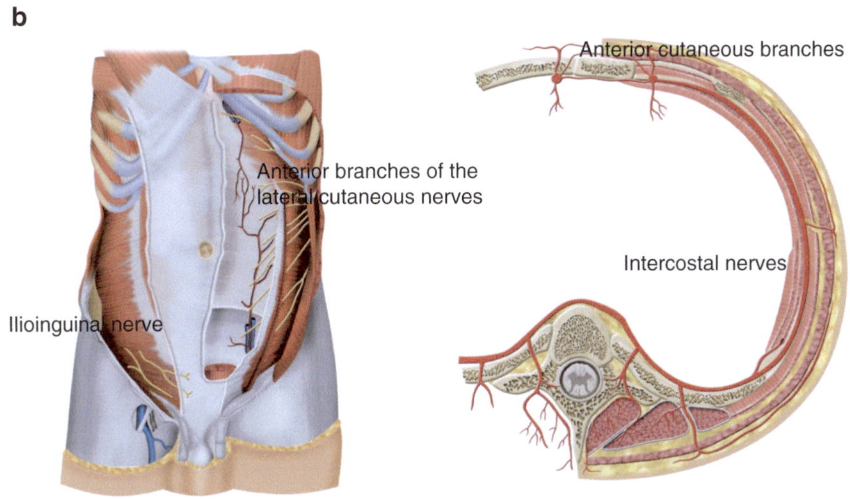

Fig. 1.29 (continued)

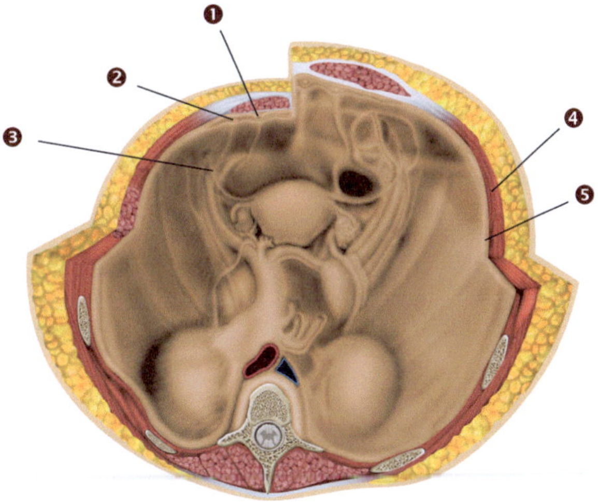

Fig. 1.30 Transverse incisions and the insertion of a lateral trocar during laparoscopy can lead to nerve damage. (1) Medial umbilical ligament, (2) inferior epigastric vessel, (3) round ligament, (4) iliohypogastric nerve, (5) ilioinguinal nerve

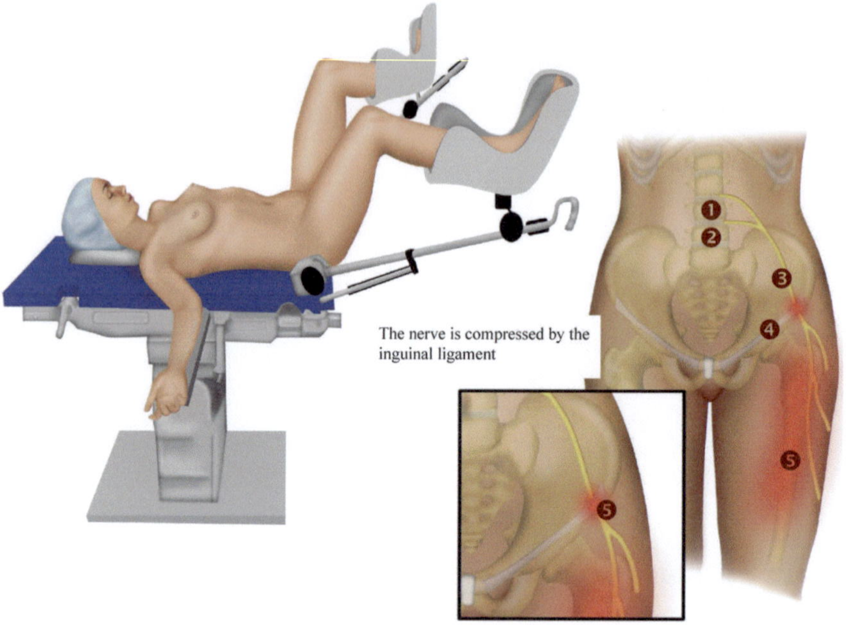

Fig. 1.31 The femoral cutaneous nerve can be compressed either by the use of a retractor or by exaggerated flexion of the thigh during lithotomy positioning. (1) L2 vertebra; (2) L3 vertebra; (3) lateral femoral cutaneous nerve; (4) inguinal ligament; (5) affected area

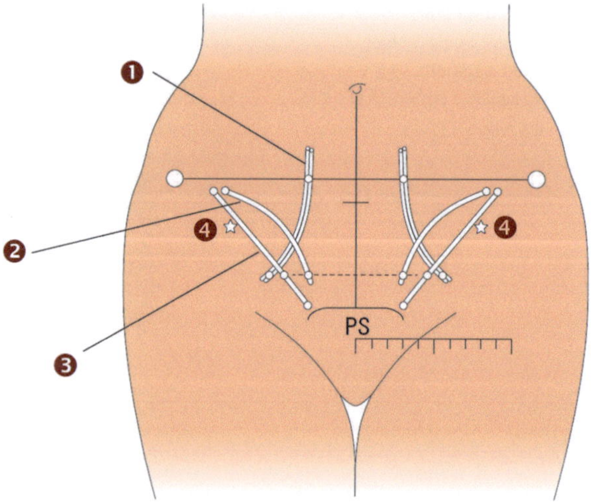

Fig. 1.32 Positioning of the lateral trocars to minimize nerve and vascular injuries. (1) Inferior epigastric vessels; (2) iliohypogastric nerve; (3) ilioinguinal nerve; (4) lateral trocar ideal positioning (5 cm above symphysis pubis, 8 cm from midline). *PS* pubic symphysis

Bibliography

1. Baggish MS, Karram MM. Atlas of pelvic anatomy and gynaecologic surgery. 3rd ed. St Louis, MO: Elsevier Saunders; 2011. p. 156.
2. Bhatti AF, Iqbal S, Lee TC. Variation in surface marking of superior epigastric vessels: a guide to safe laparoscopic port insertion. Surgeon. 2008;6(1):50–2.
3. Epstein J, Arora A, Ellis H. Surface anatomy of the inferior epigastric artery in relation to laparoscopic injury. Clin Anat. 2004;17(5):400–8.
4. Hurd WW, Bude RO, DeLancey JO, Gauvin JM, Aisen AM. Abdominal wall characterization with magnetic resonance imaging and computing tomography. J Reprod Med. 1991;36(7):473–6.
5. Hurd WW, Bude RO, DeLancey JO, Pearl ML. The relationship of the umbilicus to the aortic bifurcation: implications for laparoscopic technique. Obstet Gynecol. 1992;80(1):48–51.
6. Hurd WW, Pearl ML, DeLancey JO, Quint EH, Garnett B, Bude RO. Laparoscopic injury of abdominal wall blood vessels: a report of three cases. Obstet Gynecol. 1993;82(4 Pt 2 Suppl):673–6.
7. Joy P, Prithishkumar IJ, Isaac B. Clinical anatomy of the inferior epigastric artery with special relevance to invasive procedures of the anterior abdominal wall. J Min Access Surg. 2017;13(1):18–21.
8. Moore KL, Dalley AF, Agur AMR. Anatomia orientada para a clínica. 7th ed. Rio de Janeiro: Guanabara Koogan; 2014.
9. Netter FH. Atlas de anatomia humana. 3rd ed. Porto Alegre: Artmed; 2003.
10. Nezhat F, Brill AI, Nezhat CH, Nezhat A, Seidman DS, Nezhat C. Laparoscopic appraisal of the anatomic relationship of the umbilicus to the aortic bifurcation. J Am Assoc Gynecol Laparosc. 1998;5(2):135–40.
11. Rahn DD, Phelan JN, Roshanravan SM, White AB, Corton MM. Anterior abdominal wall nerve and vessel anatomy: clinical implications for gynecologic surgery. Am J Obstet Gynecol. 2010;202(3):234.e1–5.
12. Rock JA, Jones HW. Te Linde's operative gynecology. 10th ed. Philadelphia: Wolters Kluwer, Lippincott Williams & Wilkins; 2008.
13. Saber AA, Meslemani AM, Davis R, Pimentel R. Safety zones for anterior abdominal wall entry during laparoscopy: a CT scan mapping of epigastric vessels. Ann Surg. 2004;239(2):182–5.
14. Tinelli A, Gasbarro N, Lupo P, Malvasi A, Tsin DA, Davila F, et al. Safe introduction of ancillary trocars. JSLS. 2012;16(2):276–9.
15. Wallwiener D, Diedrich K. Atlas de cirurgia ginecológica. 7th ed. Porto Alegre: Artmed; 2012.
16. Palmer R. Safety in laparoscopy. J Reprod Med. 1974;13(1):1.
17. Hurd WW, Bude RO, DeLancey JO, Newman JS. The location of abdominal wall blood vessels in relationship to abdominal landmarks apparent at laparoscopy. Am J Obstet Gynecol. 1994;171(3):642–6.

Chapter 2
Abdominopelvic Organs

Mariano Tamura, Raquel Silveira da Cunha Araújo, Ricardo de Almeida Quintairos, Rômulo Müller dos Santos Melo, and Paulo Ayroza Ribeiro

Overview

The female genital tract consists of an internal and an external portion. The internal organs consist of the ovaries, uterine tubes, uterus, and vagina. The external ones are composed of the pubis, labia majora, labia minora, vestibule of the vagina, clitoris,

M. Tamura
Federal University of São Paulo (UNIFESP), Albert Einstein Hospital, São Paulo, Brazil

Uterine Myoma Outpatient Clinic, Escola Pau-list de Medicina da Universidade Federal de São Paulo (EPM/UNIFESP), São Paulo, Brazil

R. S. da Cunha Araújo
Federal University of Paraíba (UFPB), João Pessoa, Brazil

Brazilian Federation of Gynecology and Obstetrics Associations (FEBRASGO), São Paulo, Brazil

Faculty of Medical Sciences, Santa Casa de Misericórdia de São Paulo (SCMSP), São Paulo, Brazil

R. de Almeida Quintairos
Brazilian Federation of Gynecology and Obstetrics Associations (FEBRASGO), São Paulo, Brazil

R. M. dos Santos Melo
Brazilian Federation of Gynecology and Obstetrics Associations (FEBRASGO), São Paulo, Brazil

Fundação Santa Casa de Misericórdia do Pará (FSCMPA), Belém, Brazil

P. Ayroza Ribeiro (✉)
Brazilian Federation of Gynecology and Obstetrics Associations (FEBRASGO), São Paulo, Brazil

Department of Obstetrics and Gynecology, School of Medical Sciences, Santa Casa de Misericórida São Paulo (SCMSP), São Paulo, Brazil

H. Salomão Ayroza, P. Ayroza Ribeiro (eds.), *Atlas of Laparoscopic Gynecological Anatomy*, https://doi.org/10.1007/978-3-031-63520-5_2

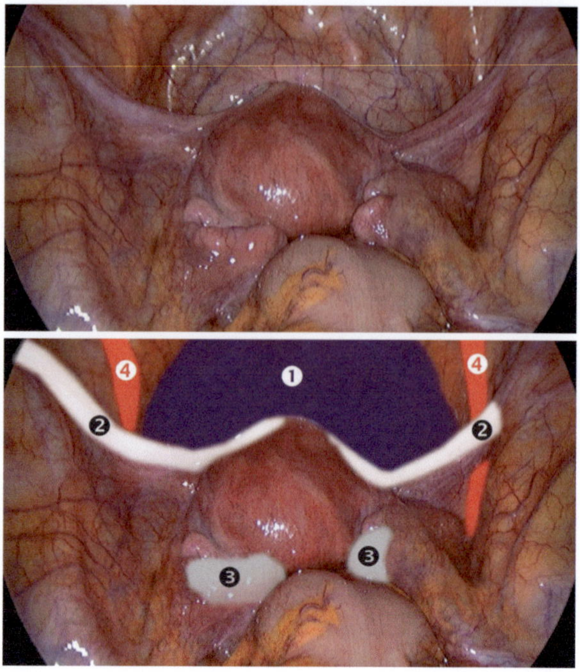

Fig. 2.1 General arrangement of the pelvic organs

bulb of the vestibule, and vestibular major glands (or Bartholin glands). The ovaries and the tubes together are called the appendages.

This chapter discusses in detail the female pelvic organs, as described below.

In Fig. 2.1, you can see the general arrangement of the organs in the female pelvis.

Uterus

It is a central organ, hollow and of firm and elastic consistency, originating in the Müller's canals in the eighth week of the embryonic development, completing its formation in the 12th week; from that moment on, only its anatomic-structural differentiation will occur until the 40th week of gestation.

The uterus is divided, from the structural point of view, into three parts: body, isthmus, and cervix. It has three layers (respectively, from outside to inside): serous, muscular, and mucous, the latter being called endometrium, where the cyclic hormonal changes occur, the menstruation.

In the uterine muscular layer occur the most common pathologies of this organ, which are the uterine myomas and adenomyosis, responsible for the largest surgical indications in gynecology. Not less important, malignant diseases such as endometrial adenocarcinoma and cervical squamous cell carcinoma are particularly common in gynecology in Brazil.

Its dimensions depend on age and parity; in general, in nulliparous women, it comprises approximately 6.5 cm in length, 4 cm in width, and 2 cm in thickness. It is positioned in anteversoflexion with discrete dextrotorsion due to the sigmoid on its left side. Its weight varies from 50 to 90 g.

According to Kamina and Gouazé, the cervix is perpendicular to the posterior surface of the vagina, and the body and isthmus/cervix form an open angle of 100–120° of flexion; its apex is located at the level of the uterine isthmus.

Anatomical Landmarks of the Uterus

When we report the anatomical landmarks, it is important to stress the divergence of traditional anatomical nomenclature and that observed in surgical practice. According to Yabuki et al., since in some ligamentous structures described in traditional anatomy, such as the uterosacral ligament, ligamentous bundles are not found when dissecting, only a complex network of fascia, vessels, and nerves is seen, which means that there is no such uterosacral ligament, but only a support system (Figs. 2.1, 2.2, and 2.3).

These landmarks are fundamental for benign and oncological surgeries of the pelvis. They are

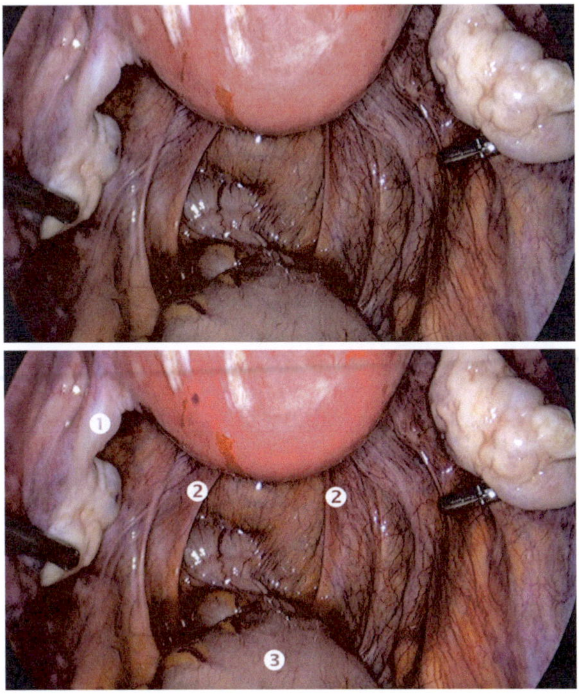

Fig. 2.2 Relation of the uterus and rectum to the uterosacral ligaments. (1) Utero-ovarian ligament. (2) Uterosacral ligament (support system). (3) Rectum

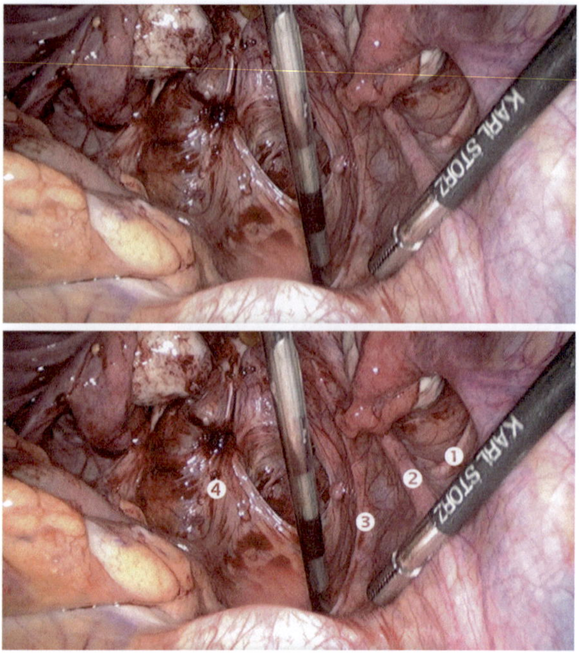

Fig. 2.3 Relations of the rectum with the right ureter and the right hypogastric nerve. (1) Obliterated umbilical artery, (2) ureter, (3) hypogastric nerve, (4) rectum

1. Bladder
2. Round ligament
3. Uterine tube
4. Uterovarian ligament
5. Obliterated umbilical artery
6. Ureter
7. Hypogastric nerve
8. Uterosacral ligament (support system)
9. Rectum

Pelvic Connective Tissue

According to Yabuki et al., the pelvic connective tissue is divided into a musculofascial bundle, or suspensor system, and a vasculonervous bundle, or support system. The suspensor system is composed of the pubovesical ligament, the superficial layer of the vesicouterine ligament, the rectouterine ligament, and the rectococcygeal ligament; the support system is divided into two parts: one cranial, composed by the mesoureter (ureter and pelvic autonomic nerves), and the other caudal, composed by the deepest layer of the vesicouterine ligament.

Vascularization

The uterus receives arterial blood from several arteries; the main one is the uterine, a branch of the hypogastric artery also called internal iliac artery. It is located by initial identification of the obliterated umbilical artery, because it consists of the first branch emerging after this anatomical landmark. The uterine artery, on reaching the uterus, crosses the ureter superiorly and divides into two branches, corporal and vaginal.

The infundibulopelvic ligament (IP ligament), in particular the ovarian artery, which is a direct branch of the abdominal aorta, has an important participation in the uterine vasculature. The artery of Sampson, within the round ligament, also contributes to this arterial blood supply. For this reason, by connecting the uterine artery or the hypogastric artery, even if permanently, uterine necrosis will not occur, since the uterus will receive supply from the ovarian and Sampson arteries, besides having the flow reversal of the posterior trunk of the internal iliac artery (superior gluteal, iliolumbar, and lateral sacral).

The identification of the uterine artery in laparoscopy is important because it offers comfort to the surgeon and safety to the patient by preventing heavy bleeding during a laparoscopic myomectomy procedure (Fig. 2.4).

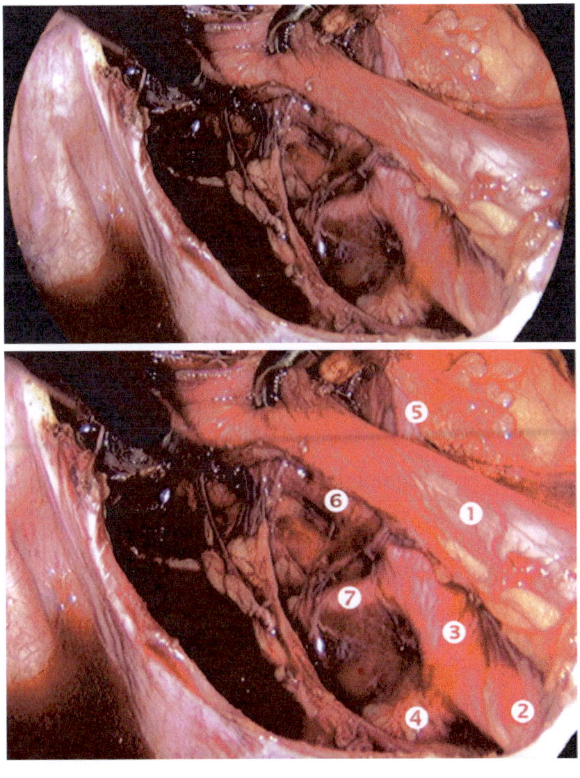

Fig. 2.4 Identification of the uterine artery and its anatomical landmarks. (1) Ureter, (2) internal iliac artery, (3) anterior trunk of the hypogastric artery, (4) posterior trunk of the hypogastric artery, (5) obliterated umbilical artery, (6) uterine artery, (7) vaginal artery

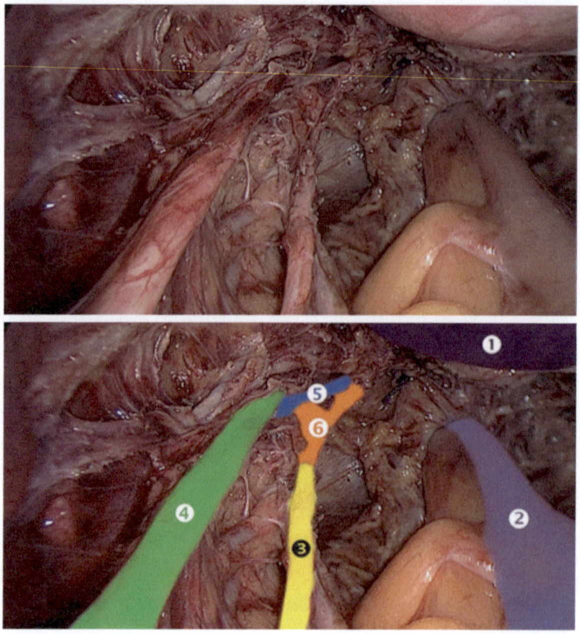

Fig. 2.5 Anatomical relations of the left deep uterine vein to the uterus, rectum, ureter, and pelvic nerves. (1) Uterus, (2) rectum, (3) left hypogastric nerve, (4) left ureter, (5) left deep uterine vein, (6) left inferior hypogastric plexus

Venous Drainage

The venous drainage of the uterus is relatively simple, because the arteries are homonymous, but the deep uterine vein is an important anatomical landmark for gynecological surgeries of deep endometriosis of the posterior and lateral compartments, as well as for oncological surgeries. This vein serves as the lower limit of dissection for the purpose of neuropreservation, because below it, we find the pelvic splanchnic nerves that will join the hypogastric nerve and form the pelvic plexus (or inferior hypogastric plexus) (Fig. 2.5).

Lymphatic Drainage

The uterine lymphatic drainage is done by a complex network of primary and secondary lymph nodes. The primary ones are parametrial, paracervical, obturator, internal iliac, external iliac, and sacral; the secondary ones are common iliac, periaortic, and inguinal.

It is important to emphasize that the pelvic lymphadenectomy has as its inferior limit the obturator nerve, which can be accessed through the paravesical space, the lateral pararectal space (Latzko), or the lumbosacral fossa (Fig. 2.6).

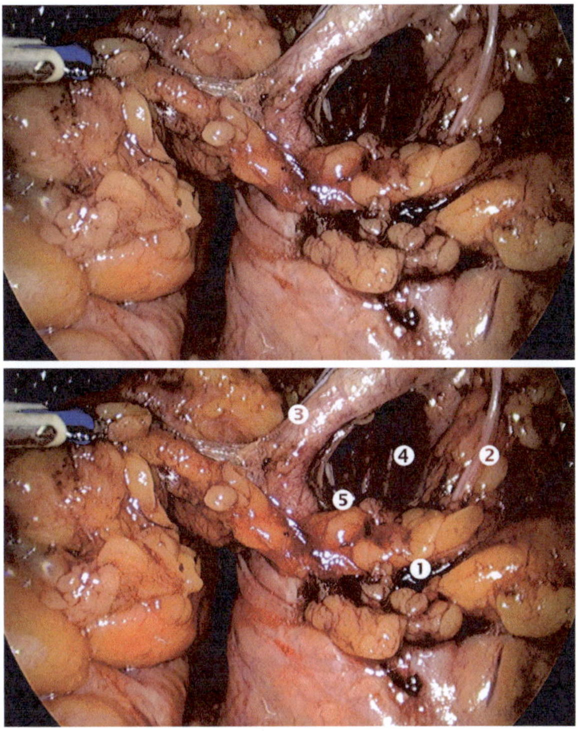

Fig. 2.6 Lumbosacral fossa and its anatomical relationships. (1) External iliac lymph nodes, (2) genitofemoral nerve, (3) external iliac artery, (4) lumbosacral fossa, (5) obturator nerve

Avascular Spaces

The uterus lies in the center of the pelvic floor, fixed by the uterine retinaculum of Martin, which, by the traditional anatomic nomenclature, is composed of three pairs of ligaments (anterior parametrium, uterosacral ligaments, and cardinal ligaments or lateral parametrium), which originate from four central avascular spaces (retropubic, vesicovaginal, rectovaginal and retrorectal or presacral) and four lateral spaces (two paravesical and two pararectal) (Fig. 2.7).

The obliterated umbilical artery, besides being the anatomic mark for the identification of the uterine artery, divides the pararectal space into medial and lateral.

The pararectal space is divided into two; this visualization is due to the mesoureter (ureter and autonomic nerves), forming the medial, also called Okabayashi space, and the lateral, known as Latzko space.

Finally, we must remember the paravaginal space, or fourth Yabuki space, an important point of reference for ureteral tunneling in oncologic surgeries, in which the retrovesical portion of the ureter makes up the roof of this space, easily identified after the section of the vesical pillar (anterior parametrium) (Fig. 2.8).

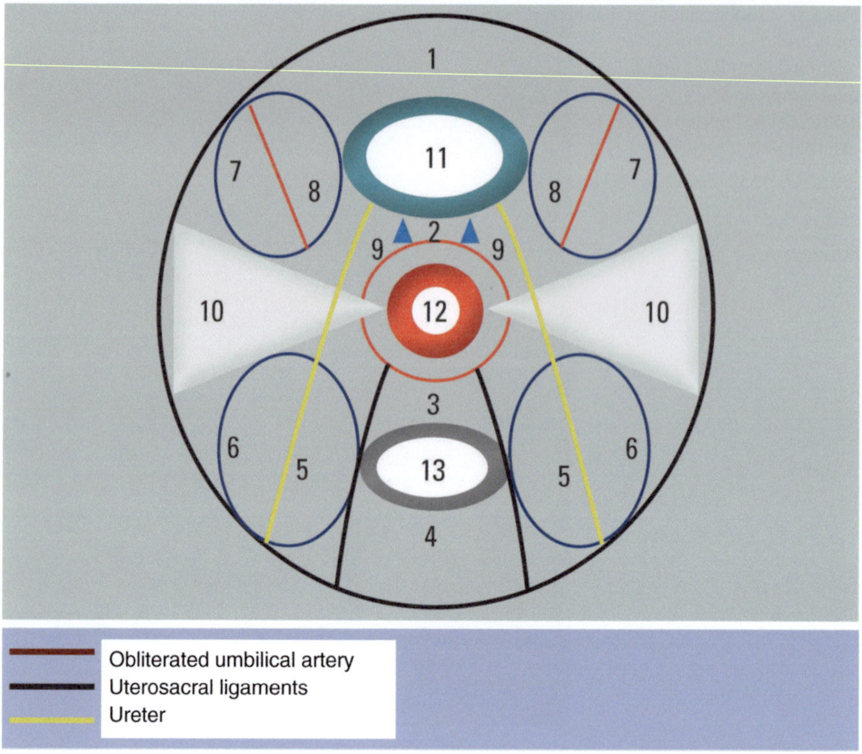

Fig. 2.7 Pelvic organs and their relationships to the pelvic spaces. (1) Retzius space, (2) vesicovaginal space, (3) rectovaginal space, (4) presacral or retrorectal space, (5) medial pararectal space (Okabayashi), (6) lateral pararectal space (Latzko), (7) lateral paravesical space, (8) medial paravesical space, (9) paravaginal space (fourth Yabuki space), (10) lateral parametrium (cardinal) containing uterine artery, (11) bladder, (12) uterine cervix, (13) rectum

Uterine Innervation

The uterine innervation, since it is a viscera, is composed of an autonomic nervous system, comprised of the superior and the inferior hypogastric plexus. The superior hypogastric plexus is responsible for most nociceptive afferent fibers, coming from the pelvic organs, and receives preganglionic sympathetic fibers from the aortic plexus and the sympathetic nerves of L2 and L3; parasympathetic preganglionic fibers from S2 and S3 also contribute to its formation. This plexus is located at the height of L5–S1, right below the bifurcation of iliac arteries, and right after it runs the bifurcation of this plexus into right and left hypogastric nerve (sympathetic).

The inferior hypogastric plexus is the junction of the hypogastric nerves and the pelvic splanchnic nerves and is responsible for most of the motor efferent fibers, arising from the parasympathetic fibers from S2 to S4. In the dissection of pelvic splanchnic nerves, it is necessary to open the hypogastric fascia in the pararectal

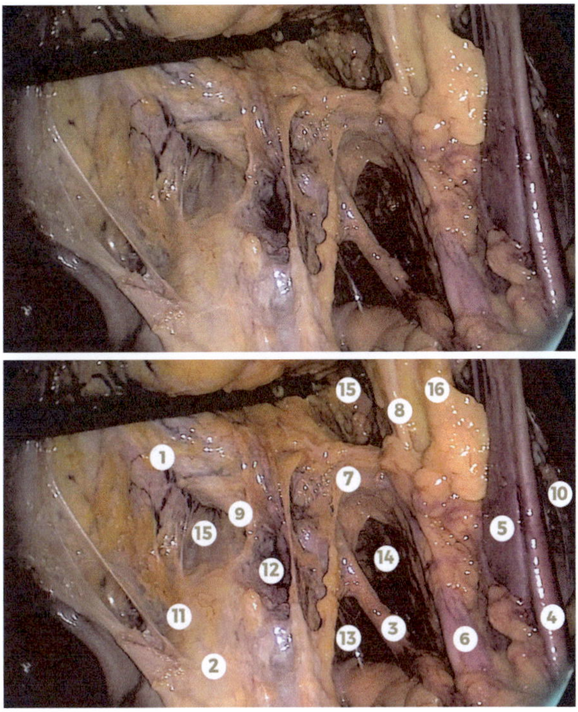

Fig. 2.8 Yabuki's fourth space and its anatomical relationships. (1) Bladder, (2) uterus, (3) ureter, (4) external iliac artery, (5) external iliac vein, (6) external iliac artery, (7) uterine artery, (8) umbilical obliterated artery, (9) vesicouterine ligament, (10) femoral nervous system, (11) vesicovaginal space, (12) paravaginal space or fourth space of Yabuki, (13) pararectal medial space or Okabayashi, (14) pararectal lateral space or Latzko, (15) paravesical medial space, (16) paravesical lateral space

space or the presacral fascia in the retrorectal space; at this point, we observe the exit of these nerves from the sacral roots, which will join the ipsilateral hypogastric nerve, forming the inferior hypogastric plexus or pelvic plexus (parasympathetic) (Fig. 2.9).

Ovaries

The female gonads, organs responsible for the production of sex cells, are called ovaries, which are also glands of the endocrine system, responsible for the production of sex hormones. The embryogenesis of the ovaries is independent of that of the genital apparatus, although its influence is indispensable for the differentiation of the internal genitalia to occur properly. In the reproductive years of a woman's life, the ovaries usually have a smooth surface, while in menopause, the surface is irregular due to residual signs of development and follicular rupture.

The ovaries are organs of pelvic location and are present bilaterally, one on the right and the other on the left side of the pelvis. They are oval and flattened, similar to the shape of almonds, about 3 cm long, 2 cm wide, and 1 cm thick. In the ovary, we can identify two distinct portions: the medulla of the ovary, which consists of

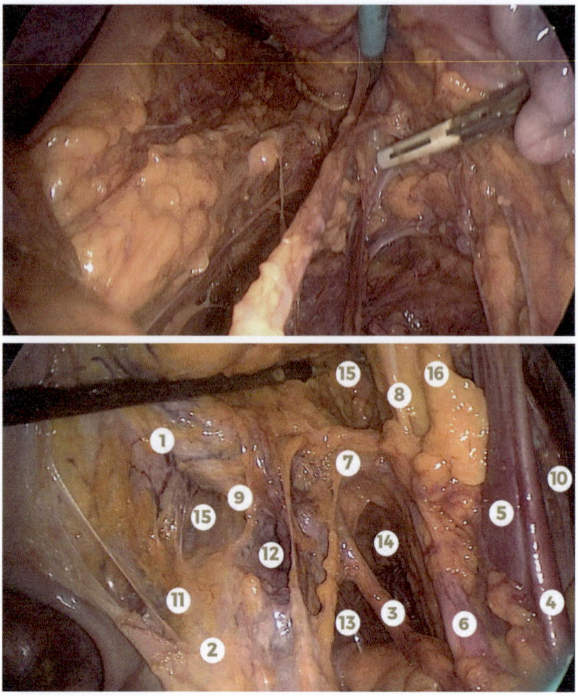

Fig. 2.9 Identification and dissection of the pelvic splanchnic nerves. (1) Hypogastric nerve, (2) sacral nerve S2, (3) sacral nerve S3, (4) splanchnic nerves, (5) inferior hypogastric plexus, (6) rectum

loose connective tissue, rich in blood vessels and blood cells (interstitial), and the cortex of the ovary, rich in ovarian follicles, corpus luteum, and interstitial cells.

The ovaries are located in spaces called ovarian fossae, near the lateral walls of the lesser pelvis, on each side of the uterus, below and behind the fallopian tubes, with variable positioning. As for the relations, the ovaries have two faces, two edges, and two extremities. The lateral face occupies the ovarian fossa, lying over the internal iliac vessels and the ureter. The medial side is related to the fimbriae of the uterine tube and the intestinal loops.

The anterior border, or hilum, is adhered to the broad ligament by the mesovarium and the tubovarian ligament. The mesovarium is a double-peritoneal fold that joins the hilum to the posterior leaflet of the broad ligament, not covering the other surfaces of the ovary, which makes it a loose-moving organ. The upper extremity is attached to the suspensory ligament of the ovary.

The lower extremity is attached to the uterus by the ovarian ligament or the ovarian ligament itself. The ovary is not covered by peritoneum, but the lateral face comes in contact with the parietal peritoneum in the ovarian fossae.

The mesovarium and the tubovarian, ovarian suspensor, and ovarian ligaments are responsible for attaching the ovaries to the uterus and pelvic cavity. The anatomical relations of the ovary are shown in Fig. 2.10.

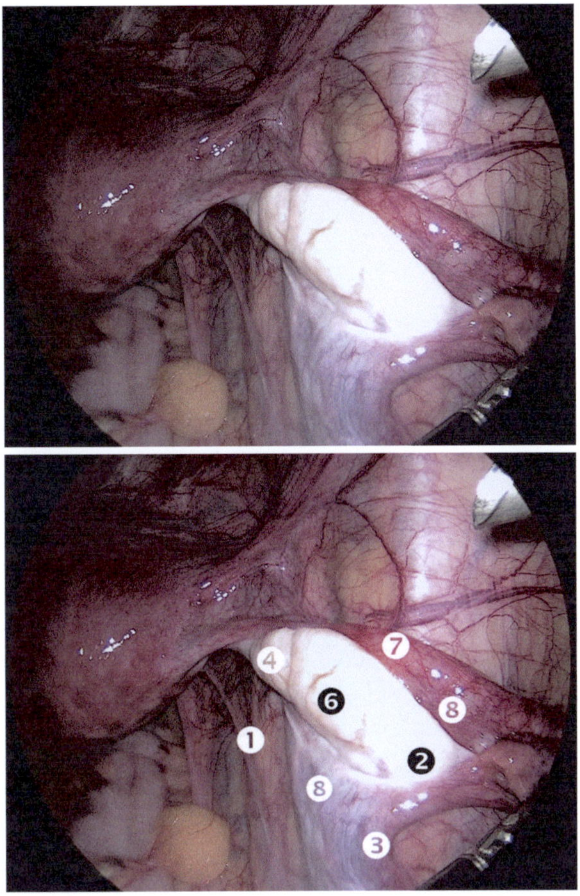

Fig. 2.10 Overview of the female pelvis with special attention to the ovary and its anatomical relationships. (1) Ovarian fossa, (2) cranial end of right ovary, (3) right suspensory ligament of ovary (infundibulopelvic ligament), (4) caudal end of right ovary, (5) right utero-ovarian ligament, (6) free face of ovary, (7) right ovary tube, (8) mesovarium

Vascularization

Arterial: Ovarian artery, collaterals of the aorta, branches of the uterine artery

The ovarian arteries originate in the anterior wall of the abdominal aorta. Their path follows the psoas major muscle, where they follow a descending oblique path, medial to the ureter. Next, they cross the ureter anteriorly and the inferior portion of the external iliac arteries, ending up bifurcating at the upper extremity of the ovary, giving rise to the external tubal and external ovarian arteries. In its retroperitoneal course, accompanied by veins, lymphatics, and nerves, these arteries form, with the parietal peritoneum that covers them, the suspensor ligament of the ovary (Fig. 2.11).

The internal ovarian artery, the terminal branch of the uterine artery, joins the external ovarian artery; together, they form a transverse arcade along the mesovarium, which gives rise to the helical arteries toward the ovary.

Venous Drainage: Ovarian Veins

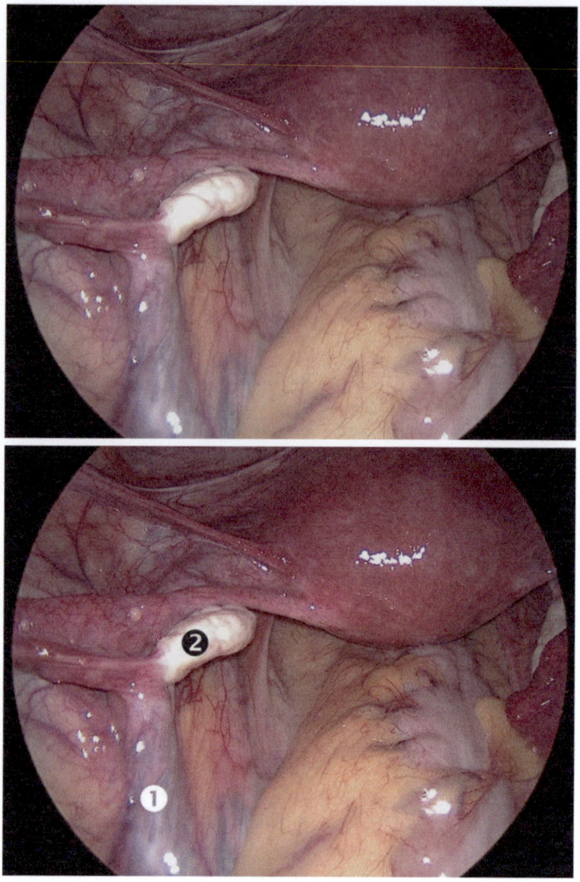

Fig. 2.11 Ovarian suspensor ligament and its anatomical relationships. (1) Left ovarian suspensory ligament, (2) left ovary

The venous drainage occurs through the pampiniform plexus, located in the mesovarium, which effects the blood drainage to the external ovarian vein. The internal ovarian vein drains into the uterine vein. To the right, the ovarian vein drains to the inferior vena cava, and to the left, the ovarian vein drains to the left renal vein.

Lymphatic System

It drains to the lumbar lymph nodes (vena cava and aorta). There is a main route, along the ovarian suspensor ligament, which drains the lymph to the lymph nodes lateral to the vena cava and aorta, and an accessory route that follows the uterine vessels to the internal iliac nodes.

Innervation

Ovarian Plexus

The sympathetic innervation of the ovaries comes from the celiac plexus; as for the path, the nerves walk with the ovarian vessels in the ovarian suspensor ligament. The ovaries also receive nerve branches from the inferior hypogastric plexus. The parasympathetic innervation comes from the inferior hypogastric plexus, which has nerve fibers arriving there through the pelvic splanchnic nerves originating from the roots of S2, S3, and S4.

In procedures for the treatment of ovarian endometriomas that are adhered to the ovarian fossa, it is essential to perform dissection for identification and removal of the ureter, since the ureter is immediately below the peritoneum that covers the ovarian fossa, where ovaries rest and in which there are sometimes adhesions adjacent to the ureter, with the risk of ureteral risk of ureteral injury.

Tips and Tricks
In surgeries that involve removal of the ovaries, it is important to pay attention to a good hemostasis in the region of the ovarian suspensor ligament before the cut, aiming to avoid excessive bleeding, since the vessels originate directly from the aorta. In this same region, there is the risk of injury to the ureter, given its relationship with the ovarian vessels. Therefore, a good presentation is indispensable, with anterior elevation of the ovarian suspensor ligament, in order to move away, from the ureter, the ovarian vessels that will be ligated and sectioned. It is also possible to open the broad ligament before performing the annexectomy, in order to identify and separate the ureter.

Tubes

The uterine tubes are the organs responsible for conducting the ovules from the ovaries to the uterus, and it is inside them that fertilization occurs. They allow the connection between the uterus and the abdominal cavity through openings in their two extremities, one lateral, close to the superior extremity of the ovary, and the other medial, in the uterine cornual region. The fallopian tubes extend laterally, where they curve in the direction of the pelvic wall and fall on the ovaries. They are located between the round ligaments of the uterus anteriorly and the ovaries posteriorly.

As to its structure, the tube is constituted by four concentric layers of tissue, being, from periphery to depth, tunica serosa, tunica subserosa, tunica muscularis, and tunica mucosa.

As far as topography is concerned, the uterine tube is divided into four parts, which in the lateromedial direction are the following (Fig. 2.12):

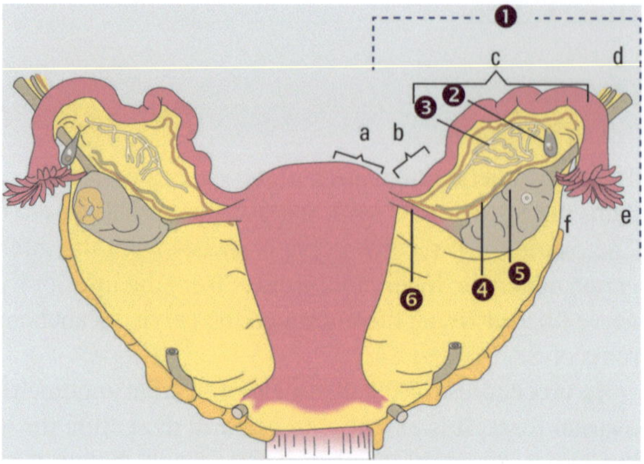

Fig. 2.12 Anatomy of the tube with its portions, vessels, and ligaments. (1) Tuba (a) intramural, (b) isthmus, (c) ampulla, (d) infundibulum, (e) fimbria. (2) Vesicle appendix (Morgagni hydatid). (3) Mesosalpinx (with epoophoron). (4) Mesovarium. (5) Ovary. (6) Ovarian ligament

1. Infundibulum: It is the most distal part of the tube, enclosing itself in folds that constitute the fimbriae, which lean over the ovary and connect to it by means of a more elongated fimbria, called the ovarian fimbriae. The infundibulum communicates with the peritoneal cavity through the abdominal tubal ostium.
2. Ampulla: It is the place where the fertilization of the ovum by the spermatozoid normally occurs. It extends from the isthmus to the infundibulum; it is the most mobile part of the tube and can reach 1 cm in diameter.
3. Isthmus: It is located between the ampulla and the uterine horn, about 2 mm in diameter.
4. Uterine part (intramural or interstitial): It is located in the thickness of the uterine wall; it measures 1 mm in diameter and is approximately 1 cm long.

Arterial Vascularization

Internal and External Tubal Arteries

The arterial irrigation of the Fallopian tubes comes from the anastomosis between the external tubal artery (branch of the ovarian artery) and the internal tubal artery (terminal branch of the uterine artery), as shown in Fig. 2.13.

Venous drainage: Internal and external tubal veins

Venous drainage is done to a plexus located in the mesosalpinx, which drains the internal and external tubal veins.

Lymphatic system: It drains to nodes lateral to the vena cava and aorta, at the origin of the ovarian arteries or following the uterine vessels to the internal iliac nodes.

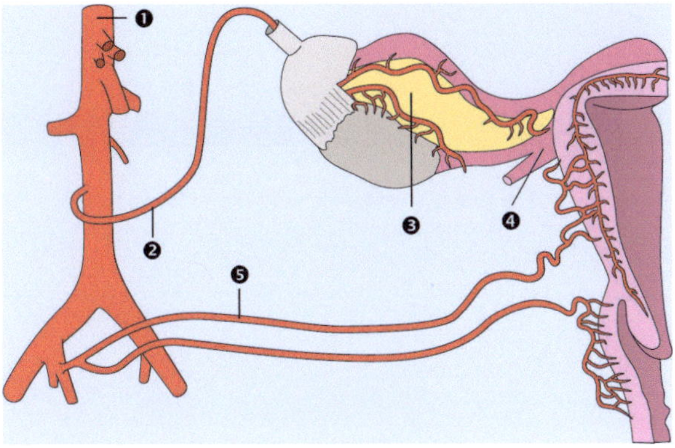

Fig. 2.13 Ovarian tube vascularization. (1) Aorta artery, (2) ovarian artery (branch of the aorta), (3) external tubal artery (branch of the ovarian artery), (4) internal tubal artery (branch of the terminal uterine artery), (5) uterine artery (branch of the internal iliac artery)

Innervation

It is similar to that of the ovaries, with the sympathetic innervation coming from the celiac plexus; as for the path, the nerves walk with the ovarian vessels in the ovarian suspensor ligament. The uterine tube also receives branches from the inferior and superior hypogastric plexus. The parasympathetic fibers come from the inferior hypogastric plexuses, to which they arrive through the pelvic splanchnic nerves, originating from the roots of S2, S3, and S4.

Bibliography

1. Fujii S, Takakura K, Matsumura N, Higuchi T, Yura S, Mandai M, et al. Anatomic identification and functional outcomes of the nerve sparing Okabayashi radical hysterectomy. 2. Gynecol Oncol. 2007;107(1):4–13.
2. Kamina P, Gouazé A. Anatomie clinique: organes urinaires et genitaux, pelvis, coupes du tronc. 2nd ed. Educa Books; 2014. Tome 4
3. Karram B. Atlas de anatomia pélvica e cirurgia ginecológica. 3rd ed. Revinter; 2012.
4. Yabuki Y, Sasaki H, Hatakeyama N, Murakami G. Discrepancies between classic anatomy and modern gynecologic surgery on pelvic connective tissue structure: harmonization of those concepts by collaborative cadaver dissection. Am J Obstet Gynecol. 2005;193(1):7–15.

Chapter 3
Fascias and Ligaments

Adriano Silva Farah, Daniel Bier Caraça, Mariana Carpenedo Tomasi, Sérgio Podgaec, and Paulo Ayroza Ribeiro

Supplementary Information The online version contains supplementary material available at https://doi.org/10.1007/978-3-031-63520-5_3.

A. S. Farah · M. C. Tomasi
Santa Casa de Misericórdia de São Paulo (SCMSP), São Paulo, Brazil

Brazilian Federation of Gynecology and Obstetrics Associations (FEBRASGO), São Paulo, Brazil

D. B. Caraça
Hospital Israelita Albert Einstein (HIAE), São Paulo, Brazil

Faculty of Medicine, University of São Paulo (FMUSP), São Paulo, Brazil

Hospital das Clínicas of the Medical School of the University of São Paulo (HCF-MUSP), São Paulo, Brazil

S. Podgaec
Department of Gynecology and Obstetrics, School of Medicine, University of São Paulo (FMUSP), São Paulo, Brazil

Albert Einstein Hospital and School of Medicine Education, São Paulo, Brazil

P. Ayroza Ribeiro (✉)
Brazilian Federation of Gynecology and Obstetrics Associations (FEBRASGO), São Paulo, Brazil

Department of Obstetrics and Gynecology, School of Medical Sciences, Santa Casa de Misericórida São Paulo (SCMSP), São Paulo, Brazil

Department of Obstetrics and Gynecology, Santa Casa de São Paulo School of Medical Sciences, São Paulo, Brazil

H. Salomão Ayroza, P. Ayroza Ribeiro (eds.), *Atlas of Laparoscopic Gynecological Anatomy*, https://doi.org/10.1007/978-3-031-63520-5_3

Overview

Fascias and ligaments are structures composed of fibrous connective tissue that covers, connects, or supports other tissues and organs. Knowing their anatomy is of utmost importance for the gynecologic surgeon, since it is often necessary to approach these structures or visualize these anatomical landmarks in order to safely access certain sites of the pelvis.

Fascia

Umbilico-Prevesical Fascia

The umbilico-prevesical fascia is triangular in shape. Its anterior edges contain the medial umbilical ligaments and the umbilical arteries (Fig. 3.1). At its base, it fuses with the prevesical fascia. In women, it reaches the upper fascia of the urogenital diaphragm. It forms the inner boundary of the retropubic space caudally and of the paravesical space laterally.

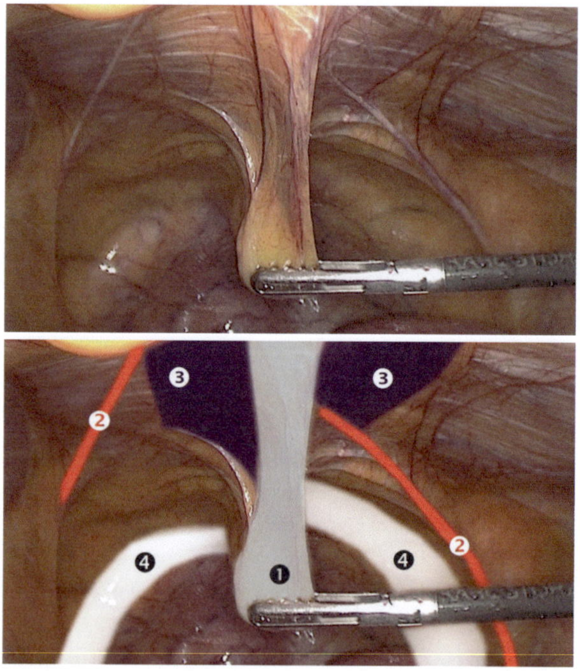

Fig. 3.1 Access to the umbilico-prevesical fascia. (1) Forceps tractioning the umbilical-prevesical fold, (2) obliterated umbilical artery, (3) peritoneum, (4) pubis

Vesicouterine Fascia

The vesicouterine fold, or vesicouterine recess, is a thick fold of peritoneum reflected from the anterior aspect of the junction between the cervix of the uterus and the body of the uterus to the posterior aspect of the bladder. It is attached to the anterior surface of the uterus and cervix and to the posterosuperior surface of the bladder. It creates the superficial vesicouterine pouch.

The surgeon must be aware of the main local structure: the bladder. The dissection of this region must be done with care, pulling the bladder caudally away, exposing the anterior surface of the body and the cervix of the uterus.

The extent of dissection depends on the surgical intention.

Here are some examples:

1. Myomectomy: Usually, access to the vesicouterine fascia in myomectomies applies to large anterior or cervical myomas. The caudal dissection should encompass full exposure of the myoma.
2. Hysterectomy: The exposure and dissection of the vesicouterine fold (Fig. 3.2) are part of the surgical time of any hysterectomy. The caudal extension depends on the type of hysterectomy performed: the subtotal, which maintains the uterine cervix, must be done up to the isthmocervical transition; the total must be done up to the vaginal dome.

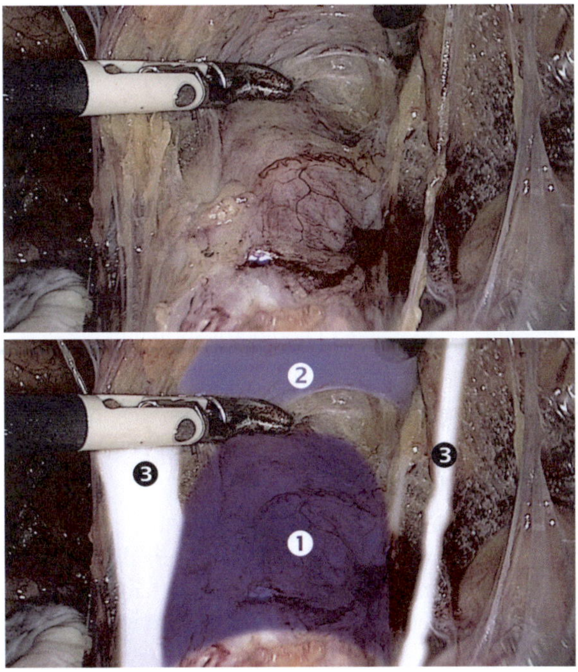

Fig. 3.2 Dissection of the vesicouterine space. (1) Uterine cervix, (2) bladder, (3) bladder pillars

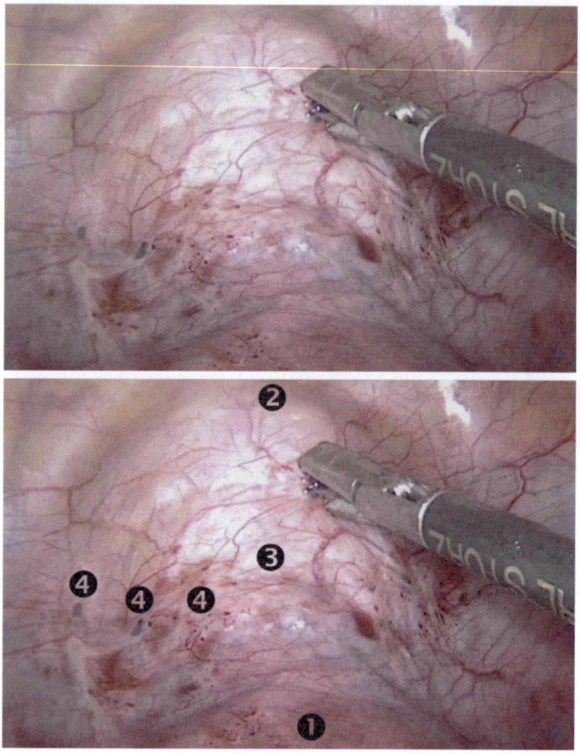

Fig. 3.3 Identification of the vesicouterine fascia with superficial endometriosis lesions. (1) Uterus, (2) bladder, (3) vesicouterine fascia, (4) superficial endometriosis lesions

3. Surgery to treat endometriosis: This depends on the degree of infiltration of the disease. In superficial peritoneal endometriosis (Fig. 3.3), the opening is usually focal, with removal of the lesion only (Fig. 3.4). Deeper lesions may require more extensive dissection, and bladder opening may be necessary (Fig. 3.5).

Tips and Tricks 1
By finding the main anatomical landmarks of the fascia (lateral umbilical ligaments and umbilical arteries) and tractioning them posteroventrally to identify the fascia, the Retzius space is easily found (Fig. 3.6). This space is used in Burch surgery, in the approach to bladder endometriosis and in ureteral reimplantation.

Tips and Tricks 2
The vesicouterine fold is an anatomical landmark frequently addressed in gynecological surgeries, such as myomectomies, hysterectomies, and surgeries to treat endometriosis.

Tips and Tricks 3
The first assistant tractions the rectum cranially for presentation of the rectovaginal fascia; at the same time, the second assistant should traction the uterus cranially and anteriorly, for visualization and identification of the fascia (Figs. 3.7 and 3.8).

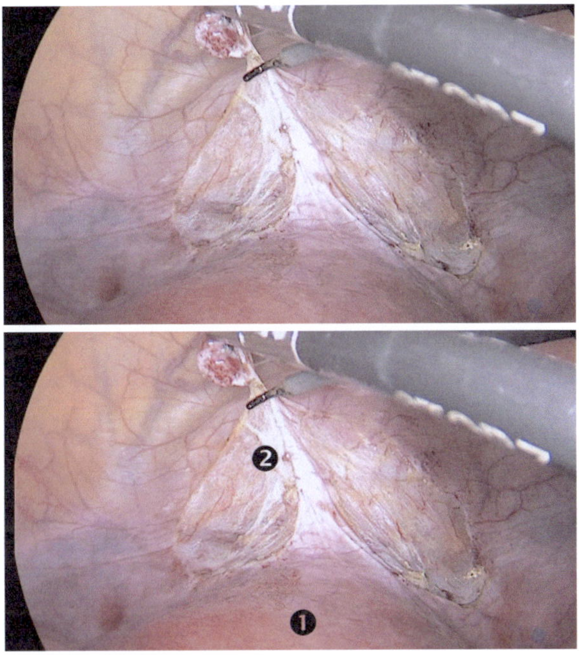

Fig. 3.4 Resection of a superficial endometriosis lesion of the vesicouterine fascia. (1) Uterus, (2) resection of peritoneal endometriotic lesion

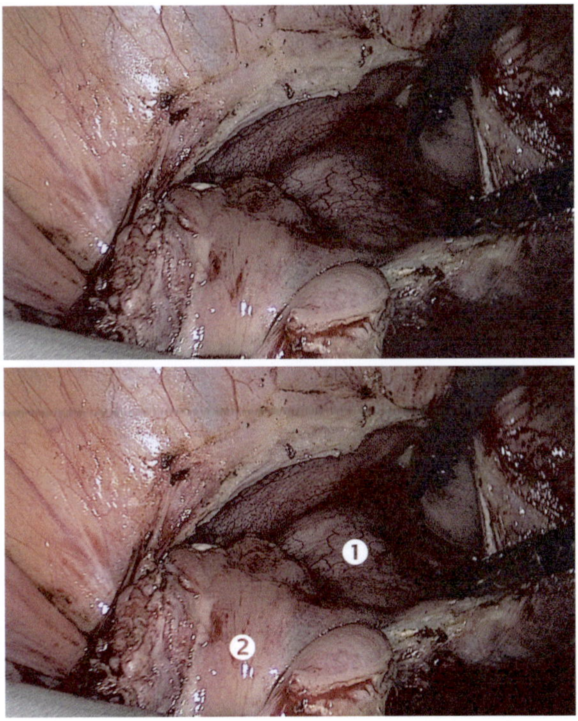

Fig. 3.5 Resection of bladder endometriosis with its opening. (1) Bladder trigone, (2) endometriosis lesion

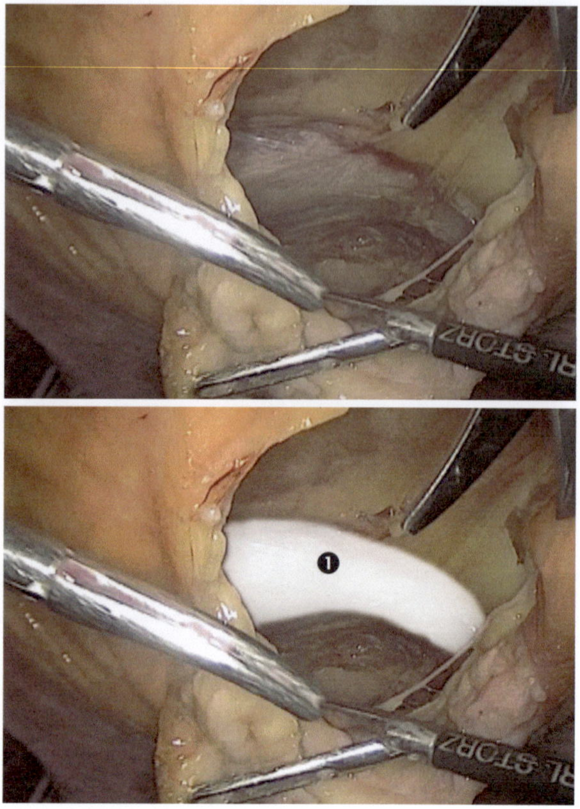

Fig. 3.6 Opening of the umbilico-prevesical fold and visualization of Retzius space. (1) Pubis

Tips and Tricks 4
The rectovaginal space, and therefore the rectovaginal fascia, can be accessed by bidigital touch (Fig. 3.9).

Rectovaginal Fascia

The rectovaginal fascia is a thick fold of peritoneum reflected from the posterior vaginal fornix to the anterior surface of the rectum. It adheres to the posterior surface of the vagina and to the anterior surface of the rectum, creating the deep recto-uterine pouch.

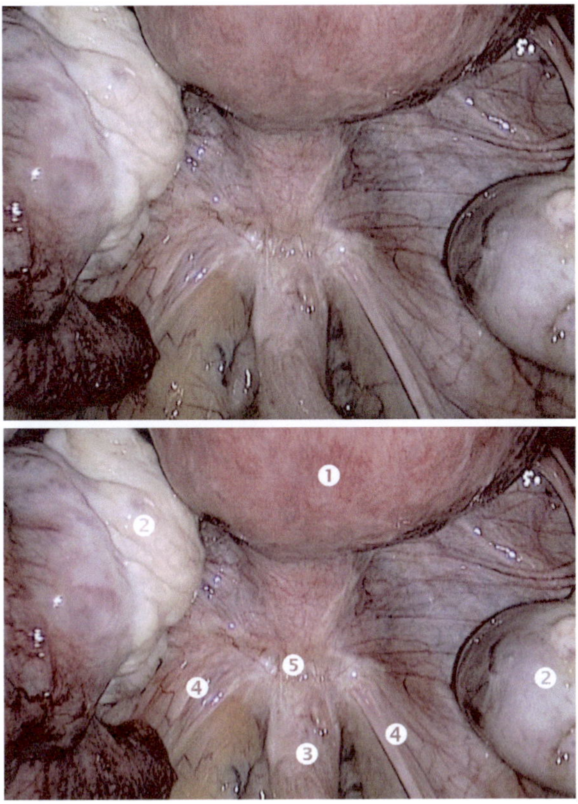

Fig. 3.7 Patient with deep endometriosis presenting with involvement of the rectum and retrocervical region. (1) Uterus, (2) ovaries, (3) rectum, (4) uterosacral ligaments, (5) rectovaginal fascia with endometriosis

Presacral Fascia

The pelvic presacral fascia is the continuation of the abdominal fascia. It is curved and covers the pelvic walls laterally and the sacrum dorsally and then fuses ventrally with the parametrium and paracervix, laterally and dorsally with the uterosacral and rectovaginal ligaments, and caudally with the rectosacral fascia. The presacral fascia supports the rectum; the attached vessels; the ureter, splanchnic, hypogastric, and sacral nerves; the inferior hypogastric plexus, and the efferent branches. The perirectal fat contained between the presacral fascia and the visceral peritoneum is called the mesorectum. Within the presacral fascia is a thin, sagittally oriented mesentery surrounding the ureter, which is called the mesoureter (Fig. 3.10).

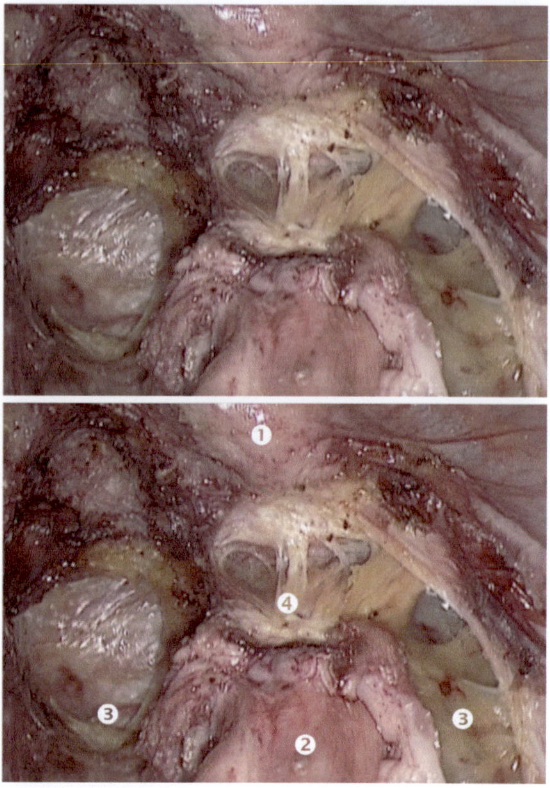

Fig. 3.8 Same patient as in Fig. 3.7 after dissection of the pararectal fossae; identification of the levator ani muscle (puborectal bundle), and identification of the fossae with the rectovaginal fascia to be explored. (1) Uterus, (2) rectum, (3) pararectal fossa bilateral (contains the wing of the rectum), (4) rectovaginal fascia

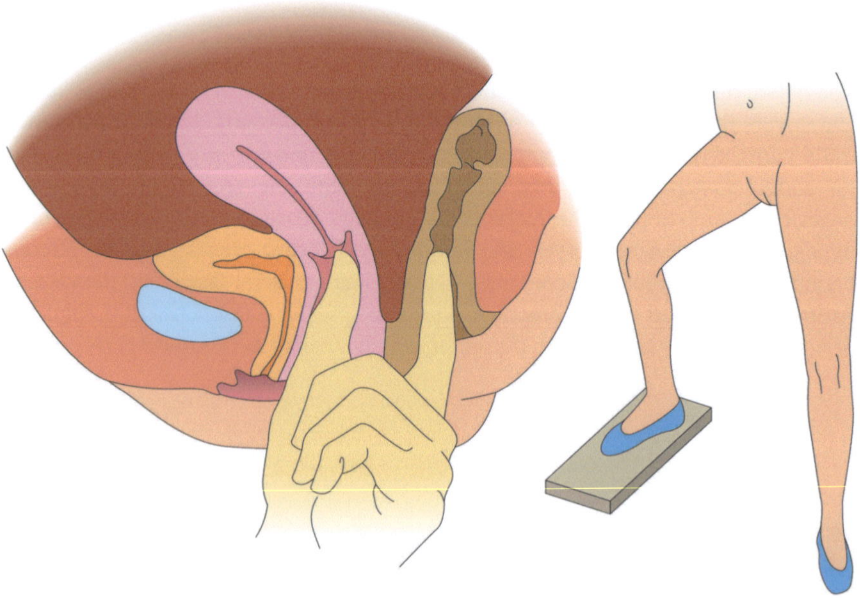

Fig. 3.9 Bidigital (rectovaginal) touch to help identify the rectovaginal space and fascia

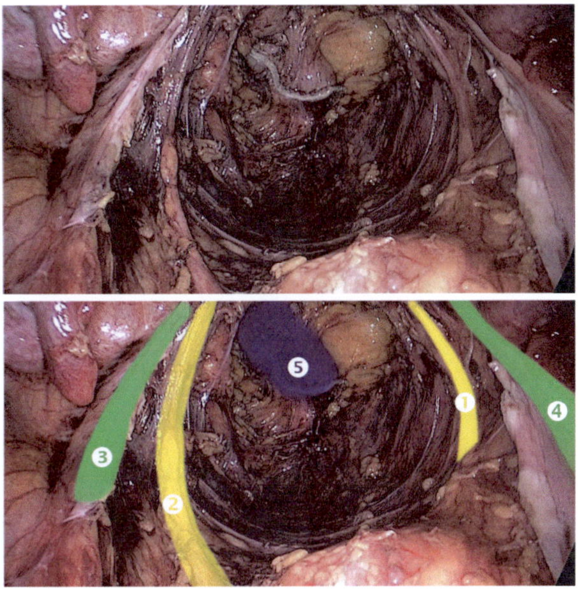

Fig. 3.10 Deep endometriosis surgery with segmental resection of the rectosigmoid. Note the amputated rectum after dissection of the pararectal spaces. The ureter and mesoureter are clearly visible and preserved. The hypogastric nerves and fascia are also preserved. (1) Right hypogastric nerve, (2) left hypogastric nerve, (3) left ureter, (4) right ureter, (5) rectum

Fascia Propria of the Rectum

The rectus fascia propria is a condensation of the endopelvic fascia that forms an involute to the mesorectum and continues distally to make up the lateral rectal wings (anterolateral structures containing the middle fetal artery).

The rectal wings are in close proximity to the autonomic nerves (sympathetic and parasympathetic), and sectioning these structures near the lateral wall of the pelvis may result in bladder dysfunction (Figs. 3.8 and 3.10).

Ligaments

Round Ligaments of the Uterus

The round ligaments are structures composed mainly of smooth muscle and connective tissue. They are a pair of narrow, flat bands approximately 10–12 cm long that originate from the anterolateral fundus of the uterus, just below the uterine horn. This ligament extends ventrally and laterally—with blood vessels, lymphatic vessels, and nerves—to the anterior abdominal wall, entering the inguinal canal and terminating in the fat on either side of the labia majora.

Exposure of extraperitoneal structures can be achieved by opening the top of the ligamentum flavum, between the round ligament and the pelvic infundibulum,

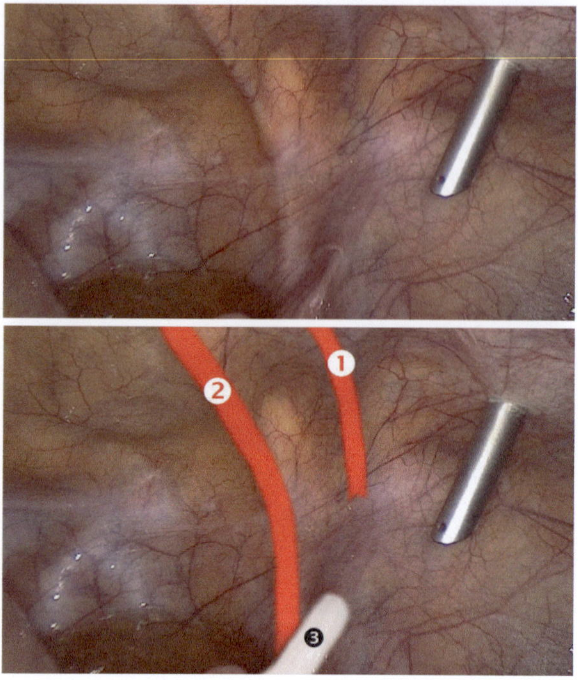

Fig. 3.11 Surgical image demonstrating the round ligament and its importance as an anatomical landmark during insertion of the auxiliary trocars. (1) Epigastric vessels, (2) obliterated umbilical artery, (3) round ligament

lateral to the external artery. This site provides easy access to both lateral walls and retroperitoneal spaces, exposing the ureter and uterine vascular supply (Fig. 3.11).

Tips and Tricks 5
The round ligament, especially in its abdominal insertion, is an important anatomical landmark, helping the surgeon in the placement of accessory trocars. The inferior epigastric artery, derived from the external iliac artery and that supplies the anterior abdominal wall, should always be identified, thus avoiding puncture accidents. It is seen, under laparoscopic vision, medially to the insertion of the round ligament in the deep inguinal ring, forming a fold of peritoneum. In gynecological surgeries, the accessory trocars, when inserted, should be positioned laterally to these vessels (Figs. 3.11 and 3.12).

Uterosacral Ligaments

The uterosacral ligaments are formed by two leaflets of visceral peritoneum that have a thin band of dense connective tissue and smooth muscle fibers. They also contain fibers of pelvic autonomic nerves, predominantly sympathetic, originating from the thoracolumbar and superior hypogastric plexus. They extend from the posterior part of the isthmus, passing through the posterior cervix and fornix of the vagina, until they attach to the anterior surface of the sacrum and form the lateral limits of the posterior Douglas fundus.

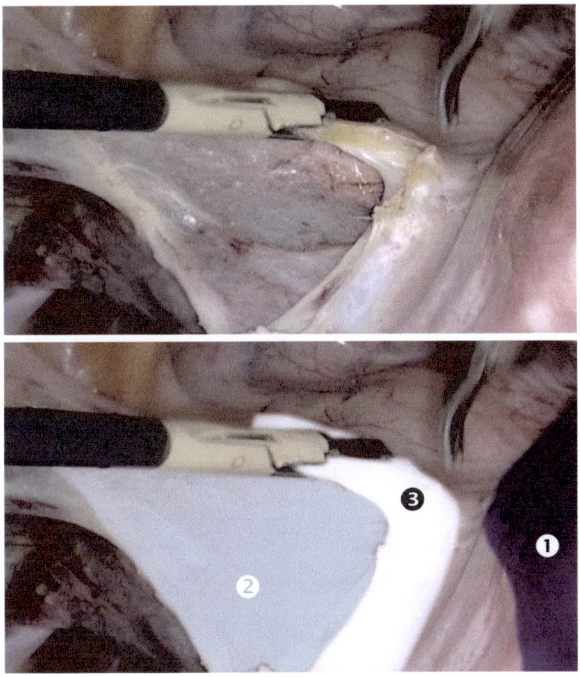

Fig. 3.12 The round ligament and the anterior leaflet of the broad ligament have already been sectioned at the beginning of a hysterectomy. (1) Uterus, (2) posterior leaflet of broad ligament (gray avascular area), (3) anterior leaflet of broad ligament

The rectum lies in a medial position, and the ureters and vessels of the lateral walls run lateral to the uterosacral ligaments.

With the rectovaginal ligament, the uterosacral ligaments form a fascial block that, together with the fascia of the pelvic organs, supports the intrapelvic position of the uterus.

Surgical Application

- In intrafascial hysterectomy, the colpotomy must be performed without detaching the uterosacral ligaments from the pericervical ring in order to maintain pelvic support (Fig. 3.13). In radical hysterectomies, the uterosacral ligaments are sectioned and sutured together.
- In endometriosis surgeries, it is very common to have adhesions with the ureter, nerves, and bowel (Fig. 3.14). To perform the excision of this ligament, the ureter must be identified and lateralized; furthermore, the nerves and the pararectal spaces (Latzko and Okabayashi) must be identified.
- In a sacrocolpofixation surgery, or in McCall's surgery, the uterosacral ligaments are identified, and the fixation of the vaginal dome is done in the intermediate portion to avoid kinking or obstruction of the ureters.

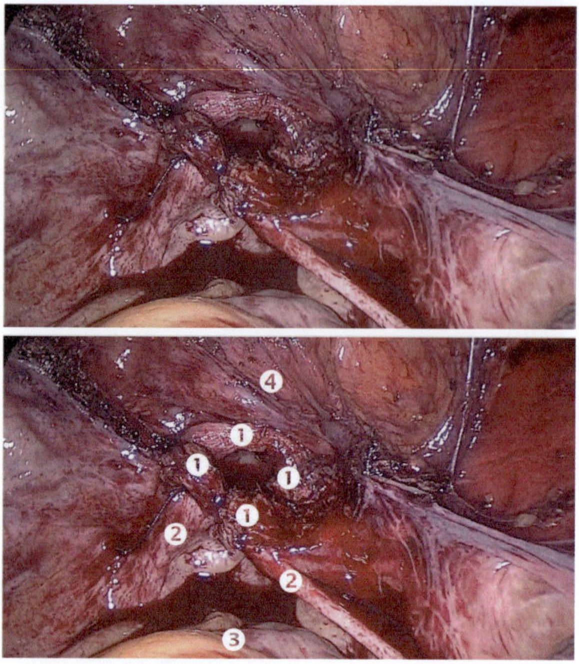

Fig. 3.13 Hysterectomy by intrafascial technique preserving the pericervical ring, without cutting the uterosacral ligaments. On the left, an X-stitch has been performed. (1) Pericervical ring, (2) uterosacral ligaments, (3) rectum, (4) bladder

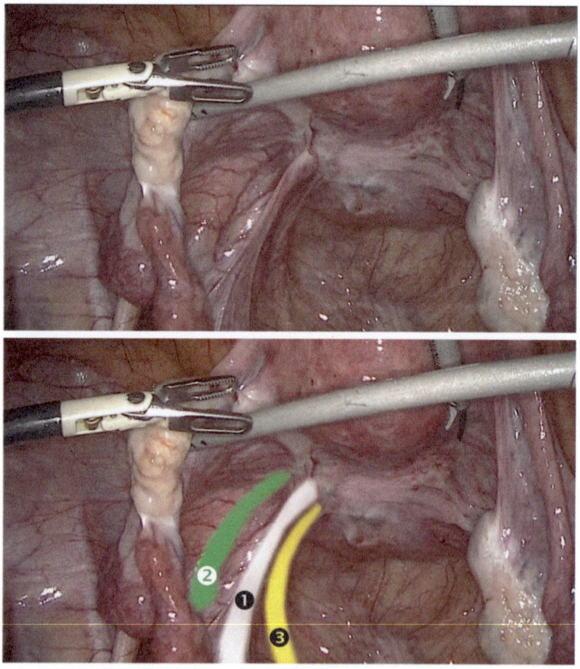

Fig. 3.14 Surgical image showing the focus of endometriosis in left uterosacral ligament and retrocervical region. (1) Uterosacral ligament with darkened uterine lesion, (2) left ureter, (3) left hypogastric nerve (vaginal, rectal, and vesical branches)

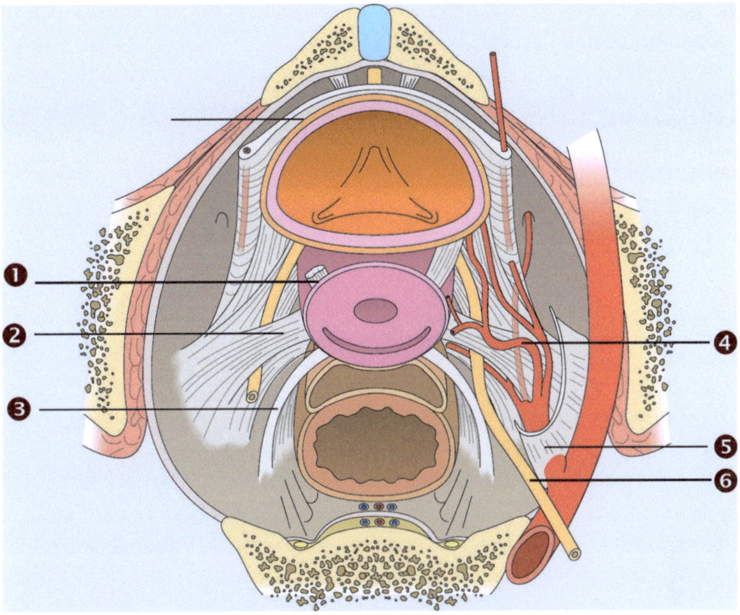

Fig. 3.15 Supporting structures of the uterus. (1) Bladder pillar, (2) cardinal ligament, (3) utero-sacral ligament, (4) uterine artery, (5) parametrium, (6) ureter

Tips and Tricks 6

1. In cases of cardinal ligament endometriosis, it is necessary to perform ureterolysis and neurolysis due to the proximity of the structures. There may be stenosis of the ureter, with functional impairment, due to the formation of a fibrotic ring.
2. For exposure of the ureter in its distal portion, after the crossing with the uterine vessels, the cardinal ligament must be dissected, a technique used in radical hysterectomies (Figs. 3.15 and 3.16).

Tendinous Arch

The tendinous arch of the pelvic fascia is a thickened linear component of the obturator fascia between the ischial spine and the pelvic surface of the pubis (Fig. 3.17). It is formed by the fusion of the pubocervical fascia with the pelvic parietal fascia, covering the obturator muscle.

The tendinous arch of the levator ani muscle fuses with the tendinous arch of the pelvic fascia coming from the ischial spine halfway up, where it joins the inferior pubic ramus to form the levator ani muscles (Fig. 3.18).

The tendinous arch secures the vagina laterally at DeLancey level 2. When there is downward pressure on the anterior wall of the vagina toward the introitus, it is the

Fig. 3.16 Radical hysterectomy after uterine artery dissection and ureterolysis. (1) Ureter, (2) uterosacral ligaments, (3) uterine artery, (4) vesicouterine fascia

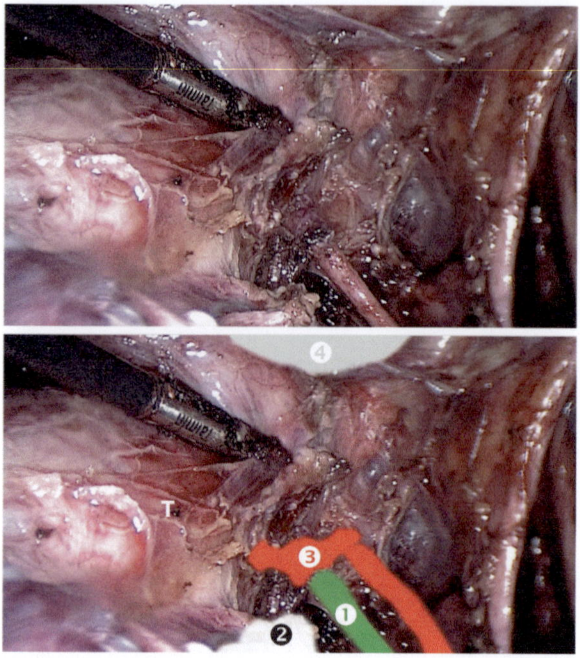

Fig. 3.17 Right side of Retzius space (from cadaver) with the partially torn tendinous arch of the pelvic parietal fascia. (1) Tendinous arch, (2) bladder, (3) pubis

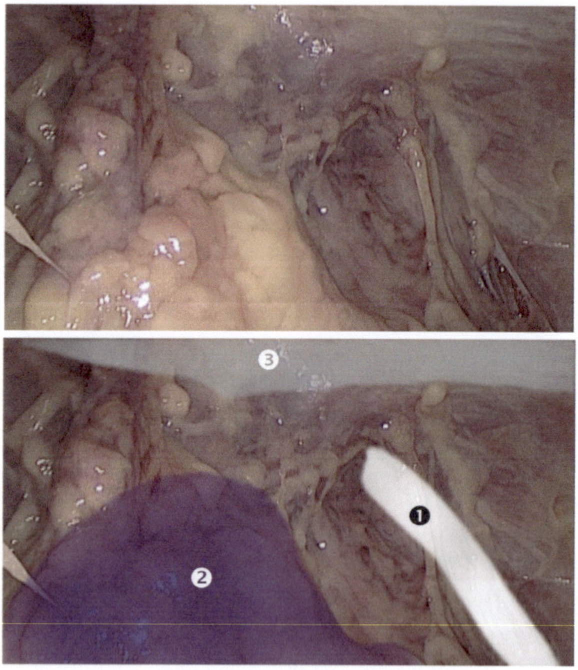

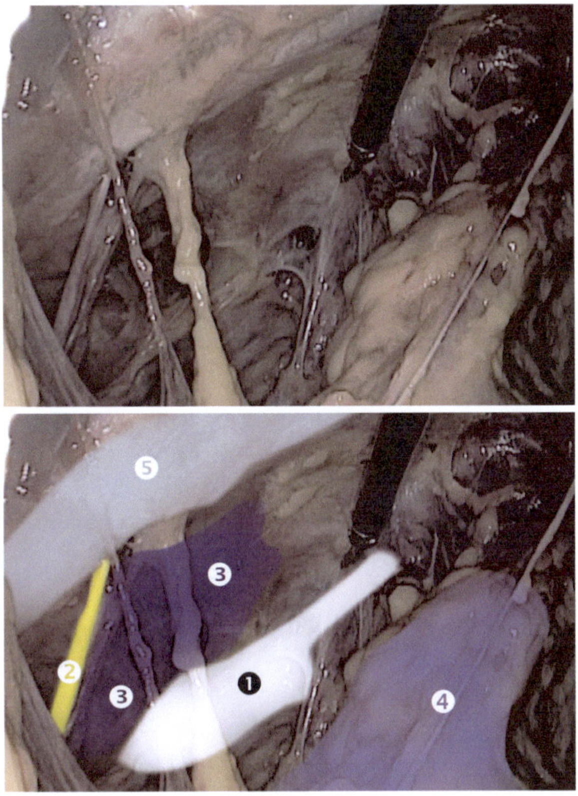

Fig. 3.18 Left side of Retzius space. (1) Tendinous arch of the levator ani muscle shown in the scissor tip, (2) obturator nerve, (3) obturator muscle, (4) bladder, (5) pubis

tendinous arch of the pelvic (pubocervical) fascia that supports it. When there is upward pressure on the posterior wall of the vagina toward the introitus, it is the tendinous arch of the levators of the anus (rectovaginal) that supports it.

Tips and Tricks 7
Patients with damage to the connective tissue that connects the vagina and the pelvic floor muscles present descent of the pelvic structures according to their location. Clinically, the mucosa of the vagina shows a rough surface due to the defect in the lateral wall. If the mucosa of the external vagina is smooth, the fascia defect is central. The correction of the cases therefore depends on the type of defect.

Bibliography

1. Baggish MSK, Karram MM. Atlas de anatomia pélvica e cirurgia ginecológica. 3rd ed. Rio de Janeiro: Revinter; 2011. p. 179–206.
2. Crispi CP, Oliveira FMM, Damian Junior JC, Oliveira MAP, Ribeiro PAG. Tratado de endoscopia ginecológica: cirurgia minimamente invasiva. 3rd ed. Rio de Janeiro: Revinter; 2012.

3. Ercoli A, Delmas V, Fanfani F, Gadonneix P, Ceccaroni M, Fagotti A, et al. Terminologia Anatomica versus unofficial descriptions and nomenclature of the fasciae and ligaments of the female pelvis: a dissection-based comparative study. Am J Obstet Gynecol. 2005;193(4):1565–73.
4. Hoffman BL, Schorge JO, Schaffer JI, Halvorson LM, Bradshaw KD, Cunningham FG. Ginecologia de Williams. 2nd ed. São Paulo: Artmed; 2014.
5. DeLancey JO. Anatomic aspects of vaginal eversion after hysterectomy. Am J Obstet Gynecol. 1992;166(6 Pt 1):1717–28.
6. Kamina P. Anatomie clinique. 2nd ed. Paris: Maloine; 2002.
7. Schleip R, Jäger H, Klingler W. What is 'fascia'? A review of different nomenclatures. J Bodyw Mov Ther. 2012;16(4):496–502.

Chapter 4
Pelvic Floor

Andresa Maria Felipe de Paiva, Graziele Vidoto Cervantes, Marina de Paula Andres, Mauricio Simões Abrão, and Priscila de Almeida Barbosa

Supplementary Information The online version contains supplementary material available at https://doi.org/10.1007/978-3-031-63520-5_4.

A. M. F. de Paiva
Ob/Gyn Department, Santa Casa de São Paulo School of Medical Sciences, São Paulo, Brazil

Brazilian Federation of Gynecology and Obstetrics Associations (FEBRASGO), São Paulo, Brazil

G. V. Cervantes (✉)
Ob/Gyn Department, Santa Casa de São Paulo School of Medical Sciences, São Paulo, Brazil

Brazilian Federation of Gynecology and Obstetrics Associations (FEBRASGO), São Paulo, Brazil

Santa Casa de Misericórdia de São Paulo (SCMSP), São Paulo, Brazil

M. de Paula Andres
Endometriosis Department, University of São Paulo School of Medicine Hospital das Clínicas (HC-FMUSP), São Paulo, Brazil

Hospital Beneficência Portuguesa of São Paulo (HBPSP), São Paulo, Brazil

M. S. Abrão
Hospital Beneficência Portuguesa of São Paulo (HBPSP), São Paulo, Brazil

Department of Obstetrics and Gynecology, School of Medicine, University of São Paulo (FMUSP), São Paulo, Brazil

P. de Almeida Barbosa
Faculty of Medicine, University of São Paulo (FMUSP), São Paulo, Brazil

Invasive Gynecologic Surgery Program, Hospital Beneficência Portuguesa of São Paulo (HBPSP), São Paulo, Brazil

H. Salomão Ayroza, P. Ayroza Ribeiro (eds.), *Atlas of Laparoscopic Gynecological Anatomy*, https://doi.org/10.1007/978-3-031-63520-5_4

Overview

The pelvic floor is responsible for controlling important functions such as urination, evacuation, or continence of urine and feces, acting as a sphincter. All these functions are performed in a voluntary manner, in a harmony between the systems of suspension and sustentation.

The suspension is performed by the smooth musculature and connective tissue, being anterior bundles (pubocervical ligament), lateral bundles (Mackenrodt's or cardinal ligaments), and posterior bundles (uterosacral ligaments, which connect the uterus to the sacrum, taking the structures upwards and backwards). The pelvic diaphragm presents dynamic functionality in the pelvic floor and divides the perineum from the pelvic cavity. It consists of the coccygeal (or ischiococcygeal) muscle and the levator ani muscles (pubococcygeal, pubovaginal, puborectal, and iliococcygeal).

The urogenital diaphragm, in turn, is responsible for the static functionality of the pelvic floor, composed of the bulbocavernosus, ischiocavernosus, transverse perineal muscles (superficial and deep), and external sphincteral muscle.

Pelvic Diaphragm

Coccygeal Muscle

This is also called ischiococcygeus. Together with the levator ani muscles, it forms the pelvic diaphragm. It assists in controlling intra-abdominal pressure and is involved in coccygeal movement during labor and delivery.

Innervation: It is derived partially from the ventral face and part of the superior face of the ventral branches of S4.

Vascularization: Its irrigation comes mainly from the pudenda interna, inferior vesical and obturator arteries, and, as an accessory, lateral sacral artery.

Origin: It has a triangular shape; it originates from the internal surface of the ischial spine and inserts on the border of the S4 and S5 sacral vertebrae and laterally to the coccyx. It is also described as the muscular portion of the sacrospinal ligament with which it fuses in its pelvic aspect, making the muscle appear absent when the ligament is more prominent (Fig. 4.1).

Tips and Tricks 1
Regarding clinical applicability, the pelvic floor is of great importance as both a suspension and support device for the female pelvic floor. With the aging of the population, the complaint of pelvic organ prolapse is becoming more prevalent.

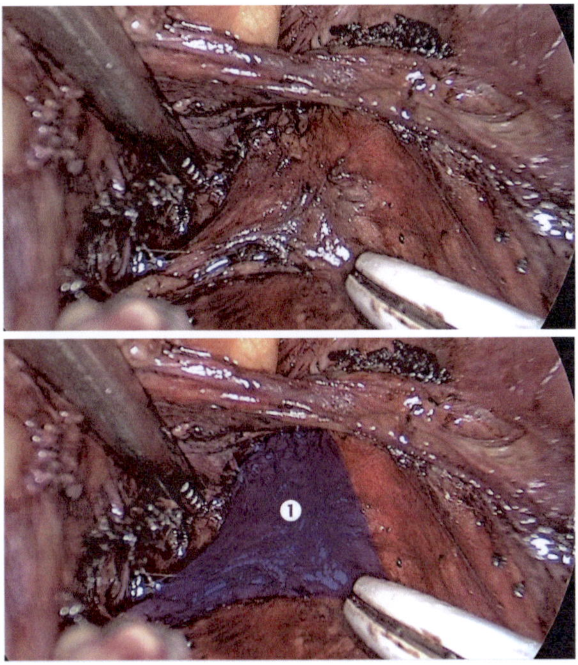

Fig. 4.1 Coccygeal muscle during laparoscopic dissection. (1) Coccygeus muscle. (Image kindly provided by Dr. Nucélio Lemos)

Elevator Ani Muscles

They are divided into bundles of muscle fibers that insert into the perineal body, rectum, vagina, urethra, and levator ani muscles (Fig. 4.2).

Innervation: The pelvic surface is innervated primarily through the third and fourth branches of the sacral vessels. It starts at the ischial spine and ends at the iliococcygeus muscle. The pudendal branch participates in the innervation of the pubovaginal muscle.

Vascularization: Its irrigation originates mainly from the pudenda interna, vesical inferior and obturator arteries, and, as an accessory, lateral sacral artery.

Pubococcygeus Muscle

The pubococcygeus muscle is found in both sexes. It has great importance in the support of the pelvic organs and in the formation of the pelvic diaphragm, being directly related to urinary incontinence in women.

Origin: On the posterior surface of the pubic bone, near the symphysis pubis, and in the anterior part of the tendinous arch, toward the coccyx. The fibers that originate from the arch of tendon insert into the anococcygeal ligament (between the coccyx and the anal canal).

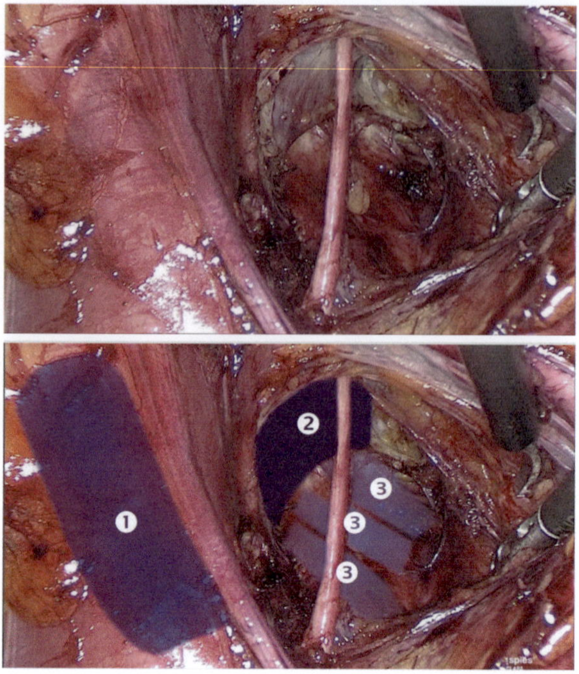

Fig. 4.2 Levator ani muscles and accessory muscles. Dissection of the pelvic floor on the left. (1) Psoas muscle, (2) internal obturator muscle, (3) levator ani muscle. (Image kindly provided by Dr. Nucélio Lemos)

Tips and Tricks 2

Kegel exercises: These are contraction and relaxation exercises designed to strengthen the pubococcygeus muscle and give voluntary control over it. Used as treatment for urinary incontinence and vaginal prolapse.

Pubovaginal or Pubovisceral Muscle

Origin: The muscle fibers originate from the pubococcygeus muscle, which comes from the posterior aspect of the body of the pubic bone and the tendinous arch toward the coccyx. In women, the fibers located medially and anteriorly extend to the vagina, the urethra, and the perineal body.

Puborectal Muscle

It is responsible for the anterior angulation of the anorectal junction, which is able to control the fecal continence effect.

Origin: Its calibrous bundle of muscular fibers also originates from the pubococcygeus muscle, which comes from the posterior aspect of the pubic bone and the arcus tendineus, but its fibers run posteriorly, forming three bundles of fibers: latero-rectal bundle, which communicates with the anal canal bundles and participates in the formation of the sphincter (internal and external) of the anus; retrorectal bundle, homologous fibers that form the anorectal junction; and coccygeal bundle, which attaches to the coccyx and the ventral sacrococcygeal ligament (Figs. 4.3, 4.4, 4.5, and 4.6).

Iliococcygeus Muscle

Represents the posterior part of the levator ani muscle (Figs. 4.7, 4.8, 4.9, and 4.10).

Origin: In the posterior region of the tendinous arch, in the thickest part, and near the obturator internus; inserts in the anococcygeal ligament and coccyx.

Tips and Tricks 3

There are several techniques for correction of pelvic organ prolapse. Currently, the most used is the laparoscopic sacrocolpopexy, with a high success rate (92.1%), which consists of the fixation of a sustentation mesh in the pelvic cavity promontory. This technique uses the fixation of the mesh to the reconstructed pericervical ring fascia (includes anterior, lateral, and posterior portions of the fascia) or to the

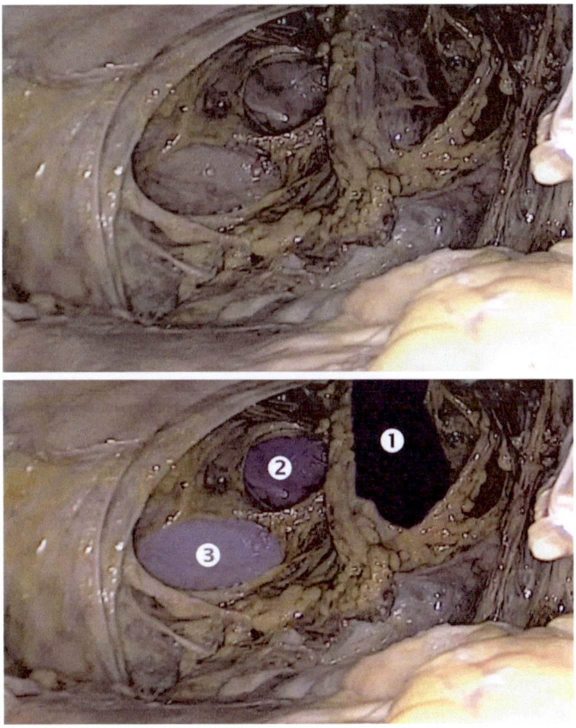

Fig. 4.3 Dissection, in a cadaver, of the left pararectal space. (1) Recto, (2) puborectalis muscle, (3) iliococcygeus muscle

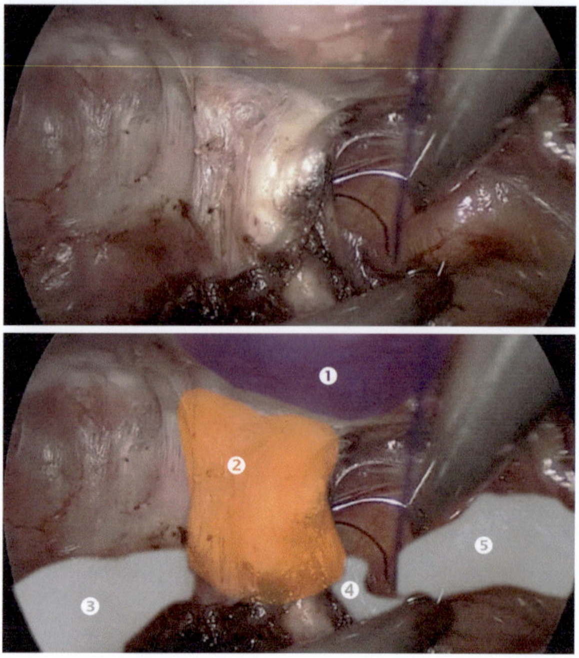

Fig. 4.4 Colposacropexy showing the passage of the needle in the puborectal muscle on the right. (1) Uterus, (2) rectouterine space, (3) rectum, (4) pararectal space, (5) puborectal muscle

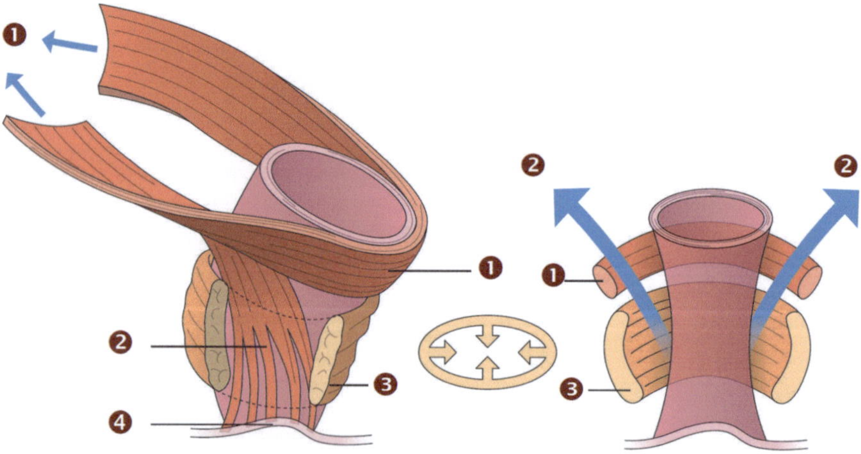

Fig. 4.5 Puborectal muscle and external anal sphincter. (1) Retrorectal fascia, (2) laterorectal fascia, (3) external sphincter of the anus muscle, (4) anus margin muscle

uterine cervix; this is done not only to reconstruct the angle and inclination of the vaginal axes but also to build a sustentation mechanism, avoiding the recurrence of the prolapse through fixation on a sustainable structure. As an alternative to laparoscopic sacrocolpopexy, laparoscopic pectopexy can be performed; according to this technique, instead of the mesh being attached to the promontory, it is attached to the pectineal ligament.

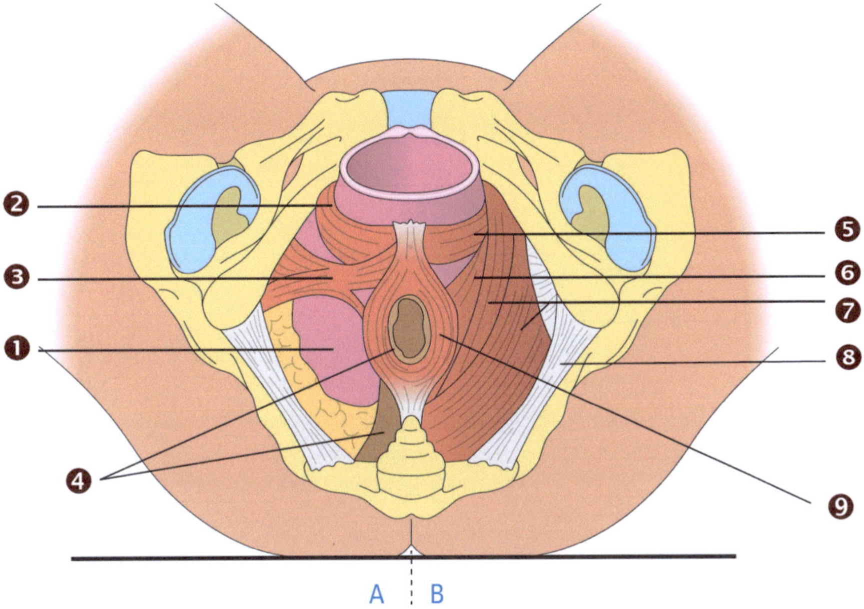

Fig. 4.6 Pubovaginal and puborectal muscles. (1) Vagina, (2) bulbocavernosus muscle, (3) superficial transverse muscle, (4) anal canal, (5) pubovaginal muscle, (6) puborectal muscle, (7) iliococcygeus muscle, (8) sacrotuberal ligament, (9) internal sphincter of the anus muscle

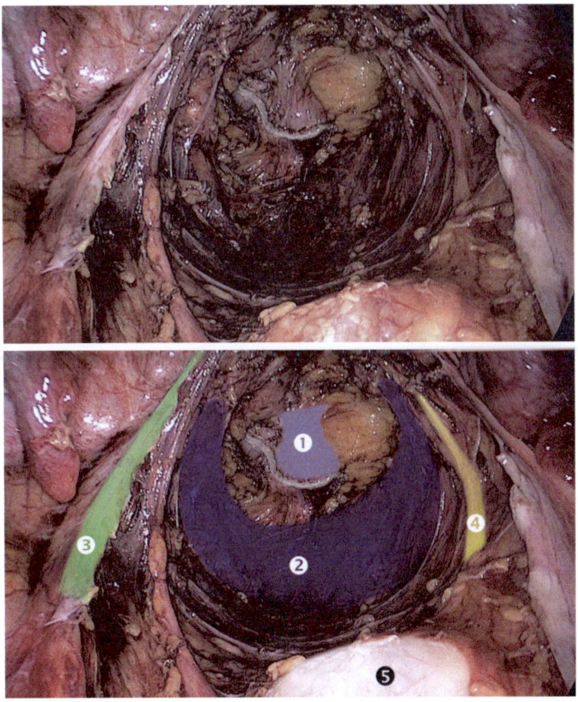

Fig. 4.7 Pararectal and retrorectal space dissection for rectosigmoidectomy for endometriotic lesion, identifying rectum, iliococcygeus muscle, left ureter, right hypogastric nerve, and promontory. (1) Rectum, (2) iliococcygeal muscle, (3) left ureter, (4) right hypogastric nerve, (5) promontory. (Image kindly provided by Dr. Maurício Abrão)

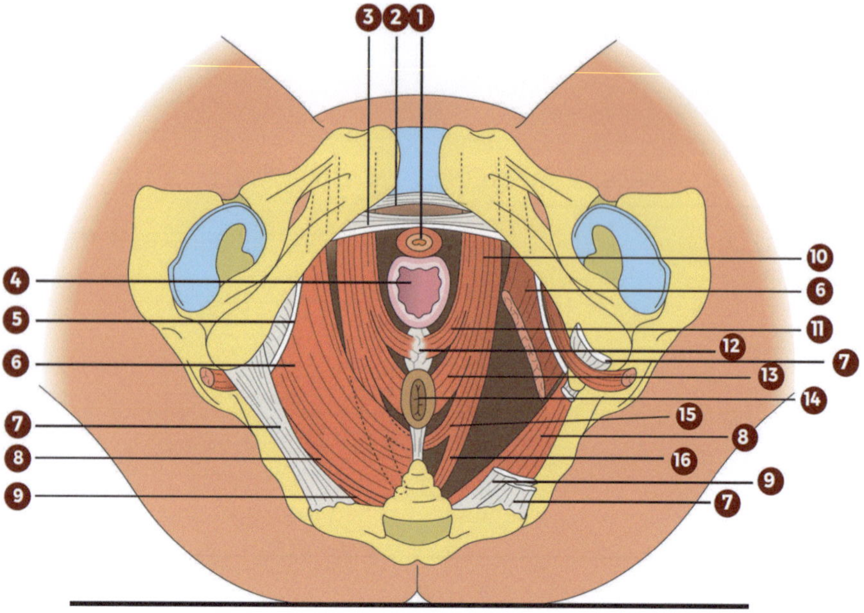

Fig. 4.8 Levator ani muscles (perineal view): (1) Urethra, (2) inferior pubis ligament, (3) transverse perineal ligament, (4) vagina, (5) tendinous arch of levator ani muscles, (6) iliococcygeal muscle, (7) sacrotuberal ligament, (8) iliococcygeal muscle, (9) sacrospinous ligament, (10) pubococcygeus muscle, (11) pubovaginal muscle, (12) perineal body, (13) puborectal muscle (laterorectal fascia), (14) anus, (15) puborectal muscle (rectoanal fascia), and (16) puborectal muscle (coccygeal fascia)

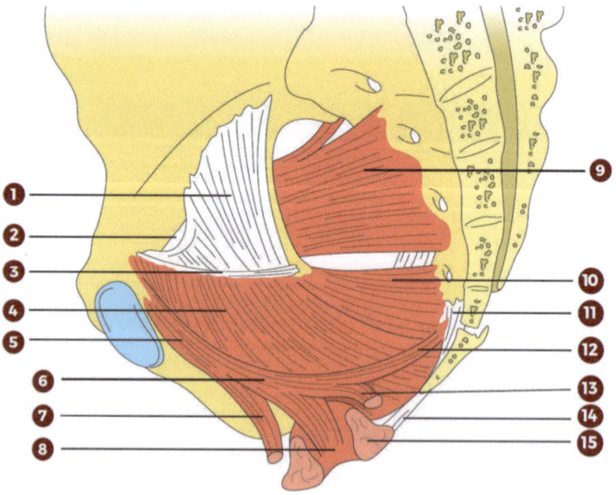

Fig. 4.9 Levator ani muscles (superomedial view): (1) fascia of the internal obturator muscle, (2) obturator canal, (3) tendinous arch of the levator ani muscles, (4) iliococcygeal muscle, (5) pubococcygeal muscle, (6) puborectal muscle, (7) pubovaginal or prostate elevator muscle, (8) puborectal muscle (laterorectal fascia), (9) piriformis muscle, (10) coccygeal muscle, (11) ventral sacrococcygeal ligament, (12) puborectal muscle (coccygeal fascia), (13) puborectal muscle (retrorectal fascia), (14) anococcygeal area, and (15) external sphincter of the anus

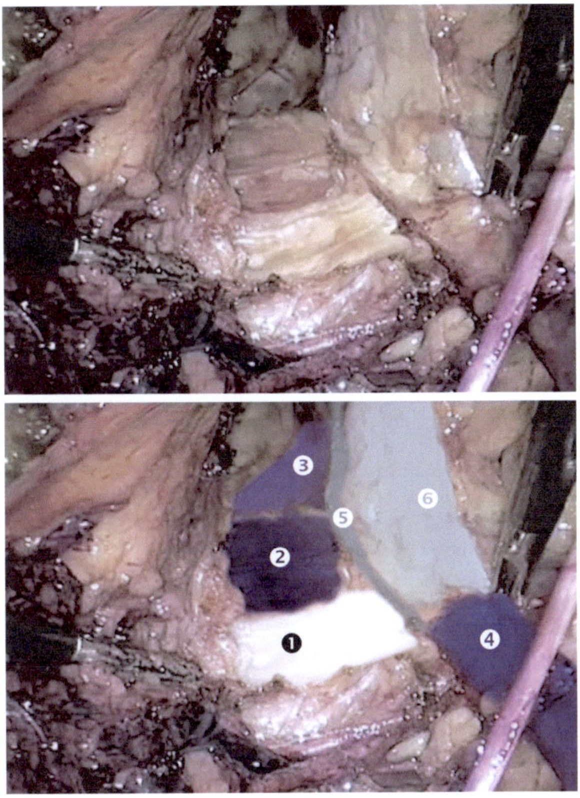

Fig. 4.10 Laparoscopic dissection, in a cadaver, of the right pararectal space. (1) Right sacrospinal ligament, (2) right coccygeal muscle, (3) ischiococcygeal muscle, (4) right internal obturator muscle, (5) levator ani muscle tendinous arch, (6) internal obturator muscle fascia. (Images kindly provided by Drs. Javier F. Magrina and Rosanne M. Kho)

Urogenital Diaphragm (Perineal Membrane)

This is a musculofascial structure located below the pelvic diaphragm. Through a traverse of fascia networks superiorly and inferiorly, this structure extends through the transverse perineal muscle or the urogenital pubic arch and continues with the ureteral muscle and the urethral sphincter (Figs. 4.11, 4.12, and 4.13).

Innervation: Perineal branch of the pudendal nerve.

Superficial Transverse Muscle of the Perineum

This muscle is poorly developed and presents similarly in both sexes. It has the function of helping the deep transverse muscle of the perineum.

Innervation: Perineal branch of the pudendal nerve.

Origin: Small muscle bundle deformed triangular located in the anterior region of the perineum and below the superficial fascia of the perineum. It originates from the inner surface of the ischial tuberosity and ends in the perineal body with the deep transverse muscle and the superficial transverse muscle of the perineum.

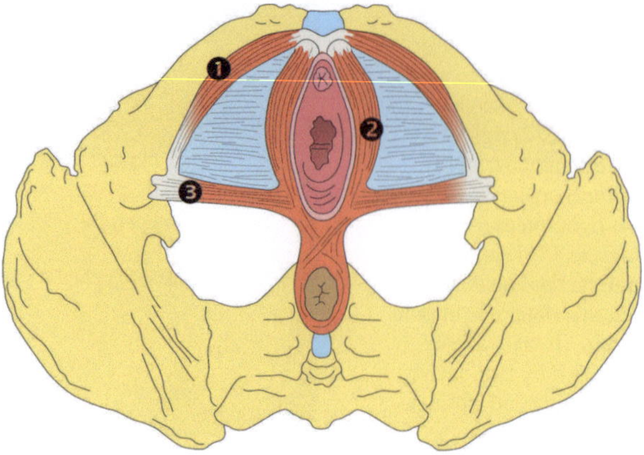

Fig. 4.11 Urogenital diaphragm in single plane: (1) ischiocavernosus muscle, (2) bulbocavernosus/bulbospongiosus muscle, and (3) superficial transverse perineal muscle

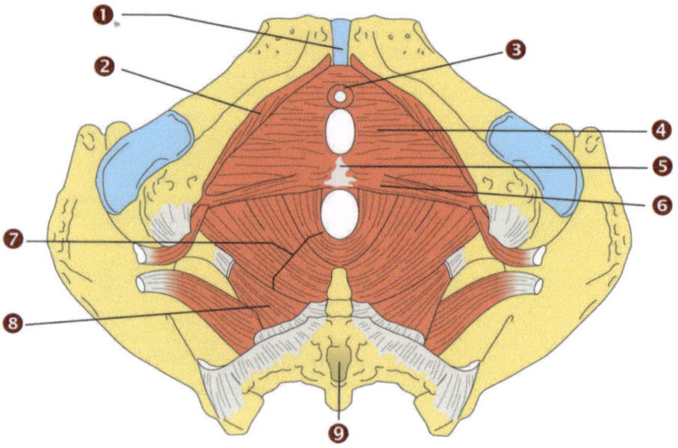

Fig. 4.12 Urogenital diaphragm visualized over pelvic diaphragm: (1) Pubic symphysis, (2) ischiocavernosus muscle, (3) external urethral sphincter muscle, (4) deep transverse perineal muscle, (5) center of the perineum, (6) superficial transverse perineal muscle, (7) levator ani muscles, (8) coccygeal muscle, and (9) coccyx

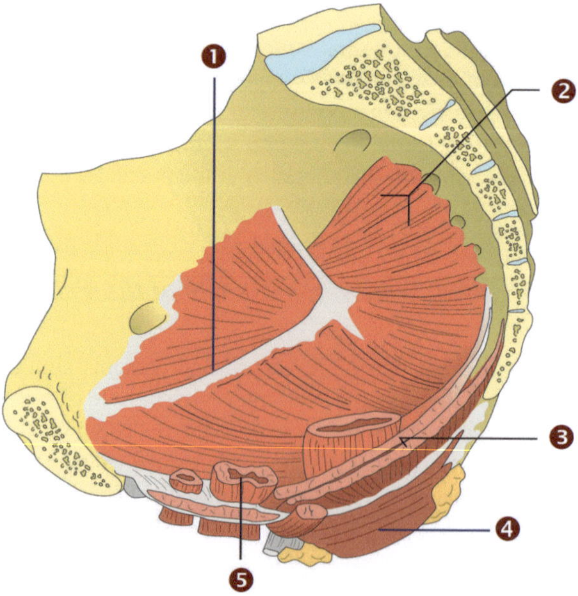

Fig. 4.13 Posterolateral view of the pelvis showing the urogenital floor muscles: (1) internal obturator muscle, (2) piriformis muscle, (3) levator ani muscle, (4) external sphincter muscle, and (5) superficial transverse perineal muscle

Deep Perineal Transverse Muscle

Innervation: Pudendal nerve.

Origin: Muscle of transverse organization, may be replaced by two muscles.

- *Urethral compressor muscle*: A group of muscle bundles originates in the ischio-pubic region and passes in the anterior plane of the urethra and inferiorly to the urethral sphincter; another group of muscle bundles, of the same origin, directs itself medially to the vagina, and some fibers may reach the perineal body and assist in the formation of the deep transverse perineal muscle itself.
- *Urethrovaginal sphincter muscle*: Thin and flat muscle group that is located anteriorly to the urethra and inferiorly to the compressor muscle of the urethra, with the purpose of urinary continence. It originates from the perineal body and is presented anterolaterally to the vagina and urethra.

Bulbospongiosus Muscle

Promotes contraction of the vagina and the veins of the clitoris, contributing to erection; assists in the secretion of the vestibular and Bartholin glands.

Innervation: Pudendal nerve.

Origin: The muscular bundles are located posteriorly to the body in the perineal muscle and make confluence with the contralateral transverse muscle and the external sphincter muscle of the anus. These bundles cover the vestibule and its glands, as well as the vaginal wall up to the body of the clitoris.

Ischiocavernosus Muscle

Innervation: Perineal branch of the pudendal nerve.

Origin: Surrounds the clitoris, assisting in its compression and erection.

Sphincter Muscle of the Urethra:

It is an external muscular layer arranged circularly in the urethra. It corresponds to the maximum capacity of urethral contractility. Its fibers extend from the vesical base to the perineal membrane. Innervation: pudendal nerve.

Origin: Its sphincter function is composed of three portions.

- Proximal portion: bundle of smooth muscle forming a ring around the urethra.

- Middle portion: muscular bundle that exerts greater pressure and contractility action.
- Distal portion: or urogenital sphincter properly, which lies close to the urogenital diaphragm and perineal membrane.

External Anal Sphincter Muscle

A bundle of striated and tubular muscles that encircles the anal canal.

Innervation: Pudendal nerve.

Origin: It is described in three portions:

- Deep portion: It has bundles diffused with the puborectal muscle and surrounds the cranial segment of the internal anal sphincter.
- Superficial portion: It is located above the subcutaneous portion and around the caudal portion of the internal sphincter, being the only part attached to bone; it has an anterior insertion in the perineal body and a posterior one in the last coccygeal segment.
- The subcutaneous portion: It is inserted anteriorly on the perineal body and posteriorly on the anococcygeal ligament. It consists of a thin muscular band 15 mm wide in the anterior layer and at the height of the anal opening, under the skin.

Tips and Tricks 4

The episiotomy, an incision made in the perineum to facilitate vaginal delivery, when necessary, includes the bulbospongiosus and superficial transverse muscles of the perineum and may extend to the levator ani muscles. The perineal correction surgeries involve the approximation of the broken portions of the bulbospongiosus and the superficial transverse muscles of the perineum and some fibers of the external anal sphincter.

In addition to the groups of fascia and muscles described above, the pelvic floor has muscles that assist in its functionality, which are discussed in the following topics.

Psoas Major Muscle

The psoas major is a large, thick muscle located mainly in the abdomen. It assists in hip flexion and mobilizes the trunk and pelvis forward. In association with the iliacus, it also acts as the medial rotator of the hip. The unilateral contraction of the muscle when fixing the thigh will produce lateral flexion of the lumbar spine to the same side.

Innervation: Muscular branch of the lumbar plexus, derived from the ventral branches of L1–L3 and occasionally L4.

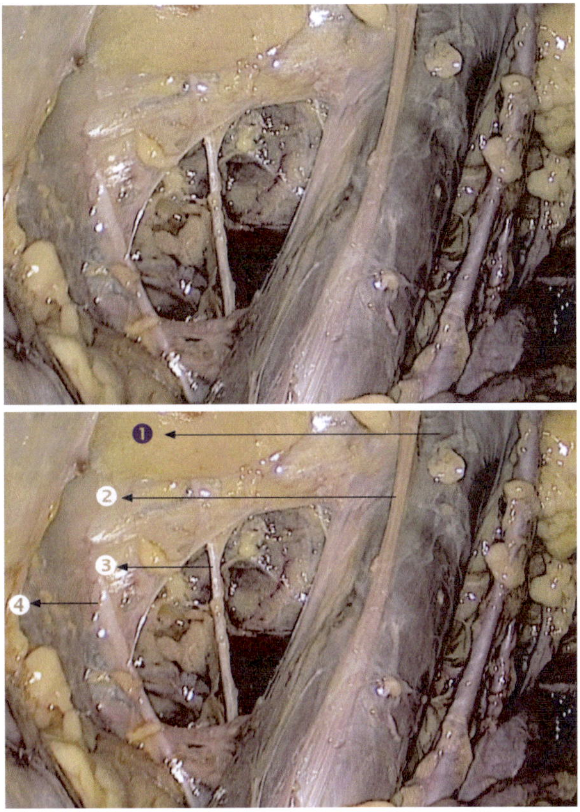

Fig. 4.14 Psoas major muscle. Dissection in cadaver and view, on the left, of the psoas major muscle, identifying the branches of L1. (1) Psoas muscle, (2) genitofemoral nerve, (3) ilioinguinal nerve, (4) iliohypogastric nerve

Origin: It has a series of glides, each of which arises from the adjacent margins of the vertebral bodies and intervertebral disks from lower border of T12 to upper border of L5; tendon arches over the narrow parts of the bodies of L1–L4; and anterior surfaces and lower margins of the transverse processes of L1–L5.

Its fibers join together and, with the help of the ilium, gradually form a tendon that runs along the pelvic border, when it becomes referred to as the joint tendon of the psoas major and iliacus. The joint tendon attaches to the apex and posterior aspect of the lesser trochanter of the femur (Fig. 4.14).

Piriformis Muscle

Described by some authors as a component or helper of the pelvic diaphragm, the piriformis muscle rotates the hip laterally, thereby abducting the flexed thigh. It is also an important muscle for holding the head of the femur in the acetabulum.

Innervation: Ventral branches of L5, S1, and S2.

Origin: Second, third, and fourth os sacral bones and its fibers pass through the greater ischial foramen and insert in the gluteal region (greater trochanter in the femur) (Figs. 4.15, 4.16, and 4.17).

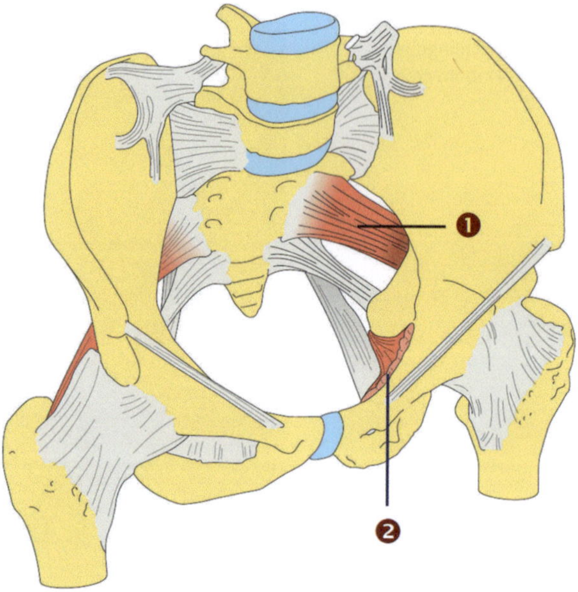

Fig. 4.15 View of the pelvis: (1) piriformis muscle, (2) obturator internus muscle

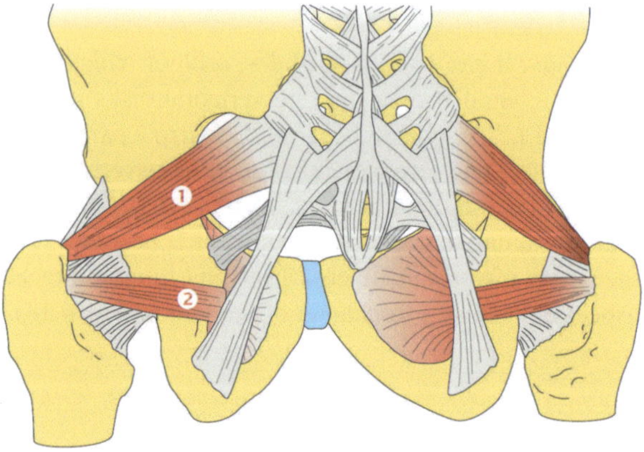

Fig. 4.16 View of the pelvis: (1) piriformis muscle originating from the second, third, and fourth sacral bones toward the ischial foramen and (2) obturator internus muscle

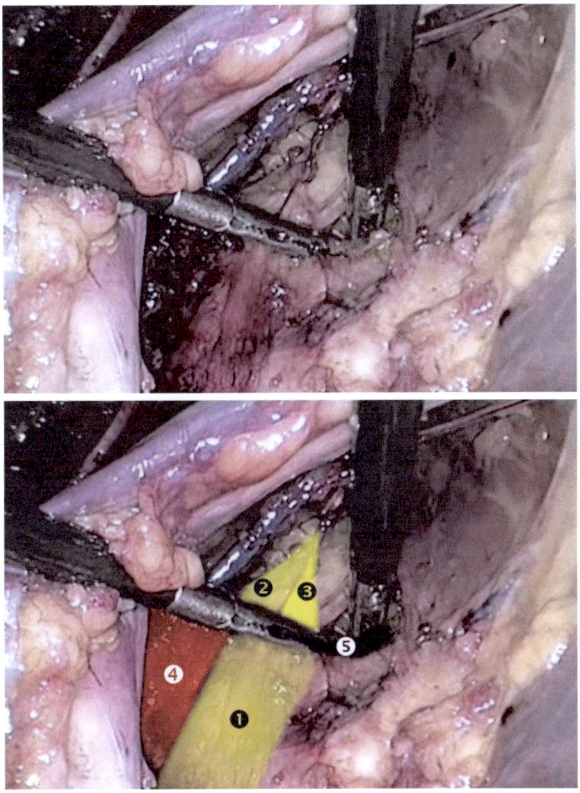

Fig. 4.17 Laparoscopic dissection in a cadaver. (1) Right lumbosacral trunk, (2) right sacral root S1, (3) right sciatic nerve, (4) right superior gluteal artery, (5) piriformis muscle. (Image kindly provided by Drs. Javier F. Magrina and Rosanne M. Kho)

Internal Obturator Muscle

Assists in abduction and rotation of the thigh.

Innervation: Internal obturator nerve.

Origin: Pelvic surface of the obturator membrane and superior and medial contours of the obturator foramen toward the greater trochanter of the femur and the trochanteric fossa (Figs. 4.12, 4.13, 4.15, and 4.18).

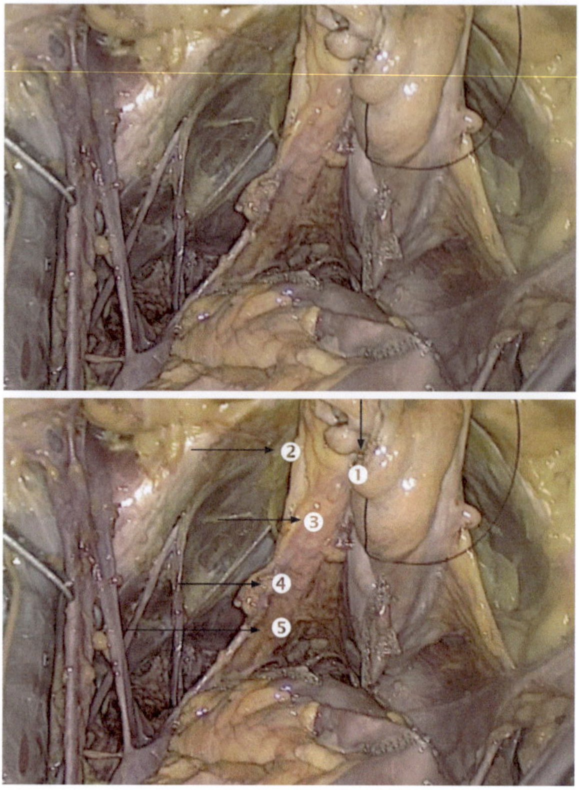

Fig. 4.18 Dissection, in a cadaver, of Retzius space and paravesical spaces (lateral and medial) on the left. (1) Pubis, (2) Cooper's ligament, (3) obturator internus muscle, (4) obturator vessels, (5) obturator nerve

Bibliography

1. Abdool Z, Dietz HP, Lindeque BG. Prolapse symptoms are associated with abnormal functional anatomy of the pelvic floor. Int Urogynecol J. 2017;28(9):1387–91.
2. Banerjee C, Noé KG. Laparoscopic pectopexy: a new technique of prolapse surgery for obese patients. Arch Gynecol Obstet. 2011;284(3):631–5.
3. Satheesha Nayak B, Rodenbaugh DW. Modeling the anatomy and function of the pelvic diaphragm and perineal body using a "string model". Adv Physiol Educ. 2008;32(2):169–70.
4. Herschorn S. Female pelvic floor anatomy: the pelvic floor, supporting structures, and pelvic organs. Rev Urol. 2004;6(Suppl 5):S2–10.
5. Hodges PW, Sapsford R, Pengel LH. Postural and respiratory functions of the pelvic floor muscles. Neurourol Urodyn. 2007;26(3):362–71.
6. Irvine LM, Shaw RW. The effects of patient obesity in gynaecological practice. Clin Obstet Gynecol. 2003;13(3):179–84.
7. Jing D, Ashton-Miller JA, DeLancey JO. A subject-specific anisotropic visco-hyperelastic finite element model of female pelvic floor stress and strain during the second stage of labor. J Biomech. 2012;3:455–60.
8. Kamina P. Anatomique clinique. 3rd ed. Poitiers-Hiver: Maloine; 2013. Tome 4.
9. Lawrence JM, Lukacz ES, Nager CW, Hsu JW, Luber KM. Prevalence and co-occurrence of pelvic floor disorders in community-dwelling women. Obstet Gynecol. 2008;111(3):678–85.

10. Levin PJ, Visco AG, Shah SH, Fulton RG, Wu JM. Characterizing the phenotype of advanced pelvic organ prolapse. Female Pelvic Med Reconstr Surg. 2012;18(5):299–302.
11. Lo TS, Jaili S, Uy-Patrimonio MC, Karim NB, Ibrahim R. Transvaginal management of severe pelvic organ prolapse in nulliparous women. J Obstet Gynaecol Res. 2017;43(3):543–50.
12. Mouritsen L, Larsen JP. Symptoms, bother and POPQ in women referred with pelvic organ prolapse. Int Urogynecol J. 2003;14(2):122–7.

Chapter 5
Pelvic Spaces

Fernanda de Almeida Asencio, Luciano Gibran, Camila Veckhaouser Calegari, and Helizabet Salomão Ayroza

Overview

In the early twentieth century, Wertheim proposed a radical surgical approach for the treatment of cervical cancer. With Cameron and Fothergill, he emphasized the functional role of the pelvic fascias in supporting and suspending the pelvic organs. Later, both anatomists and surgeons contributed to the knowledge of the anatomy (macroscopic and microscopic) of the retroperitoneal pelvic structures in women. During this period, several nomenclatures were described; in daily practice,

Supplementary Information The online version contains supplementary material available at https://doi.org/10.1007/978-3-031-63520-5_5.

F. de Almeida Asencio
Santa Casa de Misericórdia de São Paulo (SCMSP), São Paulo, Brazil

FEBRASGO (Brazilian Society of Obstetri s and Gynecology), São Paulo, Brazil

Albert Einstein Hospital, São Paulo, Brazil

L. Gibran
FEBRASGO (Brazilian Society of Obstetri s and Gynecology), São Paulo, Brazil

Faculty of Medicine, University of São Paulo (FMUSP), São Paulo, Brazil

C. V. Calegari
FEBRASGO (Brazilian Society of Obstetri s and Gynecology), São Paulo, Brazil

H. Salomão Ayroza (✉)
Obstetrics and Gynecology Department, Faculdade de Ciências Médicas da Santa Casa de Misericórdia de São Paulo (SCMSP), São Paulo, Brazil

Gynecological Endoscopy and Endometriosis Division, Santa Casa de São Paulo Hospital, São Paulo, Brazil

H. Salomão Ayroza, P. Ayroza Ribeiro (eds.), *Atlas of Laparoscopic Gynecological Anatomy*, https://doi.org/10.1007/978-3-031-63520-5_5

however, the lack of common definitions and terminologies made communication between professionals involved in the process of diagnosis and treatment of pelvic diseases difficult.

Faced with this difficulty, the Federal Commission on Anatomical Terminology (FCAT) and the International Federation of Associations of Anatomists (IFAA) developed, in 1998, an international standard for human anatomical terminology, the AT. The AT describes female anatomical structures of potential clinical and surgical interest (functional and surgical anatomy), with the objective of defining a precise and uniform nomenclature, a prerequisite for a standardized and safe clinical practice.

This chapter discusses the anatomy of the pelvic spaces, following the official nomenclature and the descriptions provided by the AT. The aim is to describe the main anatomical landmarks of each pelvic space, relating their surgical applicability and showing how to access them.

The functional organization of the pelvis is composed of dense connective structures (visceral ligaments and parietal and visceral fasciae), and the areas of looser connective tissue are reserved for the viscera and abdominal walls, which can be cleaved surgically, i.e., spaces and septa. The method of dealing with these spaces, which are virtual in terms of their physiological condition, forms the basis of surgical dissection.

As far as the septa and spaces are concerned, they are classified as follows:

Midline (central) spaces (single):

- Retzius
- Vesicovaginal
- Rectovaginal
- Retrorectal

Lateral spaces (bilateral):

- Paravesical
- Pararectal (Okabayashi and Latzko)
- Yabuki

These various spaces communicate with each other.

Unlike the term "fossa," which refers to a peritoneal depression, pelvic spaces consist of areas delimited by at least two independent and areolar connective tissue-filled fascias, which can be developed or dissected along their cleavage plane.

In the pelvis, the retroperitoneal connective tissue is organized into three main groups of fused fascia, so that their intersections delimit the pelvic spaces and form septa. These three main groups of fascia are as follows:

Pelvic parietal fascia: a dense fascial system that covers the structures that bound the pelvic cavity. It includes levator ani, obturator, coccygeal, and piriform muscles, as well as the anterior surfaces of the sacrum and coccyx and structures contiguous to the pelvic wall, such as hypogastric vessels and sacral roots.

Visceral pelvic fascia: a fascial system arising from the visceral reflection of the parietal pelvic fascia, which will envelop the pelvic organs and secure them to the pelvic wall.

Extraserosal pelvic fascia: mass of densely variable connective tissue between the parietal and visceral pelvic fascia, in which the pelvic organs are embedded. It contains the lymphovasculonervous support for the pelvic viscera.

Central Pelvic Spaces

These are virtual spaces distributed in the midline of the pelvis, easily dissected and important for the recognition of anatomical landmarks in retroperitoneal surgeries, both for benign and malignant conditions.

In all, there are four such spaces, of ventral to dorsal location, and have been mentioned previously: Retzius space or retropubic space, vesicovaginal space, rectovaginal space, and retrorectal space (Fig. 5.1).

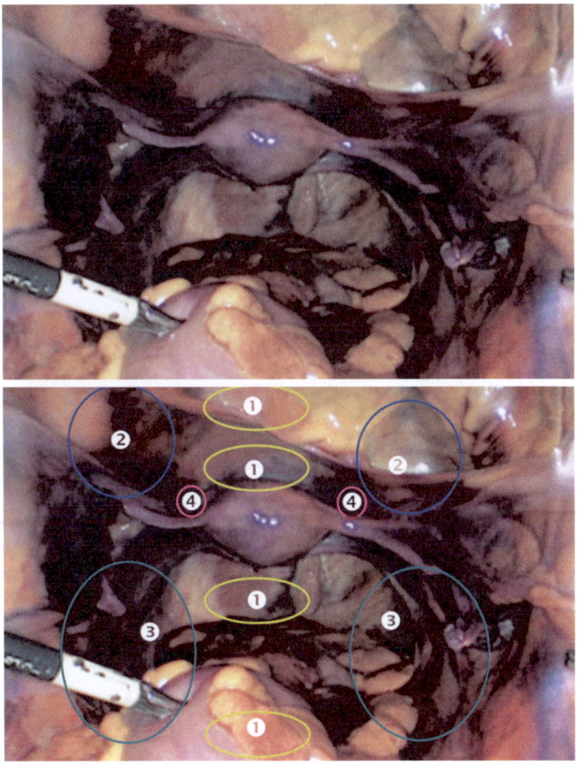

Fig. 5.1 Laparoscopic view of the pelvis, marked are the lateral pelvic spaces and the midline of the pelvis. (1) Midline spaces: Retzius spaces, vesicovaginal, rectovaginal, and retrorectal spaces, (2) paravesical spaces, (3) pararectal spaces, (4) fourth space of Yabuki

Retzius Space

Also called retropubic, this is the most ventral space of the pelvis. It is an arciform space with the concavity facing dorsally and bounded ventrally by the pubic bone. The floor of the space of Retzius is the pubocervical (paravaginal) fascia, which is inserted into the tendinous arch, a connective tissue located medially to the insertion of the musculococcygeus, in the fascia of the obturator internus (Figs. 5.2 and 5.3).

Boundaries

Anterior: posterior aspect of the symphysis pubis and tendinous arch of the pelvic fascia

Posterior: prevesical fascia or umbilico-prevesical fascia, anterior bladder wall, and pelvic urethra

Lateral: Cooper's ligament, tendinous arch of the levator ani muscle, obturator fascia, and obturator muscle

The tendinous arch of the pelvic fascia runs between the ischial spine and the caudal surface of the pubic bone and symphysis. It is formed by the fusion line of the pubocervical fascia with the pelvic parietal fascia. The tendinous arch of the levator ani muscle, on the other hand, consists of the thickening of the aponeurosis of the obturator internus muscle and at its junction with the aponeurosis of the levator ani muscle (Fig. 5.3). Figures 5.5, 5.6, 5.7, 5.8, and 5.9 show the step-by-step dissection of the space of Retzius.

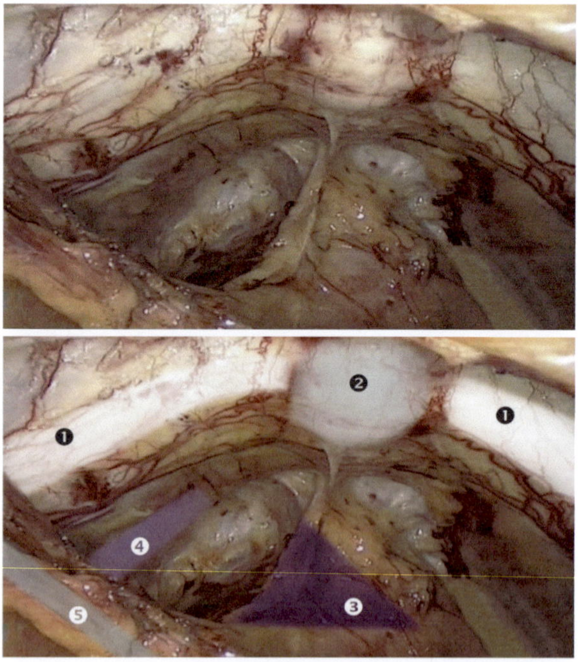

Fig. 5.2 Retzius space after dissection, with identification of the structures. (1) Cooper's ligament, (2) posterior surface of symphysis pubis, (3) anterior bladder wall, (4) obturator muscle, (5) prevesical fascia

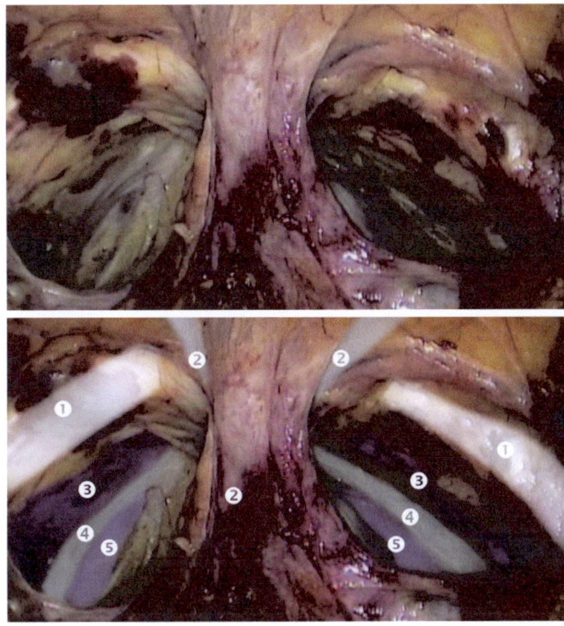

Fig. 5.3 Retzius space after dissection, with identification of the following structures: (1) Cooper's ligament, (2) posterior surface of symphysis pubis, (3) obturator muscle, (4) levator ani tendinous arch, (5) levator ani muscle

Tips and Tricks 1

The anterior peritoneum is tractioned, and the incision must be made at the level of the urachus, toward the abdominal wall, until the visualization of the prevesical fascia. The dissection must follow along a vertical plane toward the pelvic lateral wall, above the prevesical fascia.

Pneumodissection helps develop the space. The right and left Cooper's ligaments, revealed on each side, mark the lateral/superior limits of the space of Retzius. The space is completely dissected, with fine movements, until the obturator muscle, the tendinous arch of the levator ani muscle, and the most caudal vaginal dome are identified.

To perform Burch colposuspension, the lateral aspect of the vaginal dome must be exposed by a finger placed in the vaginal fornix. The suture is performed first in Cooper's ligament, in an anteroposterior direction, and then in the vagina, from the inside out, trying not to transfix the vaginal wall. Two to four sutures are needed on each side, elevating the vagina to the height of the tendon arch of the levator ani muscle. The traction should be moderate; at this point, the surgeon's experience is extremely important (Figs. 5.4, 5.5, 5.6, 5.7, 5.8, and 5.9).

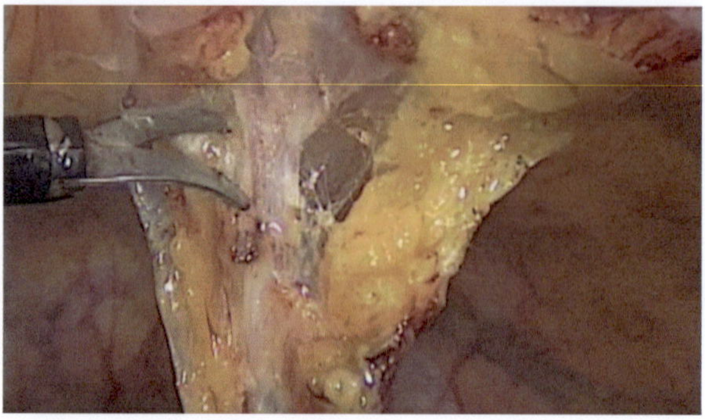

Fig. 5.4 Parietal peritoneum and opening of the peritoneum at the level of the urachus, with its section

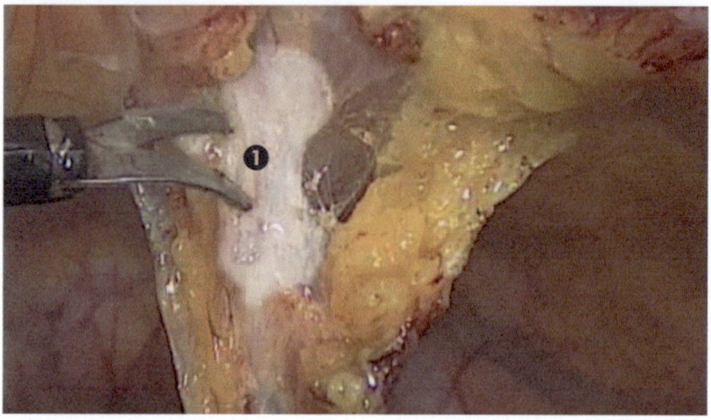

Fig. 5.5 Drawn parietal peritoneum and opening of the peritoneum at the level of the urachus, with its section and identification of the prevesical fascia. (1) Prevesical fascia

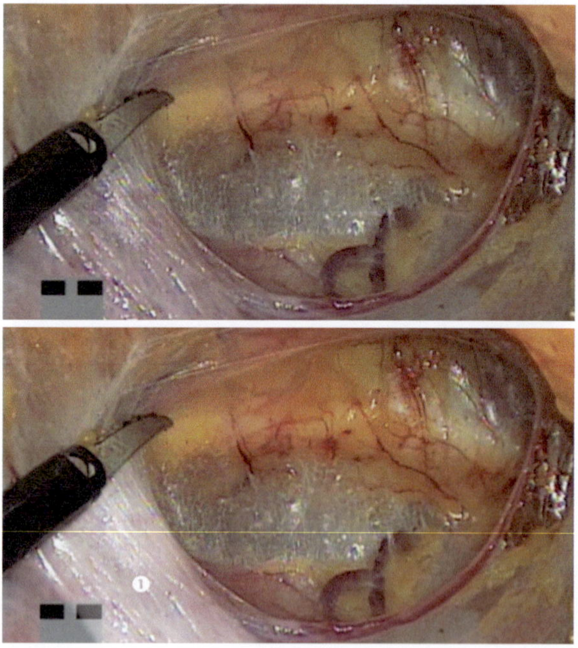

Fig. 5.6 Space development after identification of the prevesical fascia, with dissection of the areolar tissue. (1) Prevesical fascia

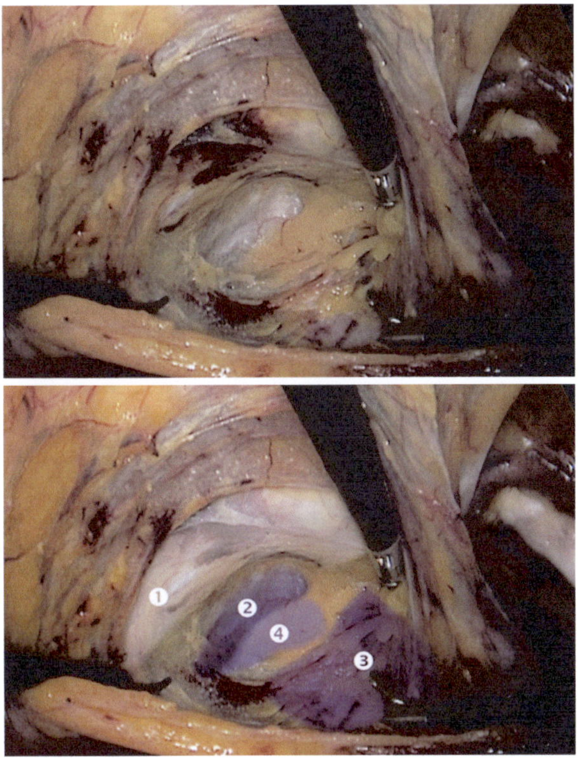

Fig. 5.7 Identification of Retzius space and its anatomical landmarks. (1) Left Cooper's ligament, (2) levator ani muscle, (3) anterior wall of the bladder, (4) left lateral vaginal wall

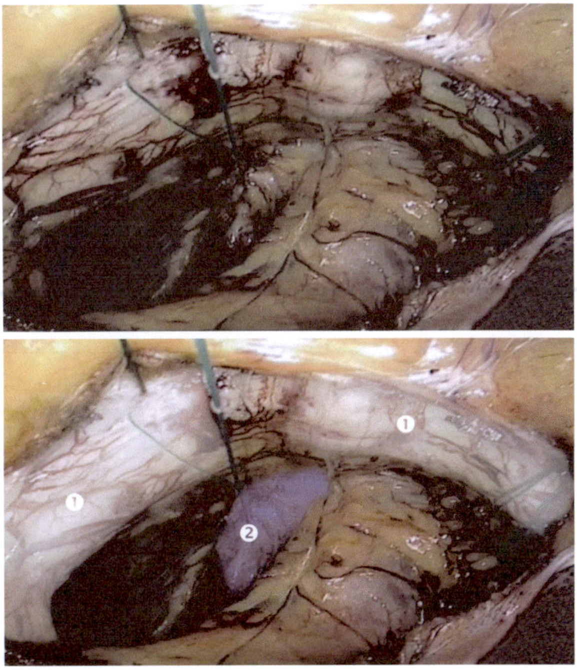

Fig. 5.8 Burch surgery. Suture with anteroposterior direction on the left side. (1) Left Cooper's ligament, (2) lateral wall of the vagina on the left

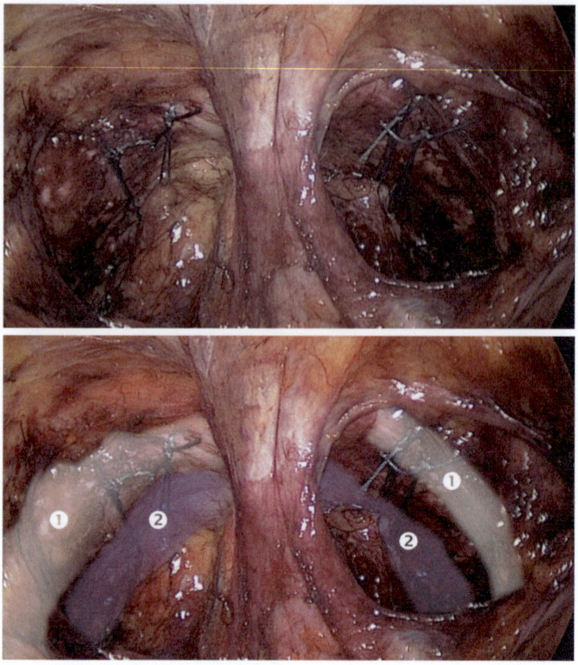

Fig. 5.9 Final view of the procedure. Bilateral suture with moderate traction. (1) Cooper's ligament, (2) lateral vaginal wall

Surgical Applicability

Burch surgery: paravaginal defect repair.

Vesicovaginal Space

Comprises the space between bladder and vagina, covered cranially by the peritoneum of the vesicouterine fold and bounded laterally by the vesicouterine ligaments or bladder pillars (Figs. 5.10, 5.11, and 5.12).

Boundaries

Anterior: posterior face of the bladder

Posterior: anterior surface of the vagina and pubocervical fascia

Lateral: vesicouterine ligaments or bladder pillars

Because of the anatomical and functional importance, emphasis should be given to the description of the lateral limit of the vesicovaginal space: the superficial and deep vesicouterine ligaments, between which we find the distal ureter exiting the parametrium toward the bladder.

The bladder innervation, through the bladder branch of the inferior hypogastric plexus, is intimately related to the distal ureter. Its path is through the deep vesicouterine ligament toward the bladder region.

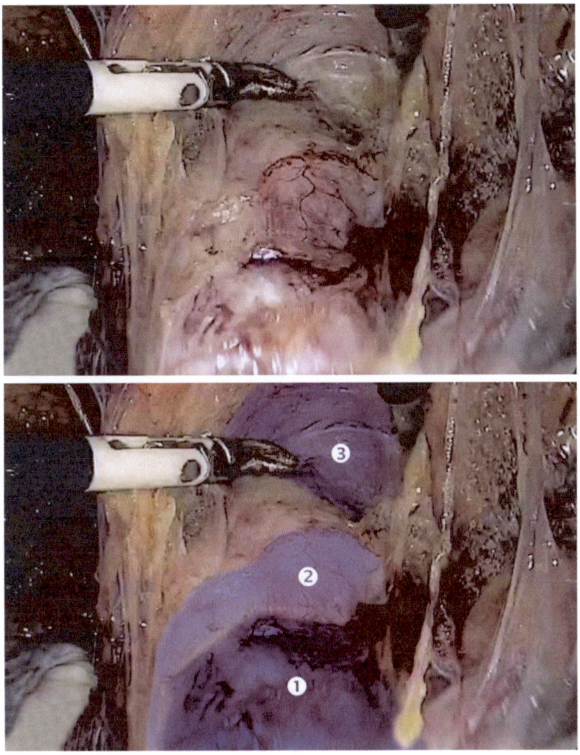

Fig. 5.10 Dissection of the vesicovaginal space, with identification of the transition. (1) Cervix, (2) vagina, (3) posterior bladder wall with prevesical fat

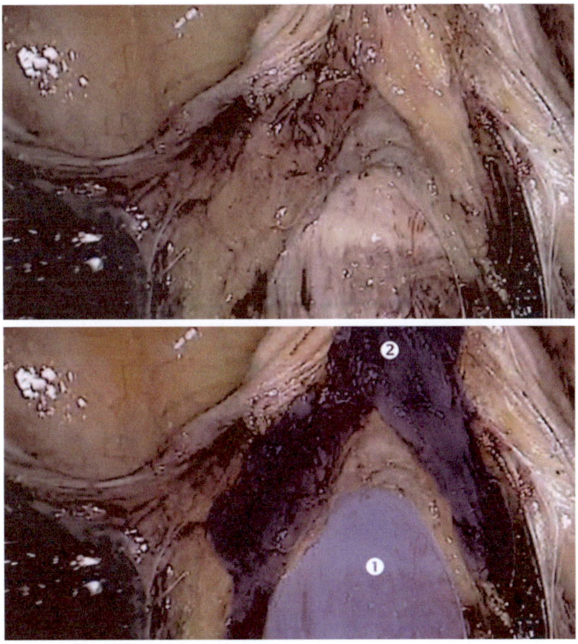

Fig. 5.11 Caudal limit of dissection of the vesicovaginal space in hysterectomy for malignant disease, with identification of the transition. (1) Vagina, (2) posterior bladder wall with prevesical fat

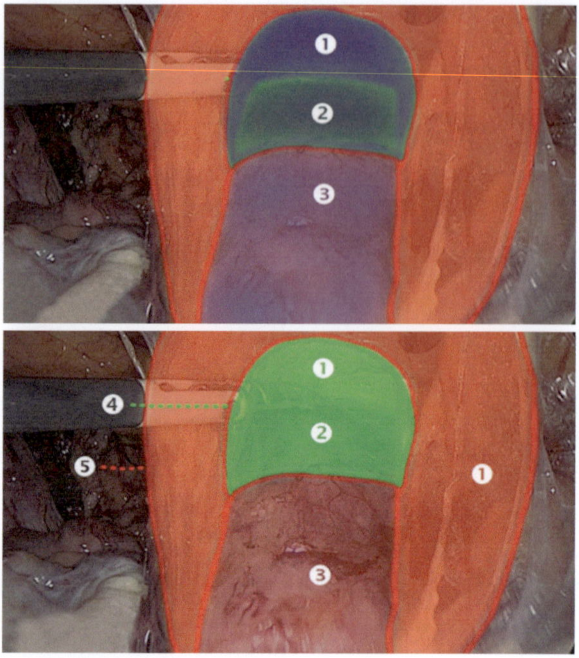

Fig. 5.12 Vesicovaginal space boundaries after dissection. (1) Bladder, (2) vagina, (3) cervix, (4) vesicovaginal space, (5) vesicouterine space

The efferent nerve fibers of the bladder plexus are postganglionic of parasympathetic and sympathetic origin. Surgical rupture of the bladder plexus can result in bladder dysfunction, including urge incontinence, stress incontinence, difficult urination, and dysuria. These are changes often found after radical hysterectomy surgery, in which the ureter is completely mobilized.

Kraima et al. (2016), after dissecting cadavers of women and fetuses, observed that the efferent fibers of the bladder plexus also run along the upper surface of the ureter, in the superficial vesicouterine ligament. The authors state that the distal ureter is a risk zone in which the bladder plexus can be surgically damaged (Fig. 5.13).

Tips and Tricks 2

For safe dissection of this space, it is important to remember that the bladder is a free and mobile organ, except in the region of the vesical trigone. Thus, for an adequate presentation, it is necessary to grasp, with atraumatic forceps, both the bladder peritoneum and the bladder wall.

Dissection of the vesicovaginal space begins with incision of the peritoneum and opening of the vesicovaginal space along the midline, with dissection in a caudal direction between the internal pillars or vesicouterine ligaments.

For total hysterectomy for benign disease, dissection of this space should be sufficient for adequate vaginal exposure in order to perform colpotomy and then colporrhaphy. In cases of anterior prolapse repair for mesh fixation, dissection should

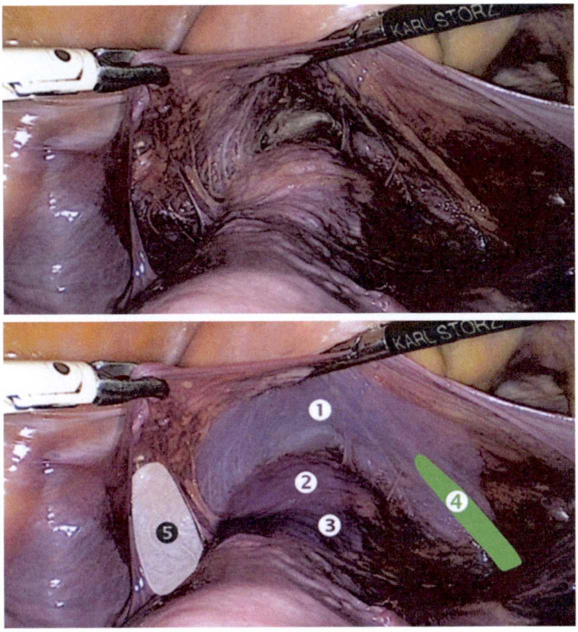

Fig. 5.13 Limits of the vesicovaginal space after dissection in a cadaver, with identification of the anatomical landmarks. (1) Bladder, (2) vagina, (3) cervix, (4) ureter, (5) vesicouterine ligament

continue as low as possible, in close proximity to the bladder neck, identified by the contour of the urinary catheter balloon, and over a surface wide enough to allow the anterior portion of the mesh to spread completely. The space in which the mesh will be installed is triangular and of variable size, with the lower point close to the bladder neck.

The anterior mesh is placed below the bladder and fixed with a non-transfixing stitch to the anterior surface of the vagina. It is essential not to have any stitches that transfix the vagina, in order to avoid any risk of contamination of the prosthesis.

In radical hysterectomy, however, the dissection of this plane continues until the exposure of the anterior vaginal fascia at 3–4 cm from the cervix. At this point, the vesicouterine ligaments can be identified as a dense connective tissue that extends from the posterior aspect of the bladder on each side to the anterior vaginal fascia, with which it is united. Lateral dissection of the anterior vaginal fascia may continue below the vesicouterine ligament until the ureter is located at its entry into the trigone.

Surgical Applicability

- Total hysterectomy
- Radical hysterectomy
- Promontofixation

Rectovaginal Space

Access to the rectovaginal space comprises the dissection of the cleavage planes between the posterior vaginal wall and the rectal fascia. The posterior vaginal wall is associated with the rectum along its entire length. It is directly related to the rectal wall only in its lower three-quarters, as in the upper quarter, the rectouterine excavation—or former Douglas bag fundus—separates the two organs.

The posterior vaginal wall can therefore be divided into two parts, a peritoneal and a rectal. In the latter, situated below the rectouterine excavation, the vagina is applied to the rectum, from which it is separated only by a thin layer of connective tissue and few vessels. Some authors maintain that the space contains a fibrous layer, the true "rectovaginal septum," corresponding to Denonvilliers' fascia in man.

The anterolateral rectum is connected to the vagina by longitudinal fibers of fibrovascular tissue, called the rectal pillars, or wing of the rectum, which form the posterior parametrium with the bilateral uterosacral and rectovaginal ligaments (Figs. 5.14 and 5.15).

Boundaries

Anterior: posterior vaginal wall

Posterior: anterior surface of the rectum and rectus fascia itself

Lateral: uterosacral ligaments

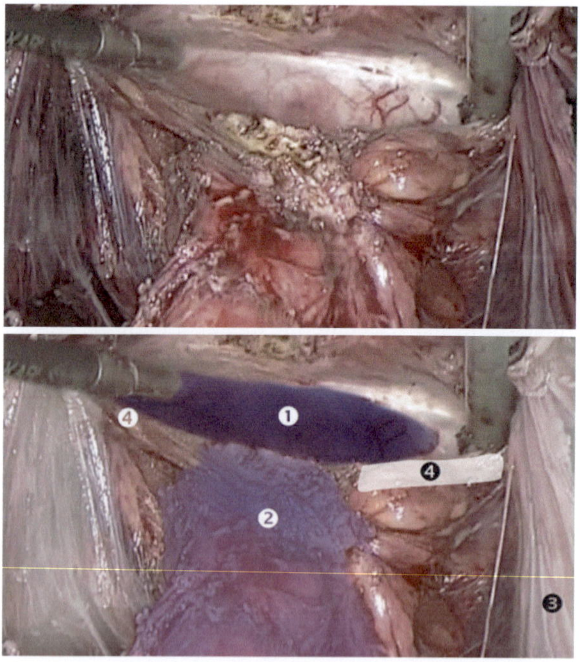

Fig. 5.14 Laparoscopic view after dissection of the rectovaginal space. (1) Posterior wall of the vagina, (2) anterior wall of the rectum and perirectal fat, (3) uterosacral ligaments, (4) rectovaginal septum

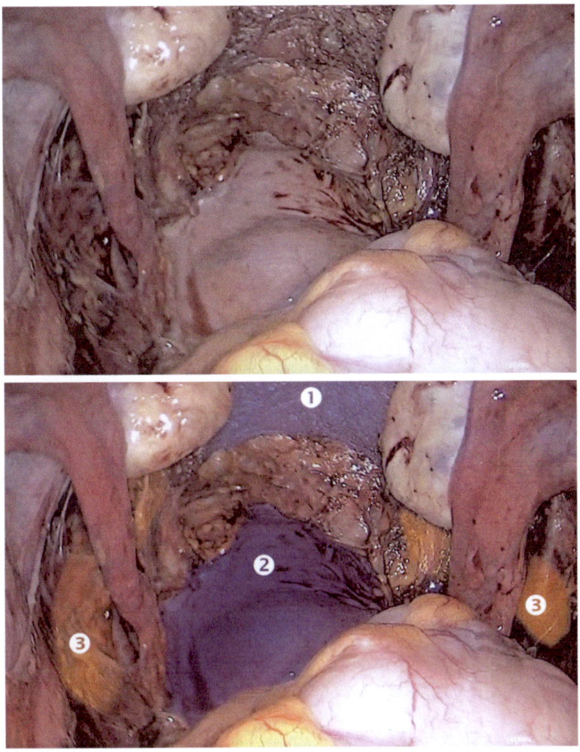

Fig. 5.15 Laparoscopic view after dissection of the pararectal spaces and the rectovaginal space. (1) Posterior wall of the vagina, (2) anterior wall of the rectum and perirectal fat, (3) pararectal space

It is important to emphasize the anatomy of the uterosacral ligaments, which are the anatomical landmark and the lateral limit of dissection of the rectovaginal space. They arise in the posterolateral face of the supravaginal part of the vaginal cervix and fornix and run posteriorly in the pelvis and laterally to the rectum, attaching to the presacral fascia at the level of the S2–S4 vertebrae (Fig. 5.16).

Surgical Applicability

- Promontofixation in the presence of rectocele
- Deep endometriosis of the posterior compartment of the pelvis

Tips and Tricks 3

Dissection of this space begins with its adequate exposure by cranial traction of the rectum and anteriorization of the uterus; at this exposure, the peritoneum resembles an arch. The peritoneum is incised about 2 cm below its uterine insertion, and the incision is extended in an inverted "V" shape between the uterosacral ligaments. The plane of cleavage is identified as close as possible to the vaginal wall and is then guided through the perirectal fat, keeping the dissection above this limit. Dissection

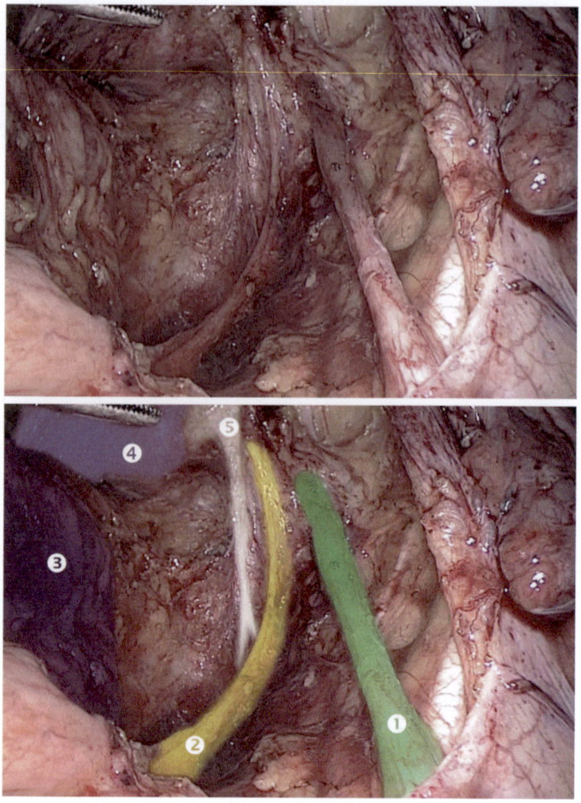

Fig. 5.16 Dissected right pararectal and rectovaginal spaces, allowing the identification of the anatomical landmarks. (1) Right ureter, (2) right hypogastric nerve, (3) rectum, (4) vaginal wall, (5) uterosacral ligament

of this plane is simple, provided that exposure has been performed correctly, and is facilitated by the gas dissection technique (pneumoperitoneum), the traction applied to the rectum, and the thrust applied to the uterus.

During pelvic prolapse surgery, the lower limit of dissection of this space will be the anorectal angle. The dissection continues laterally to the anorectal angle in depth to reveal the levator ani muscle to which the mesh will be attached. At this point, the dissection should extend far enough to allow easy access to the sutures in this space directly in contact with the pelvic floor.

Finally, the dissected space is limited laterally by the levator ani muscle and the pelvic lateral wall, the anterior vagina, and the posterior rectum.

Retrorectal Space

It comprises the space between the posterior face of the rectum and the presacral region. In this space, there are two fascias that will delimit three different planes. They are the fascia proper of the rectum and the presacral fascia, delimiting the presacral, interfascial, and transmesorectal spaces.

The presacral fascia is the pelvic continuation of the visceral abdominal fascia; that is, at the height of the sacrum bone, the visceral pelvic fascia is called presacral fascia, covering the ventral face of the sacrum and coccyx. It traces a curve that covers the pelvic walls laterally and the sacrum dorsally, fusing ventrally with the parametrium and paracervix. This fascia gives support to the rectum. The perirectal fat contained between the presacral fascia and the visceral peritoneum (fascia propria of the rectum) is called the mesorectum.

The mesorectum contains the lymphatics and the dividing branches of the rectal vessels and nerves; it surrounds the subperitoneal rectum in three-quarters at its dorsal circumference and distally, near the levator ani, becomes thinner and then ends. The parasympathetic innervation of the pelvic viscera, the rectosigmoid, and the anal canal is given by the pelvic splanchnic nerves from the anterior branches of the sacral roots from S2 to S4 (Figs. 5.17 and 5.18).

The following is a description of the spaces bounded by the rectus proprius and presacral fascia.

- *Presacral space*: It is located anterior to the sacrum near the periosteum. It contains the nerves (sacral roots) and vessels that pass through the sacral foramen. Its identification and dissection begin just below the promontory region and at the bifurcation of the great iliac vessels.
- *Interfascial space*: Dissection is performed between the presacral fascia and the rectus fascia itself. This space is formed by connective and adipose tissue, containing vessels and nerves in a cranio-caudal direction in relation to the rectal wall.

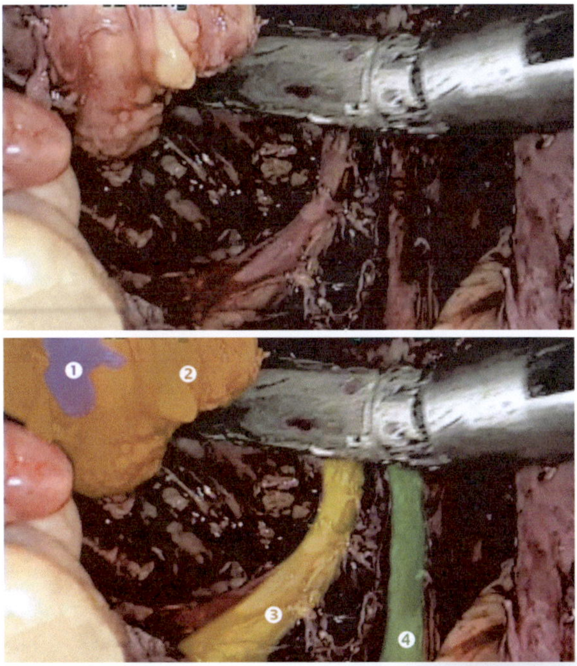

Fig. 5.17 Dissection of the right pararectal space, with surgical approach to the transmesorectal space and identification. (1) Rectal wall, (2) mesorectal adipose tissue, (3) right hypogastric nerve, (4) right ureter

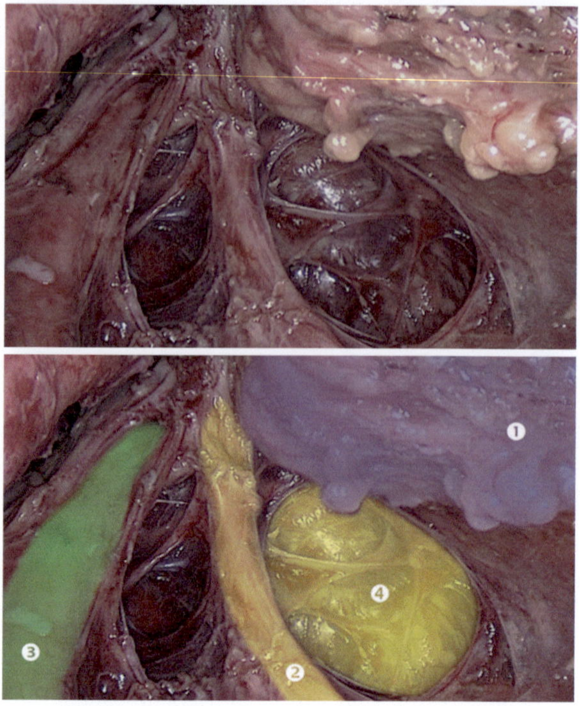

Fig. 5.18 Dissection of the left pararectal space, with a wide approach, isolating the rectal segment. (1) Rectum, (2) left hypogastric nerve, (3) left ureter, (4) pelvic splanchnic nerves

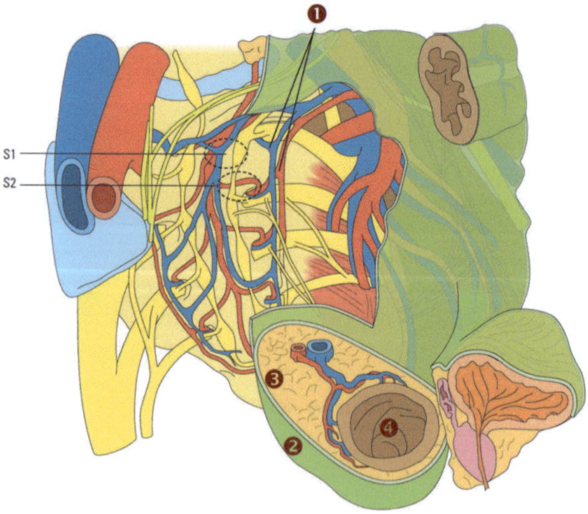

Fig. 5.19 Space posterior to the presacral fascia, with identification of: (1) vessels: artery and vein of the sacral roots from S1 to S3, with descending path anterior to the sacrum bone and lateral to the pelvis; (2) fascia propria of the rectum; (3) mesorectum; and (4) rectum

– *Transmesorectal space*: This is located anteriorly to the rectus fascia propria, containing the mesorectum. It is the plane of dissection for benign conditions, in order to spare the vasculature and innervation of the rectum (Figs. 5.19, 5.20, 5.21, and 5.22).

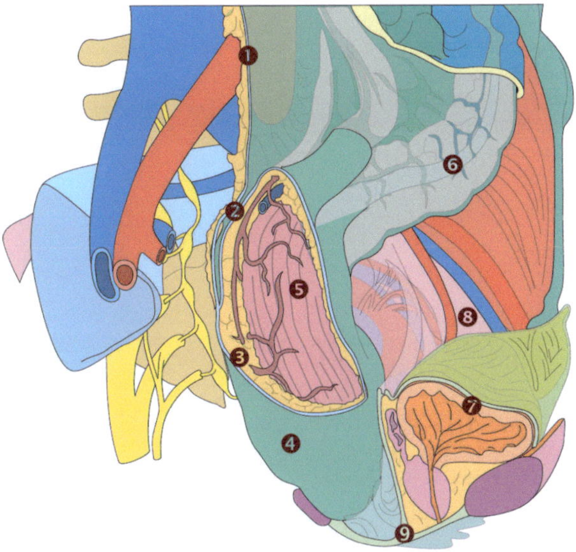

Fig. 5.20 It shows (1) Toldt's fascia, (2) presacral fascia, (3) mesorectum, (4) fascia propria of the rectum, (5) rectum, (6) sigmoid, (7) bladder, (8) parietal fascia, and (9) Denonvilliers' fascia

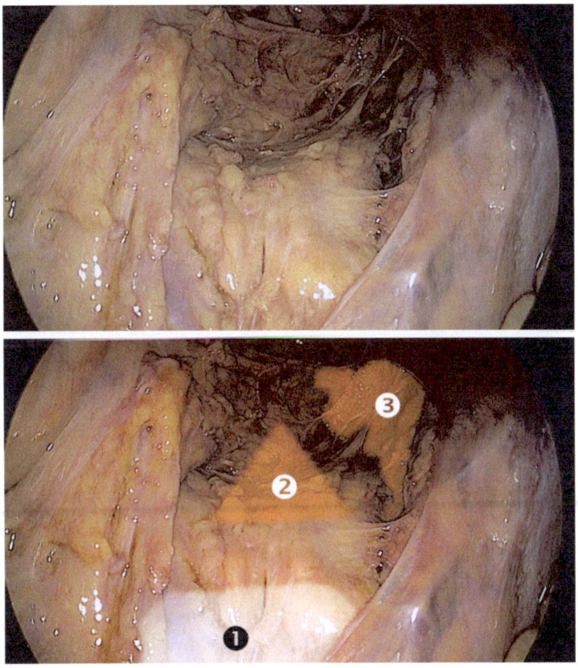

Fig. 5.21 Cadaveric dissection of the presacral space. (1) Promontory, (2) presacral space, (3) pararectal space

Boundaries

Anterior: posterior surface of the rectum covered by the rectus fascia propria

Posterior: sacrum bone covered by the presacral fascia

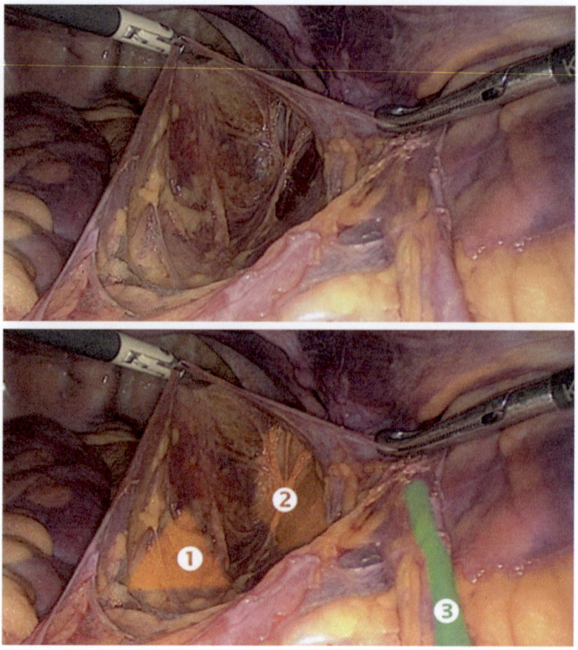

Fig. 5.22 Dissection of the presacral space, in a cadaver, toward the right pararectal space. (1) Presacral space, (2) right pararectal space, (3) right ureter

Tips and Tricks 4
The access to the transmesorectal space is latero-caudal. To achieve complete mobilization of the rectosigmoid and access the inferior mesorectum at the level of the lateral rectal ligaments, the pararectal space of Okabayashi must be dissected, identifying the main anatomical landmarks such as the left and right hypogastric nerves and following the approach to the transmesorectal space medial to the hypogastric nerve toward the rectus fascia propria. By observing this plane, it is possible to preserve the vascularization and innervation (sympathetic and parasympathetic) of the mesorectum.

Lateral Spaces

These are virtual spaces situated lateral to the organs in the midline of the pelvis, separated from the pelvic lateral wall. They are important for the recognition of anatomical landmarks in retroperitoneal surgeries, for both benign and malignant conditions, with emphasis on the treatment of deep endometriosis and pelvic lymphadenectomy. In an overview, three bilaterally distributed spaces that communicate with each other are described: paravesical space, pararectal space, and paravaginal space (or Yabuki's fourth space).

Paravesical Space

It is found laterally to the urinary bladder, medially to the pelvic wall, and anteriorly to the pararectal space. It can be divided into medial and lateral, and the anatomical landmark of this division is the obliterated umbilical artery. The paravesical and pararectal spaces can communicate. The anatomical landmarks that delimit both are the parametrium and the paracervix. Dissection of these spaces ensures ease of complete removal of the uterus and its adnexa during radical hysterectomy (Fig. 5.23).

The limit of dissection of the medial paravesical space is the pelvic floor, formed by the tendinous arch of the levator ani muscle. For the lateral paravesical space, the limit of lateral dissection is the obturator nerve.

Boundaries
Medial: bladder
Lateral: Cooper's ligament + obturator vessels and nerve
Inferior: parametrium and paracervix

Tips and Tricks 5
The paravesical space can be approached after sectioning the round ligament and pelvic infundibulum when performing hysterectomy and adnexectomy. If the uterus and ovary are preserved, the approach then uses an incision parallel to the external iliac vessels in the peritoneum stretching between the round ligament and the pelvic infundibulum. In both cases, the umbilical artery within the broad ligament is the standard reference for the entry point.

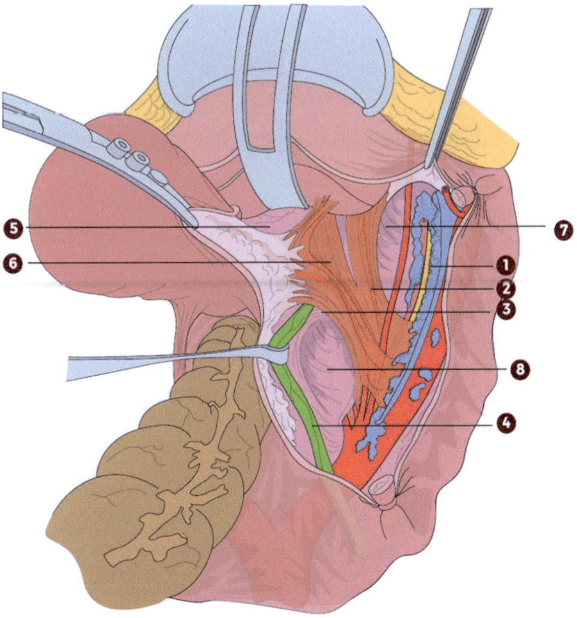

Fig. 5.23 The parametrium and paracervix can be observed with emphasis on (1) obturator nerve, (2) inferior vesical pillar, (3) lateral parametrium, (4) ureter, (5) vesicouterine space, (6) paracervix, (7) medial paravesical space, and (8) lateral pararectal space (Latzko)

The paravesical space is divided into medial and lateral by the obliterated umbilical artery. To find this artery, a traction must be applied just above the pelvis on the anterior abdominal wall in order to detach it in the broad ligament.

The paravesical space can be approached after sectioning the round ligament and opening the anterior leaflet of the broad ligament. The development of the paravesical space is initiated with the identification of the main anatomical landmark: the obliterated umbilical artery.

Dissection is continued through the areolar tissue that fills the paravesical space during pelvic lymphadenectomy and continues laterally to the obliterated umbilical artery until Cooper's ligament and the internal obturator muscle are located, as well as the endopelvic fascia at the bottom.

The development of the paravesical space allows exposure of the anterior aspect of the parametrium, which comprises connective and adipose tissue partially covered by a fibrous lamina that is not very visible and not always present.

The vesicohypogastric fascia extends from the superior vesical artery to the lateral border of the bladder and the vesicouterine ligament. At the Piver III radical level, this fascia must be sectioned to preserve the superior vesical artery (Figs. 5.24, 5.25, and 5.26).

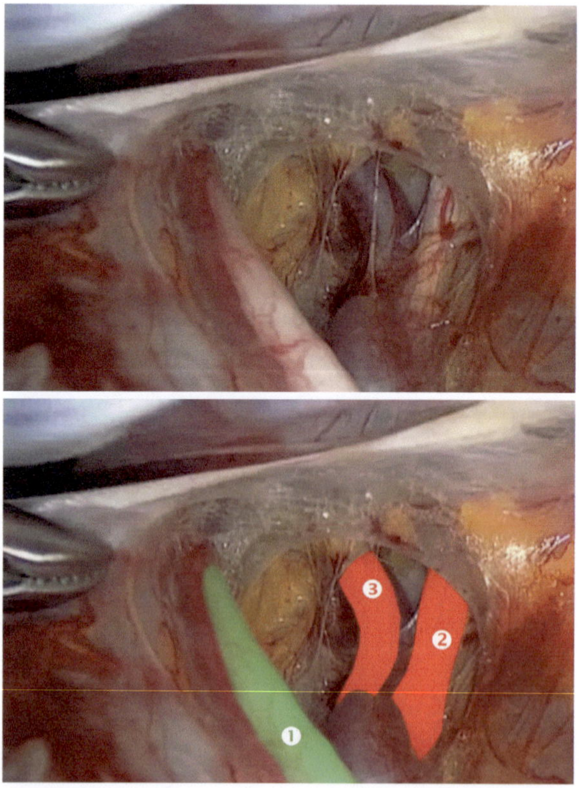

Fig. 5.24 Right medial paravesical space, identifying the main anatomical landmarks. (1) Right ureter, (2) right obliterated umbilical artery, (3) right uterine artery

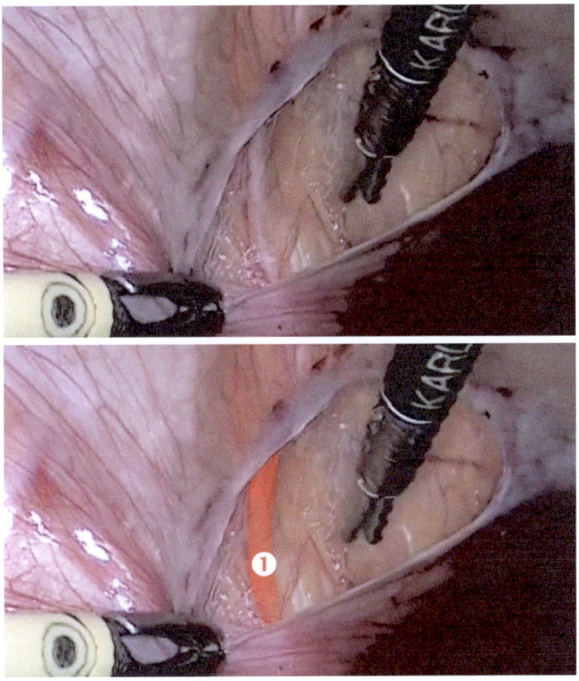

Fig. 5.25 Identification of the obliterated umbilical artery. (1) Obliterated umbilical artery

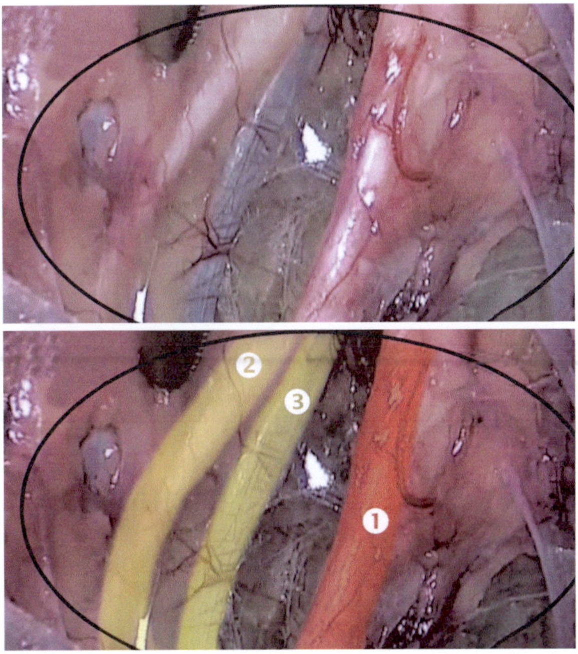

Fig. 5.26 Left lateral paravesical space dissected. (1) Obliterated umbilical artery, (2) left obturator vessels and nerve, (3) obturator vein

Surgical Applicability

- Promontofixation in the presence of rectocele
- Deep endometriosis of the posterior compartment of the pelvis

Pararectal Space

This comprises the space lateral to the rectum, bounded anteriorly by the parametrium and paracervix and laterally by the pelvic wall, with the iliac vessels prominent (Figs. 5.27, 5.28, 5.29, and 5.30).

Like the paravesical space, the pararectal space is also divided into two parts: Okabayashi space and Latzko space. The anatomical landmark of this division is the ureter. Medially to the ureter, laterally to the rectum, and posteriorly to the posterior leaflet of the broad ligament is the Okabayashi space. Laterally to the ureter, between it and the lateral pelvic wall or the iliac vessels, is the space of Latzko (Figs. 5.31, 5.32, 5.33, and 5.34).

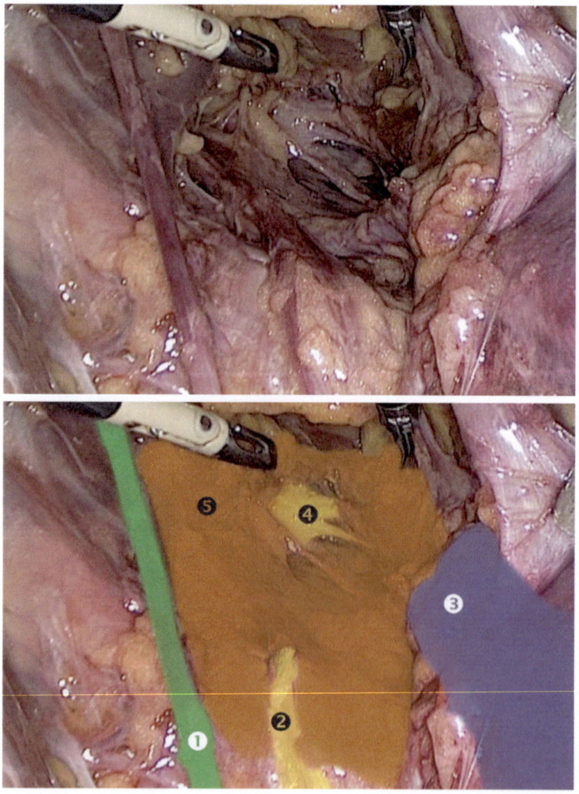

Fig. 5.27 Cadaveric dissection. Left Okabayashi space (medial pararectal) dissected. (1) Left ureter, (2) left hypogastric nerve, (3) rectum, (4) left sacral root, (5) left Okabayashi space

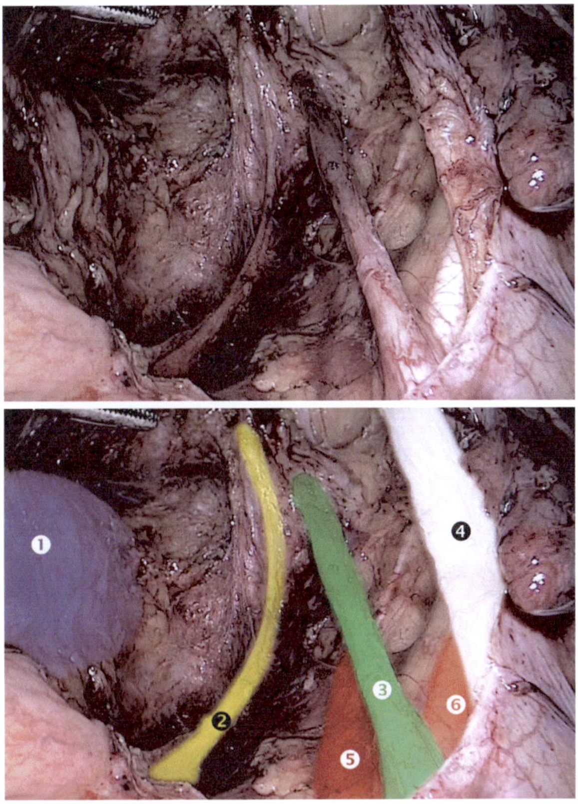

Fig. 5.28 Dissected right Okabayashi pararectal space with identification of the anatomical landmarks. (1) Rectum, (2) hypogastric nerve, (3) ureter, (4) pelvic infundibular ligament, (5) internal iliac artery, (6) external iliac artery

Boundaries

Anterior: posterior leaflet of the broad ligament, parametrium, and paracervix

Posterior: sacral region and piriform muscle

Lateral: lateral pelvic wall and iliac vessels

Medial: rectus and uterosacral ligament

During the dissection of the Okabayashi space, it is possible to identify the right and left hypogastric nerves with a path parallel and medial to the ureters, which should be lateralized; the dissection should continue medially to these structures. The right and left hypogastric nerves are branches of the superior hypogastric plexus, have a descending path in the pelvis, and, together with the pelvic splanchnic nerves, will form the inferior hypogastric plexus.

The hypogastric nerves run along the lateral surface of the rectum and have sympathetic innervation responsible for bladder compliance, among other functions. They then run along the dorsolateral part of the uterosacral ligament before their junction with the pelvic splanchnic nerves to form the inferior hypogastric plexus.

Deeper in the dorsolateral part of the pararectal space, and below the level of the middle rectal artery, are the pelvic splanchnic nerves arising from the sacral roots of

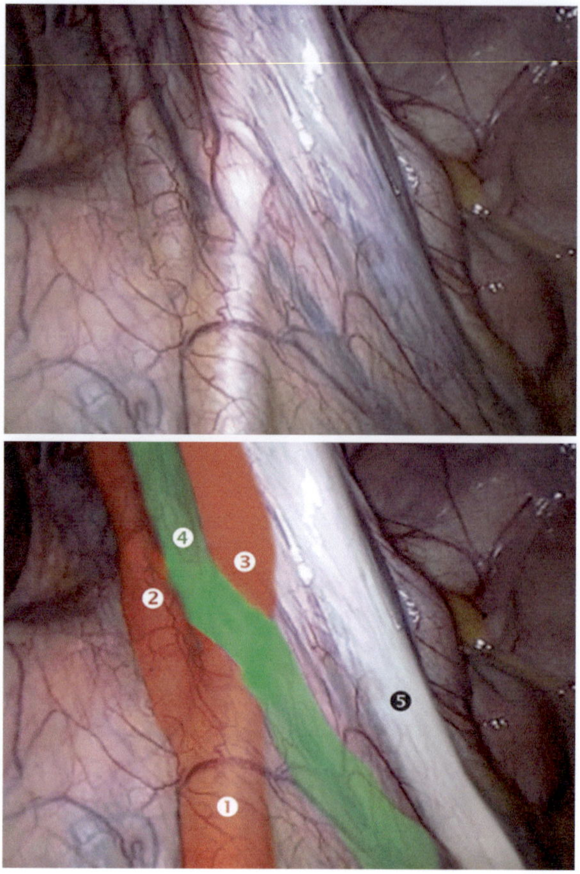

Fig. 5.29 Laparoscopic image of the pelvic transition. The bifurcation of the iliac arteries and the crossing of the right ureter anteriorly to the external iliac artery are identified through transparency. (1) Right common iliac artery, (2) right internal iliac artery, (3) right external iliac artery, (4) right ureter, (5) right infundibulopelvic ligament

S2, S3, and S4; these nerves conduct parasympathetic fibers that command detrusor contractility in relation to urination.

The inferior hypogastric plexus gives off branches that innervate rectal and bladder walls, upper third of the vagina, and uterus. The anatomic landmark for identification of the inferior hypogastric plexus is the deep uterine vein, located posterior to the ureter at the level of the paracervix (Figs. 5.34, 5.35, and 5.36).

Tips and Tricks 6

The pararectal space approach is performed on the following occasions: deep endometriosis surgery and oncologic surgery—medial and lateral approaches, respectively, in relation to the pelvic infundibulum.

In the medial approach, the incision in the peritoneum is made medial to the pelvic infundibulum. The first structure to be visualized here, under the peritoneum, is the ureter, which needs to be separated from the internal iliac artery. Following the rules of dissection, the space must be dissected parallel and lateral to the ureter, until the apex of the uterosacral ligament is reached.

By mediating the ureter, the lateral pararectal space (i.e., Latzko space) is clearly opened and dissected from its origin. The uterine artery can be easily identified and

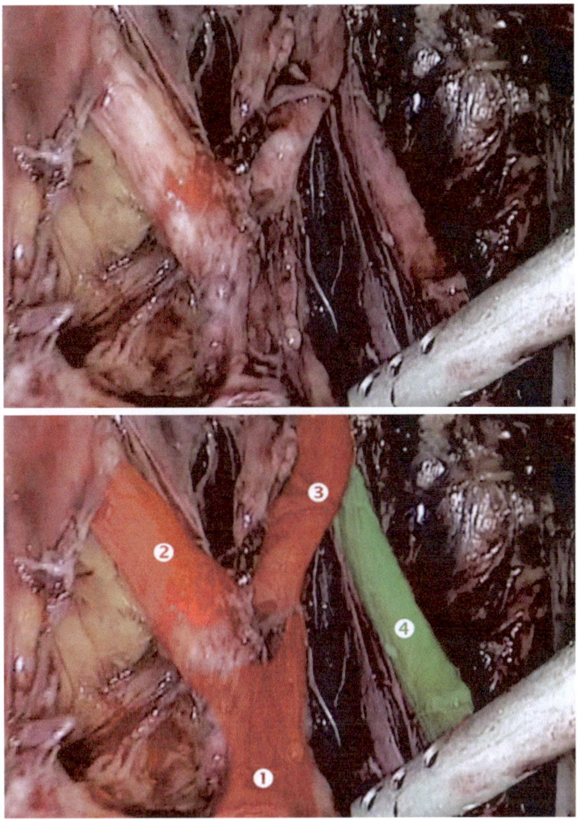

Fig. 5.30 Laparoscopic image after dissection. (1) Left internal iliac artery, (2) left umbilical artery, (3) left uterine artery, (4) left ureter

dissected. By lateralizing the ureter from the fold of the peritoneum or the posterior leaflet of the broad ligament, the Okabayashi space is clearly opened, and the parasympathetic nerves can be seen in careful dissection. This is useful in radical hysterectomy with nerve preservation. These principles are also applicable in endometriosis surgery.

In the lateral approach, the incision in the peritoneum is made lateral to the pelvic infundibulum, and here the first visible structures are the external iliac artery and vein. This area is the best place for a lymph node dissection. The internal iliac artery lies below the external iliac vein (Figs. 5.37, 5.38, and 5.39).

The classical development of the pararectal space, described by Latzko, consists of the separation of the broad ligament from the pelvic wall. This dissection must progressively advance, following the areolar tissue that fills this virtual space, bounded anteriorly by the parametrial fascia, laterally by the pelvic wall and the internal iliac vein, posteriorly by the sacrum, and medially by the mesoureter and the rectosigmoid.

Following the dissection of Latzko space for pelvic lymphadenectomy, it is possible to identify more superficially the bifurcation of iliac arteries and the obturator nerve just below this bifurcation. Following the dissection plane, dorsally to the obturator nerve, it is possible to identify the lumbosacral trunk, formed by the L4

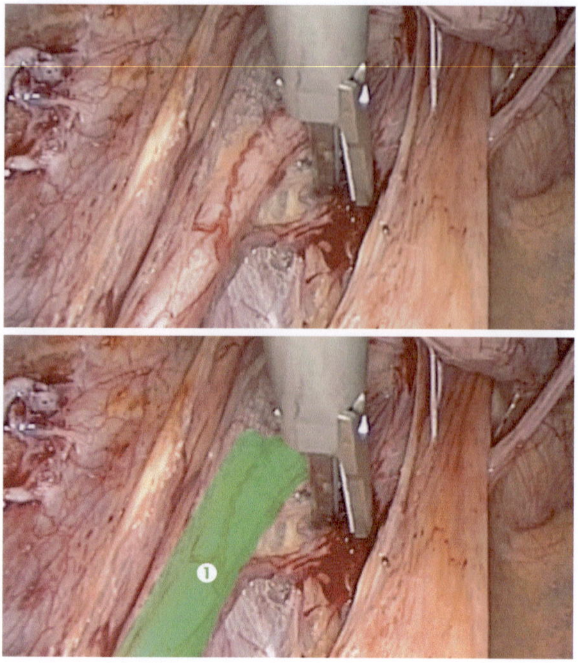

Fig. 5.31 Laparoscopic image during ureterolysis. Initial dissection of the Okabayashi space on the left. (1) Ureter

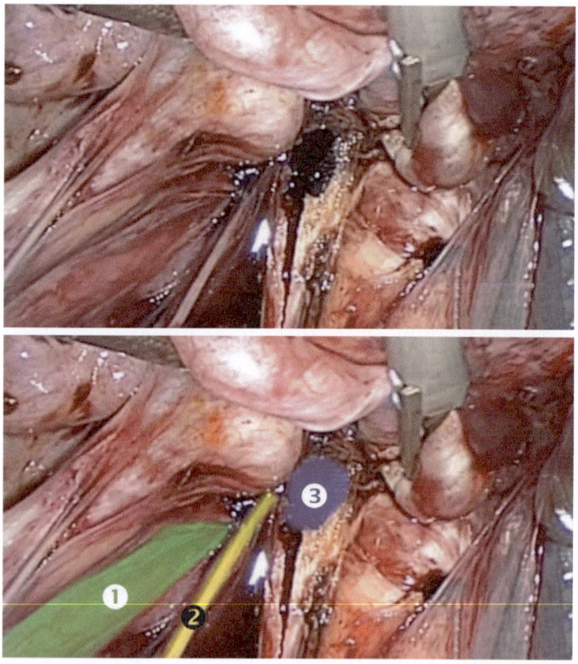

Fig. 5.32 Laparoscopic image. Okabayashi pararectal space dissection and resection of endometriosis nodule. (1) Left ureter, (2) left hypogastric nerve, (3) endometriosis nodule

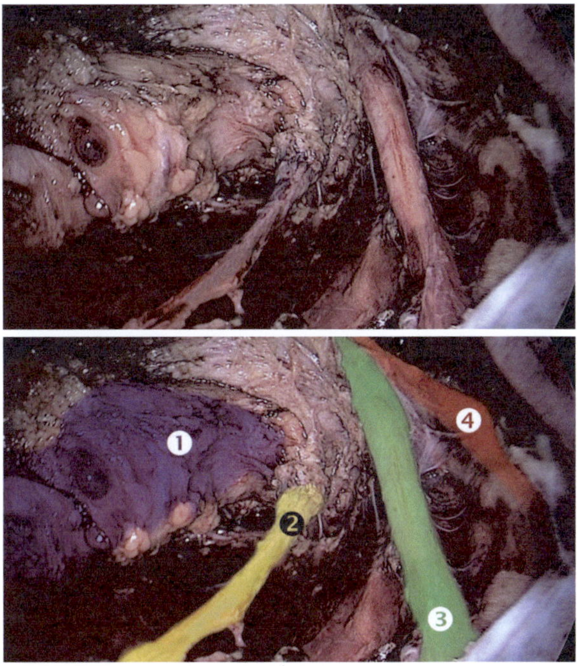

Fig. 5.33 Laparoscopic image after pararectal space dissection. Okabayashi space, medial to the ureter, and Latzko space, lateral to the ureter. (1) Rectum, (2) right hypogastric nerve, (3) right ureter, (4) right uterine artery

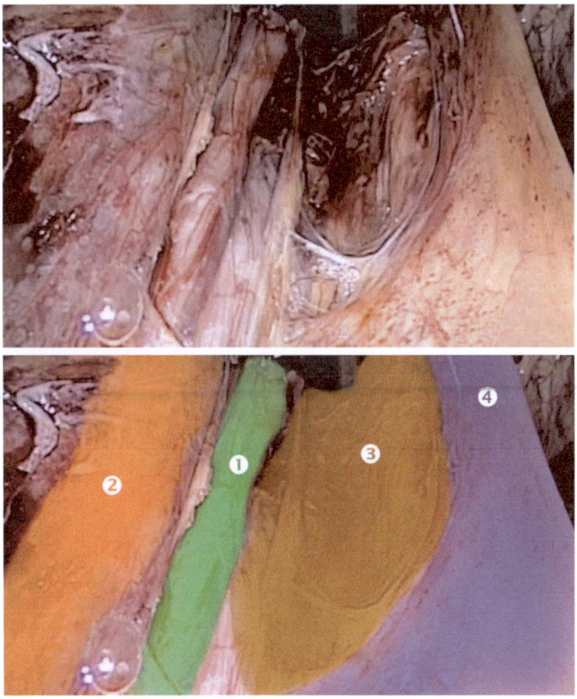

Fig. 5.34 Laparoscopic image of the pararectal space and its division. On the left, ureter, hypogastric nerves, and the two spaces (Latzko space, identified lateral to the ureter; Okabayashi space, identified medial to the ureter). (1) Left ureter, (2) Latzko space to the left, (3) Okabayashi space to the left, (4) rectum

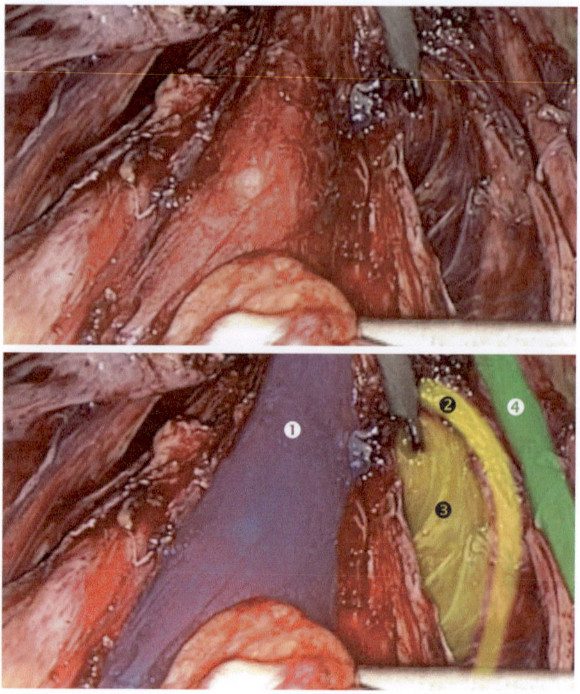

Fig. 5.35 Laparoscopic image after dissection of the right Okabayashi space. (1) Rectum, (2) right hypogastric nerve, (3) pelvic splanchnic nerves to the right, (4) right ureter

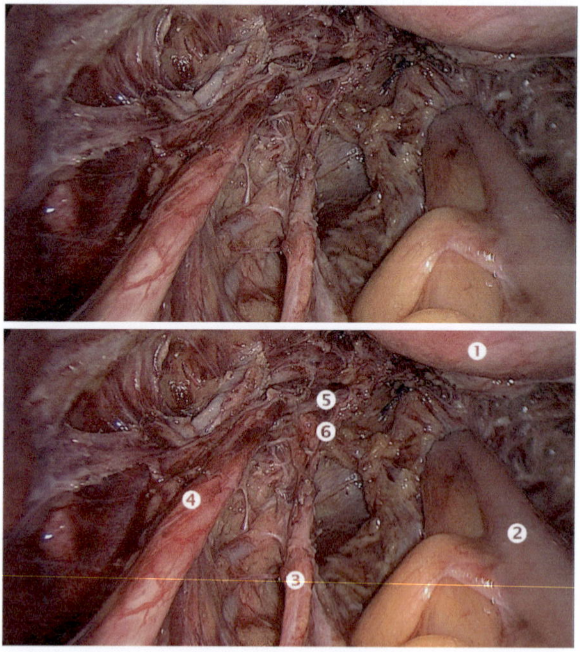

Fig. 5.36 Anatomical relations of the deep uterine vein to the uterus, rectum, ureter, and pelvic nerves. (1) Uterus, (2) rectum, (3) left hypogastric nerve, (4) left ureter, (5) left deep uterine vein, (6) left inferior hypogastric plexus

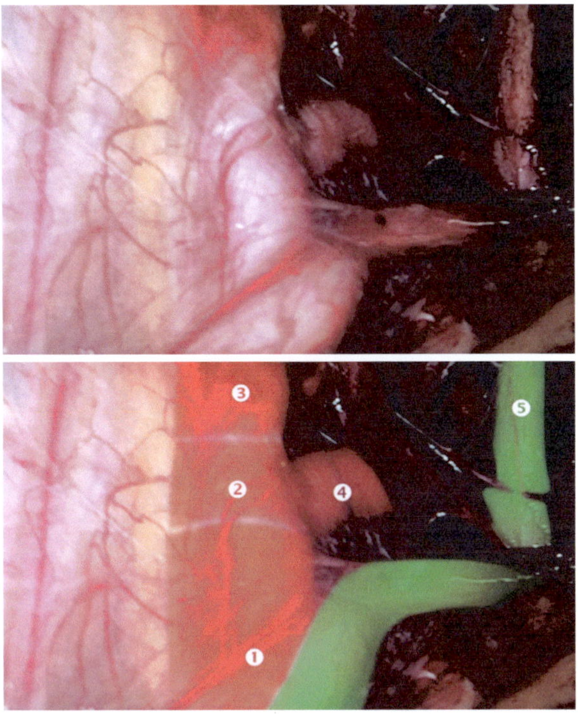

Fig. 5.37 Laparoscopic image of the left pelvic transition, identifying the bifurcation of the iliac arteries and the crossing of the left ureter anteriorly to the left common iliac artery. (1) Left common iliac artery, (2) bifurcation of iliac vessels to the left, (3) left external iliac artery, (4) left internal iliac artery, (5) left ureter

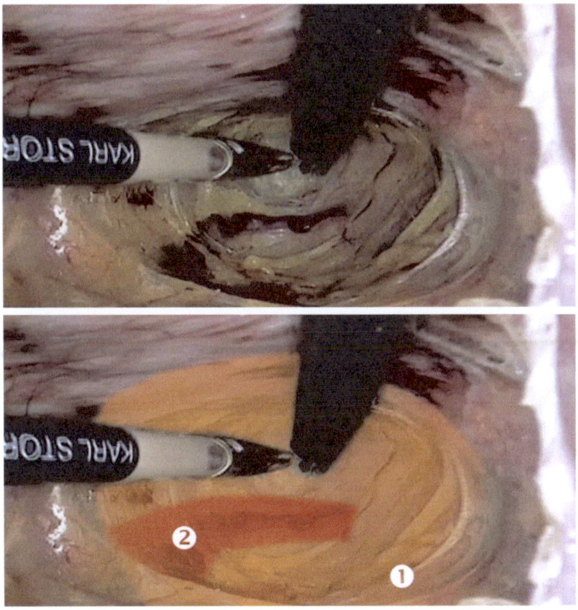

Fig. 5.38 Laparoscopic image of the left Okabayashi space. (1) Okabayashi space to the left, (2) left middle rectal artery

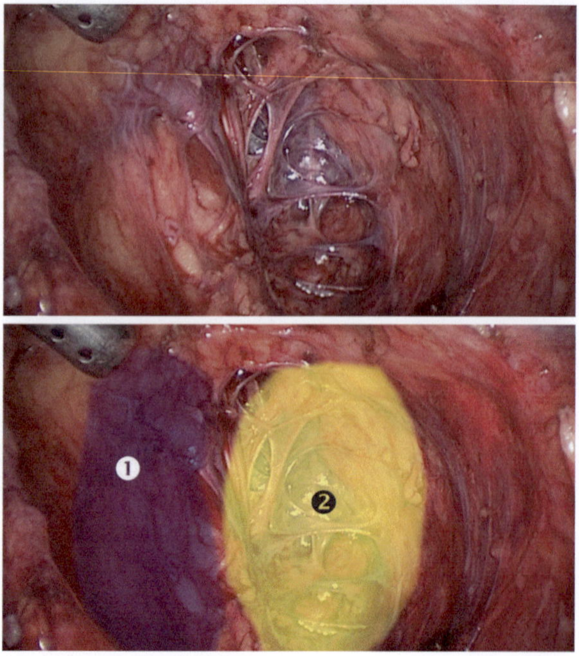

Fig. 5.39 Laparoscopic image after dissection of the Okabayashi space on the right. (1) Rectum and (2) pelvic splanchnic nerves formed by the sacral roots of S2, S3, and S4 to the right

and L5 roots. The lumbosacral trunk presents a descending path in the pelvis, along which we receive the sacral roots from S2 to S4 to form the sciatic nerve deeper (dorsally) in the pelvis. If necessary, dissection can continue dorsally until reaching the plane of the levator ani muscle, which is covered by the endopelvic fascia.

Surgical Applicability

- Pelvic lymphadenectomy
- Radical hysterectomy
- Deep paracervical endometriosis
- Rectosigmoidectomy (segmental or discoid)

Paravaginal or Yabuki Space

The Yabuki space, unlike the other pelvic spaces, is not lined by peritoneal epithelium. Also called the fourth Yabuki space or paravaginal space, it is a small midline retroperitoneal space confined to the anterior surface of the uterus, right at the insertion of the ureter into the bladder.

It is lined by the cervicovesical fascia and contains parasympathetic nerves that innervate the bladder. Careful dissection in this space assists in nerve-preserving radical hysterectomy.

The cervicovesical fascia is divided into anterior and posterior leaflets. The anterior leaflet allows the ureter to insert into the bladder. The anterior fascia wraps around the ureter to form the bladder pillars, while the posterior leaflet communicates with the endopelvic fascia at the height of the levator ani muscle (Fig. 5.40).

The fourth space of Yabuki lies between the deep vesicouterine ligament and the ureter. The vesicouterine ligament (also called the bladder pillar) forms a fibrous tract, approximately 2–3 cm wide, that extends from the posterior and lateral aspect of the bladder to the cervix, where it fuses with the anterior cervicovaginal fascia.

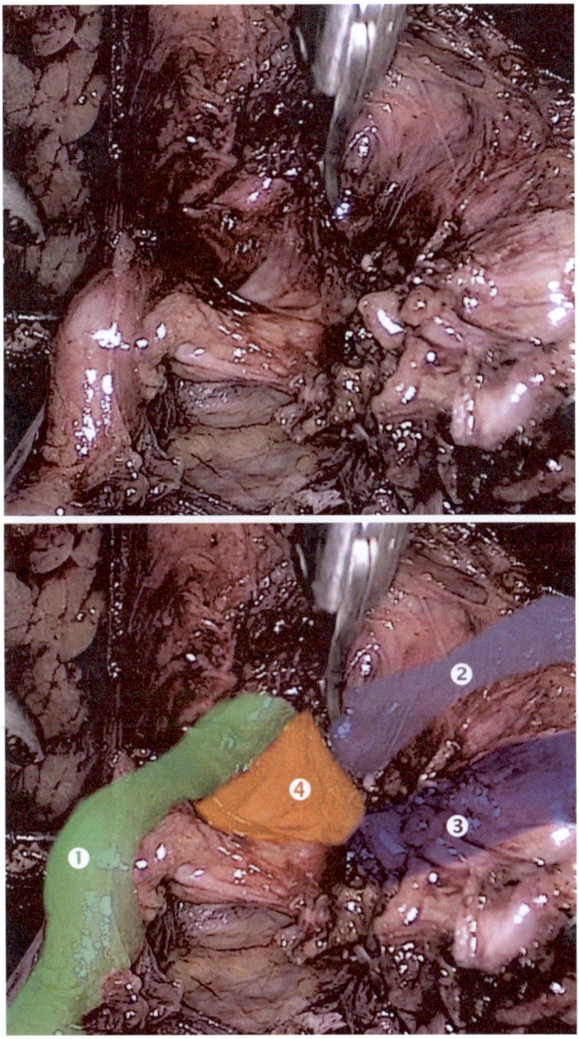

Fig. 5.40 Laparoscopic image after dissection of the left Yabuki space. (1) Left ureter, (2) vagina, (3) cervix, (4) left Yabuki space

This ligament is part of the pubocervical ligament, which is attached to the periosteum of the symphysis pubis and connected to the anterior vaginal fascia.

During the anterior parametrial dissection in radical hysterectomy, the fourth Yabuki space can be identified after sectioning the anterior vesicouterine ligament; the ureter is pulled in order to elevate the posterior leaf of the vesicouterine ligament, thus exposing the so-called fourth space.

As mentioned before, the vesical branches of the inferior hypogastric plexus are in path with the vesicouterine ligaments, hence the relevance of the description of this space (Figs. 5.40, 5.41, and 5.42).

Boundaries

Anterior: insertion of the ureter into the bladder/intravesical ureter

Posterior: parametrium and paracervix

Lateral: paravesical space

Medial: uterine cervix/lateral wall of the vagina

Tips and Tricks 7

After traction of the bladder toward the symphysis pubis and extension of the uterus in a cranial direction, the superficial layer of the vesicouterine ligament will be exposed. The middle segment of the superficial layer of the vesicouterine ligament should be grasped and pulled with forceps, and the upper part of the space needs to be coagulated and cut along the lateral margin of the vesicouterine ligament. The ureter should appear, as the goal of the dissection, and the connective tissue needs to be coagulated and cut in order to develop the fourth Yabuki space. Then the entire

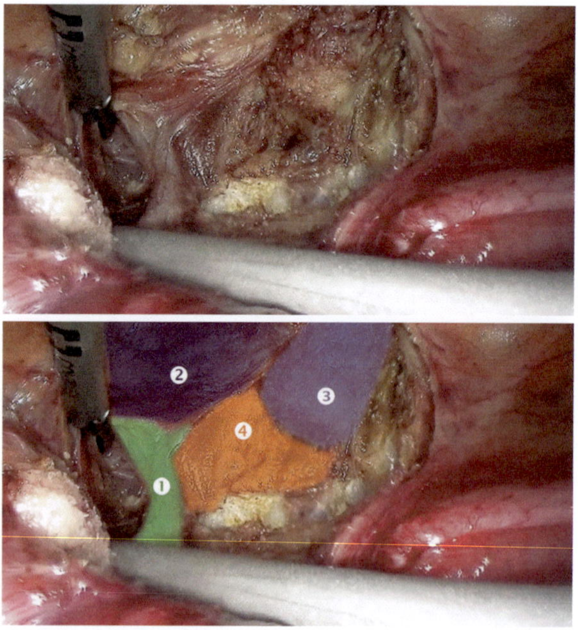

Fig. 5.41 Laparoscopic image after dissection of the left Yabuki space. (1) Left ureter, (2) vagina, (3) cervix, (4) left Yabuki space

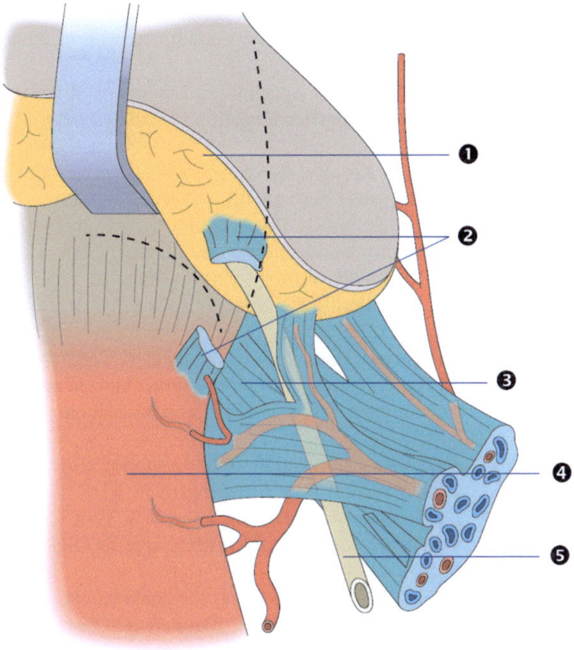

Fig. 5.42 Relationships of the uterine vesical ligament, ureter, and bladder. Shown are (1) bladder, (2) vesicouterine ligament, (3) Yabuki space, (4) cervix, and (5) ureter

upper part of the ureter, including the blood vessels, must be coagulated from the exit of the parametrial ureteral tunnel to the vesicouterine junction. Thus, you have the complete development of the fourth Yabuki space.

Then, by lifting the ureter, tension will be formed in the reflection of the lateral umbilical ligament, which must be punctured, using Kelly forceps, from the fourth space into the paravesical space, which must be coagulated and dissected. During the action, excessive bleeding will occur if the deep uterine vein that passes under the ureter is forced. With this maneuver, the ureter is completely separated from the parametrium; thus, bladder and parametrium will remain connected only by the deep layer of the vesicouterine ligament.

Bibliography

1. Ceccaroni M, Clarizia R, Bruni F, D'Urso E, Minelli L, Gagliardi ML, Roviglione G, et al. Nerve-sparing laparoscopic eradication of deep endometriosis with segmental rectal and parametrial resection: the Negrar method. A single-center, prospective, clinical trial. Surg Endosc. 2012;26(7):2029–45.
2. Ceccaroni M, Clarizia R, Roviglione G, Ruffo G. Neuro-anatomy of the posterior parametrium and surgical considerations for a nerve-sparing approach in radical pelvic surgery. Surg Endosc. 2013;27(11):4386–94.

3. Ceccaroni M, Pontrelli G, Scioscia M, Ruffo G, Bruni F, Minelli L. Nerve-sparing laparoscopic radical excision of deep endometriosis with rectal and parametrial resection. J Minim Invasive Gynecol. 2010;17(1):14–5.
4. Ceccaroni M, Pontrelli G, Spagnolo E, Scioscia M, Bruni F, Paglia A, et al. Parametrial dissection during laparoscopic nerve-sparing radical hysterectomy: a new approach aims to improve patients' postoperative quality of life. Am J Obstet Gynecol. 2010;202(3):320.e1–2.
5. Che X, Huang X, Zhang J, Xu H, Zhang X. Is nerve-sparing surgery suitable for deeply infiltrating endometriosis? Eur J Obstet Gynecol Reprod Biol. 2014;175:87–91.
6. Cibula D, Abu-Rustum NR. Pelvic lymphadenectomy in cervical cancer: surgical anatomy and proposal for a new classification system. Gynecol Oncol. 2009;116(1):33–7.
7. Díaz-Feijoo B, Bradbury M, Pérez-Benavente A, Franco-Camps S, Gil-Moreno A. Nerve-sparing technique during laparoscopic radical hysterectomy: critical steps. J Minim Invasive Gynecol. 2018;25(7):1144–5.
8. Ercoli A, Delmas V, Fanfani F, Gadonneix P, Ceccaroni M, Fagotti A, et al. Terminologia Anatomica versus unofficial descriptions and nomenclature of the fasciae and ligaments of the female pelvis: a dissection-based comparative study. Am J Obstet Gynecol. 2005;193(4):1565–73.
9. Fujii S. Anatomic identification of nerve-sparing radical hysterectomy: a step-by-step procedure. Gynecol Oncol. 2008;111(2 Suppl):S33–41.
10. Fujii S, Takakura K, Matsumura N, Higuchi T, Yura S, Mandai M, et al. Anatomic identification and functional outcomes of the nerve sparing Okabayashi radical hysterectomy. Gynecol Oncol. 2007;107(1):4–13.
11. Hampton BS, Sung VW. Improving medical student knowledge of female pelvic floor dysfunction and anatomy: a randomized trial. Am J Obstet Gynecol. 2010;202(6):601.e1–8.
12. Jiménez AM, Colomer AT. An update of anatomical references in total laparoscopic radical hysterectomy: from surgical anatomy to anatomical surgery. J Minim Invasive Gynecol. 2008;15(1):4–10.
13. Kamina P, Gouazé A. Anatomie clinique: organes urinaires et genitaux, pelvis, coupes du tronc. 2nd ed. Educa Books; 2014. Tome 4.
14. Kraima AC, Derks M, Smit NN, van de Velde CJ, Kenter GG, DeRuiter MC. Careful dissection of the distal ureter is highly important in nerve-sparing radical pelvic surgery: a 3D reconstruction and immunohistochemical characterization of the vesical plexus. Int J Gynecol Cancer. 2016;26(5):959–66.
15. Kraima AC, van Schaik JV, Susan S, van de Velde CJ, Hamming JF, Lakke EA, et al. New insights in the neuroanatomy of the human adult superior hypogastric plexus and hypogastric nerves. Auton Neurosci. 2015;189:60–7.
16. Mirilas P, Skandalakis J. Surgical anatomy of the retroperitoneal spaces part II: the architecture of the retroperitoneal space. Ann Surg. 2010;76(1):33–42.
17. Paramasivam S, Proietto A, Puvaneswary M. Pelvic anatomy and MRI. Best Pract Res Clin Obstet Gynaecol. 2005;20(1):3–22.
18. Querleu D, Morrow CP. Classification of radical hysterectomy. Lancet Oncol. 2008;9(3):297–303.
19. Sakuragi N, Todo Y, Kudo M, Yamamoto R, Sato T. A systematic nerve-sparing radical hysterectomy technique in invasive cervical cancer for preserving postsurgical bladder function. Int J Gynecol Cancer. 2005;15(2):389–97.
20. Stoker J. Anorectal and pelvic floor anatomy. Best Pract Res Clin Gastroenterol. 2009;23(4):463–75.
21. Yabuki Y, Asamoto A, Hoshiba T, Nishimoto H, Nishikawa Y, Nakajima T. Radical hysterectomy: an anatomic evaluation of parametrial dissection. Gynecol Oncol. 2000;77(1):155–63.
22. Yabuki Y, Sasaki H, Hatakeyama N, Murakami G. Discrepancies between classic anatomy and modern gynecologic surgery on pelvic connective tissue structure: harmonization of those concepts by collaborative cadaver dissection. Am J Obstet Gynecol. 2005;193(1):7–15.

Chapter 6
Pelvic Irrigation

Anna Luiza Lobão Gonçalves, Raquel Ferreira Lima, Rodrigo Fernandes, and Helizabet Salomão Ayroza

Overview

The pelvis contains numerous structures in a small space. The female pelvis is more complex because of the intracavitary presence of the reproductive organs, different from what is found in the male pelvis. The functionality of these organs, especially the uterus during pregnancy, requires greater blood support from the female pelvis.

The lymphatic drainage system is formed by transparent canaliculi along the retroperitoneal fat and is closely connected to the venous system. Along the canaliculi are found ganglion structures containing accumulations of lymph cells known

Supplementary Information The online version contains supplementary material available at https://doi.org/10.1007/978-3-031-63520-5_6.

A. L. L. Gonçalves
Gynecological Endoscopy and Endometriosis Division, Faculty of Medical Sciences, Santa Casa de Misericórdia de São Paulo (SCMSP), São Paulo, Brazil

Santa Casa de Sao Paulo School of Medical Sciences, São Paulo, Brazil

Brazilian Federation of Gynecological and Obstetrical Associations (FEBRAS-GO), São Paulo, Brazil

R. F. Lima
Brazilian Federation of Gynecological and Obstetrical Associations (FEBRAS-GO), São Paulo, Brazil

Faculty of Medical Sciences, Santa Casa de Misericórdia de São Paulo (SCMSP), São Paulo, Brazil

R. Fernandes
Cancer Institute of the State of São Paulo - University of São Paulo Medical School (FMUSP), São Paulo, Brazil

H. Salomão Ayroza (✉)
Obstetrics and Gynecology Department, Faculdade de Ciências Médicas da Santa Casa de Misericórdia de São Paulo (SCMSP), São Paulo, Brazil

Gynecological Endoscopy and Endometriosis Division, Santa Casa de São Paulo Hospital, São Paulo, Brazil

H. Salomão Ayroza, P. Ayroza Ribeiro (eds.), *Atlas of Laparoscopic Gynecological Anatomy*, https://doi.org/10.1007/978-3-031-63520-5_6

as lymph nodes. The cluster of lymphatics and nodes responsible for locoregional drainage is called the lymphatic chain. The main vascular structures of the pelvis are found in the retroperitoneum, adjacent to the posterolateral walls. The venous system is deeper and presents more anatomical variations than the arterial one.

The abdominal aorta and vena cava, although not in the pelvis, are primarily responsible for pelvic irrigation.

Abdominal Aorta Artery

Anatomical Landmarks 1

Origin: Thoracic Aorta

Origin: The descending aorta, after passing the diaphragm, penetrates the abdomen, receiving then the name of abdominal aorta.

Path: It passes through the diaphragmatic opening of the aorta, behind the median arcuate ligament. The abdominal aorta begins at the inferior border of the T12 vertebra and descends, parallel to the spine, anteriorly to the lumbar vertebrae and the anterior longitudinal ligament to end on the body of L4, dividing into right and left common iliac arteries. To the right of it is the inferior vena cava, covered anteriorly by the parietal peritoneum.

Irrigation: The aorta gives off branches intended for the irrigation of the organs and walls of the abdominal cavity. The parietal branches irrigate the abdominal wall, and the visceral branches irrigate the viscera of the abdominal cavity.

Branches: Parietal and visceral vessels originate from the abdominal aorta (Fig. 6.1).

The parietal branches/vessels are:

- Inferior diaphragmatic (phrenic) arteries
- Lumbar arteries (originate from the back of the aorta, opposite the bodies of the four upper lumbar vertebrae)
- Median sacral artery

The visceral branches/vessels are:

- Superior mesenteric arteries
- Inferior mesenteric arteries
- Middle suprarenal arteries
- Renal arteries
- Ovarian arteries (female)
- Celiac trunk

Tips and Tricks 1

In the periaortic and pericaval regions are the lymph node chains of the same name. The removal of these chains is recommended in cases of endometrial, cervical

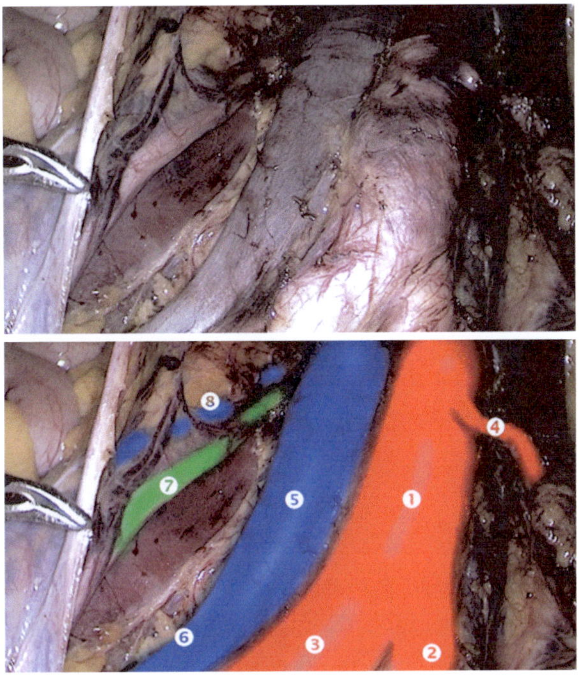

Fig. 6.1 Para-aortic lymphadenectomy. (1) Aorta artery, (2) left common iliac artery, (3) right common iliac artery, (4) inferior mesenteric artery, (5) vena cava, (6) right common iliac vein, (7) right ureter, (8) right gonadal vein

(advanced), and ovarian cancer. The limits for periaortic lymphadenectomy are the ureters, the left renal vein, and the bifurcation of the aorta. The inferior mesenteric artery divides the lymphadenectomy into supra-mesenteric and infra-mesenteric, also known as levels 3 and 4 (Figs. 6.2 and 6.3) [1].

Pelvic Arteries

The pelvic irrigation mainly originates from the internal iliac artery at the sacroiliac synostosis. Numerous branches leave from it towards the target organs and structures. Some endings may present anastomoses originating from the same system as the internal iliac artery or from distinct systems, such as external iliac, aortic, and thoracic vessels.

In the female pelvis minor, also called true pelvis (space limited by the bones of the pelvis; contains bladder, distal part of the ureters, pelvic genital organs, rectum, blood and lymphatic vessels, and nerves), there are six main arteries:

- Two internal iliac arteries
- Two ovarian arteries (arising from the aortic system)
- One median sacral artery (arising from the aortic system)
- One superior rectus artery (arising from the inferior mesenteric artery) (Fig. 6.4)

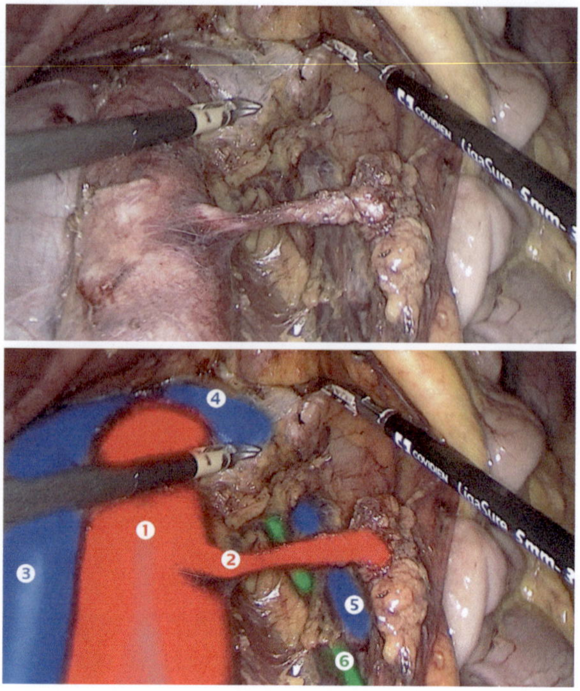

Fig. 6.2 Para-aortic lymphadenectomy. (1) Aorta artery, (2) inferior mesenteric artery, (3) vena cava, (4) left renal vein, (5) left gonadal vein, (6) left ureter

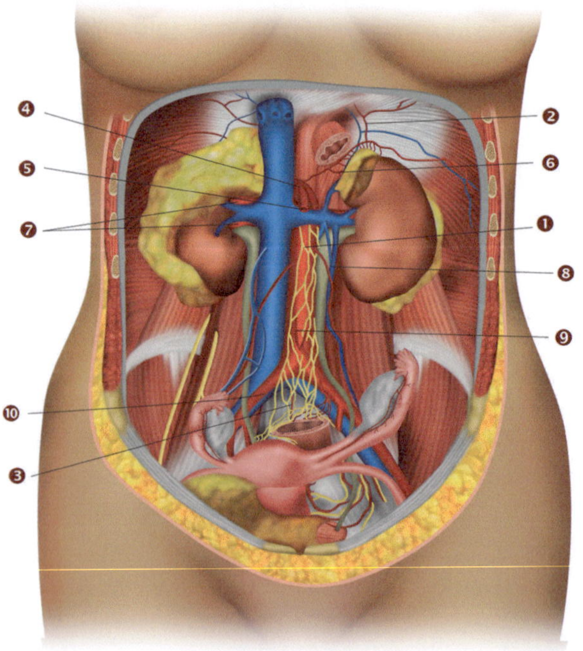

Fig. 6.3 Coronal section of abdomen and pelvis, showing the abdominal aorta and its branches. (1) Abdominal aorta, parietal branches: (2) inferior phrenic arteries and (3) median sacral artery. Visceral branches: (4) celiac trunk, (5) superior mesenteric artery, (6) middle suprarenal arteries, (7) renal arteries, (8) ovarian arteries, and (9) inferior mesenteric artery. And the terminal branches: (10) common iliac arteries

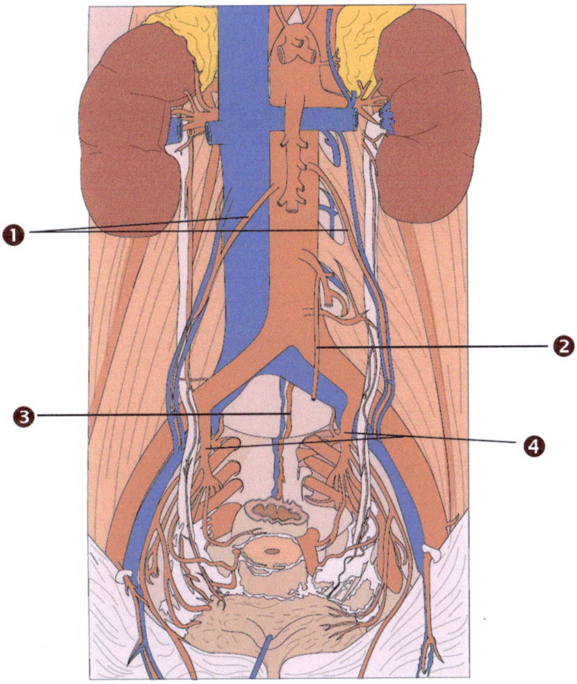

Fig. 6.4 Total view of the abdomen and pelvis with the six main arteries of the female pelvis minor: (1) ovarian arteries, (2) superior rectus artery, (3) median sacral artery, and (4) internal iliac arteries

Common Iliac Arteries

Anatomical Landmarks 2

Origin: Abdominal Aorta

Origin: Abdominal aorta. At the level of the fourth lumbar vertebra, the aorta bifurcates, originating its terminal branches: right and left common iliac arteries.

Path: They descend in an inferolateral direction until the anterior portion of the sacroiliac joints, when they bifurcate into external and internal iliac.

Branches: Internal iliac arteries and external iliac arteries.

Irrigation: Pelvis, abdominal wall, and lower limbs. They receive lymph from the common iliac lymph nodes.

Tips and Tricks 2

The common iliac arteries are directly related to major accidents of first laparoscopic puncture, because they are positioned in the same direction as the umbilical scar.

In most cases, one finds the left ureter crossing over the left common iliac artery. On the contralateral side, the ureter usually crosses over the external iliac artery. This fact is due to the sinister positioning of the arterial system in comparison to the venous.

The lymphadenectomy in the portion of the common iliac arteries and veins is also known as level 2 [1]. It is worth emphasizing the care with the left common iliac vein, which is located between the common iliac arteries and has a thin wall, with high risk for injury during the procedure (Figs. 6.5, 6.6, 6.7, and 6.8).

External Iliac Arteries

Anatomical Landmarks 3

Origin: Common iliac artery

Origin: Arise from the bifurcation of the common iliac arteries in the region of the sacroiliac synostosis.

Path: They run in an inferior and lateral direction along the medial border of the psoas major. They exit the pelvis posteriorly to the inguinal ligament, midway

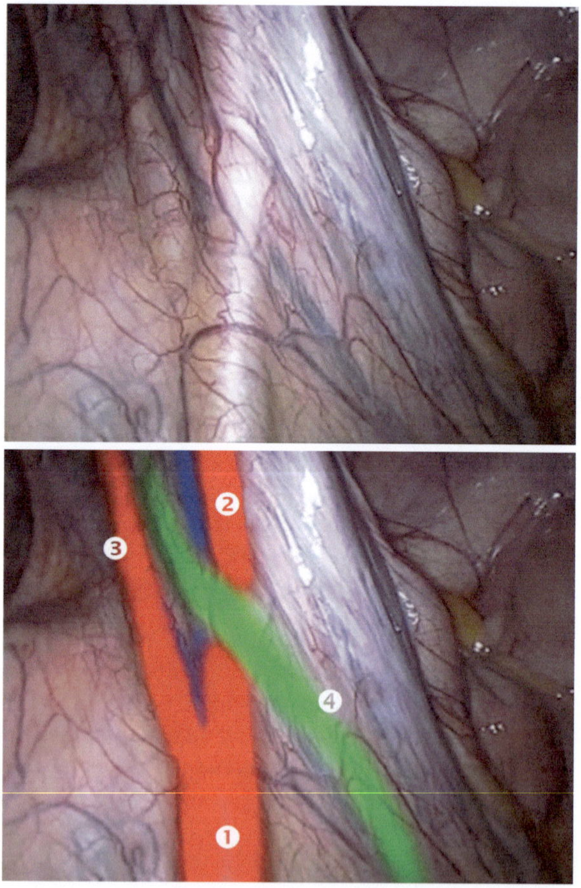

Fig. 6.5 In the right hemipelvis, the common iliac artery and its branches are identified through transparency. (1) Right common iliac artery, (2) right external iliac artery, (3) right internal iliac artery, (4) right ureter crossing the right external iliac artery

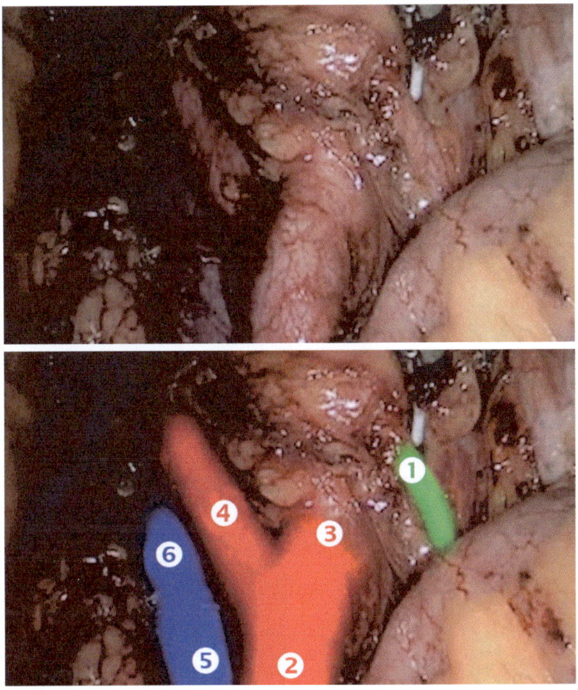

Fig. 6.6 In the right hemipelvis, the common iliac artery and its branches are identified. (1) Ureter (forceps tip), (2) right common iliac artery, (3) right external iliac artery, (4) right internal iliac artery (hypogastric), (5) right common iliac vein, (6) internal iliac vein

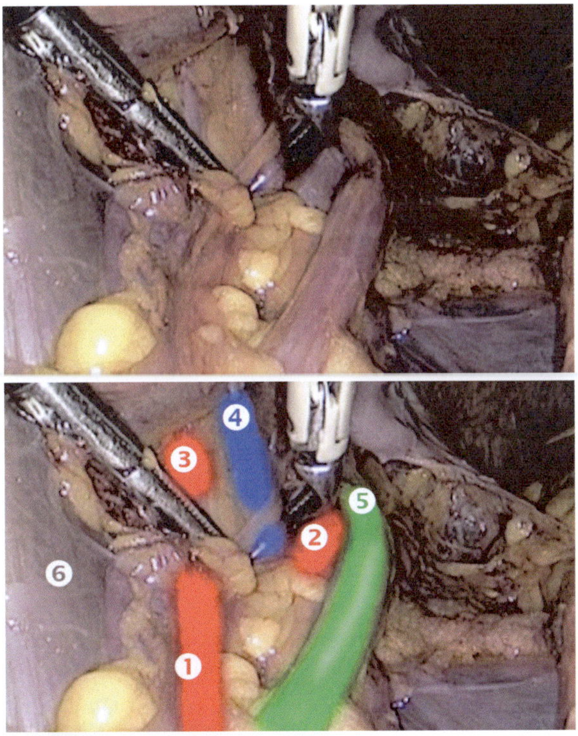

Fig. 6.7 Cadaveric dissection. On the left, the common iliac artery and its branches are identified. (1) Left common iliac artery, (2) left internal iliac artery, (3) left external iliac artery, (4) left external iliac vein, (5) left ureter crossing the left internal iliac artery, (6) psoas muscle

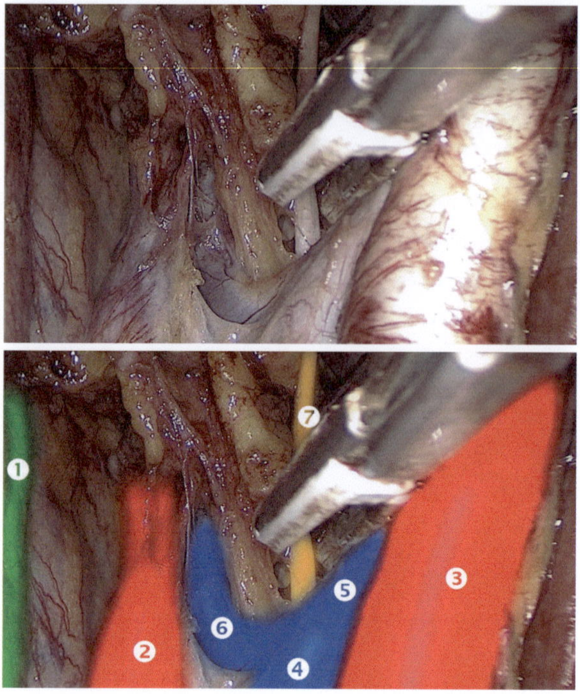

Fig. 6.8 Right pelvic lymphadenectomy. (1) Right ureter, (2) right internal iliac artery, (3) right external iliac artery, (4) right common iliac vein, (5) right external iliac vein, (6) right internal iliac vein, (7) right obturator nerve

between the anterosuperior iliac spine and the pubic symphysis, when they receive the name femoral arteries.

Branches: Deep circumflex iliac artery, inferior epigastric artery, femoral artery.

Irrigation: Abdominal wall, iliac muscle, external genitalia, and lower limbs. They receive lymph from the external iliac lymph nodes.

Tips and Tricks 3

The external iliac artery is one of the anatomical landmarks of pelvic lymphadenectomy. The genitofemoral nerve (the most cranial and lateral limit of the procedure) may be very close to the vessel, which requires extra attention during its dissection (Figs. 6.9, 6.10, and 6.11).

Anatomical Landmarks 4

Origin: External iliac artery.

Origin: First branch of the external iliac artery.

Path: It follows the deep side of the anterior wall of the abdomen, parallel to the inguinal ligament.

Branches: None.

Irrigation: Iliac muscle, deep wall of the abdomen in the inguinal region, and iliac fossa.

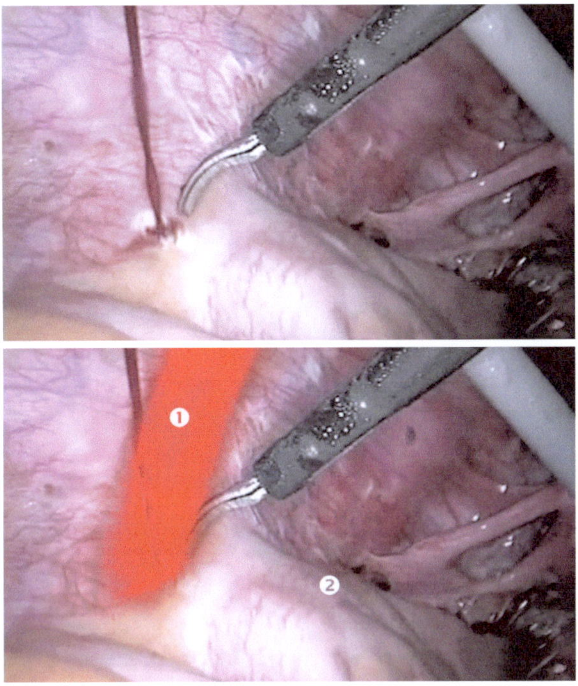

Fig. 6.9 Accidental injury to the left external iliac artery during release of the sigmoid from Toldt's fascia. (1) Left external iliac artery during sigmoid release, (2) sigmoid

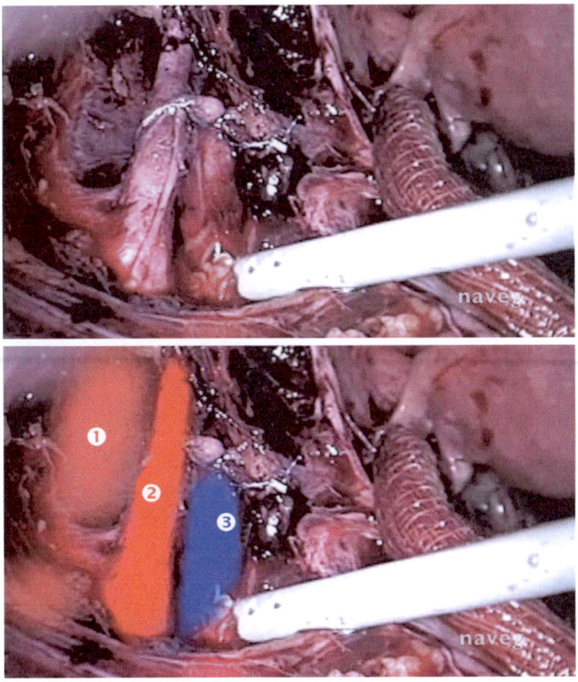

Fig. 6.10 Dissection of the left external iliac vessels during a lymphadenectomy. (1) Left psoas muscle, (2) left external iliac artery, (3) left external iliac vein

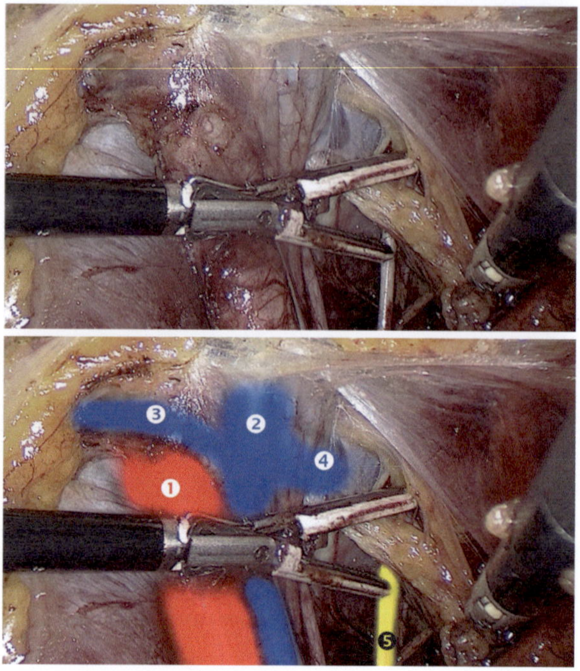

Fig. 6.11 Left pelvic lymphadenectomy. (1) Left external iliac artery, (2) left external iliac vein, (3) left deep circumflex iliac vein, (4) left corona mortis, (5) left obturator nerve

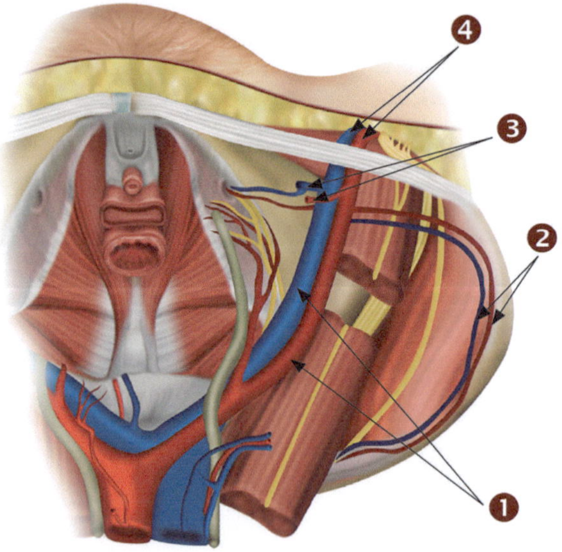

Fig. 6.12 In the right hemipelvis, the external iliac vessels and their branches are identified. (1) External iliac vessels, (2) deep circumflex iliac vessels, (3) inferior epigastric vessels, and (4) femoral vessels

Tips and Tricks 4
This artery should be remembered in cases of endometrioma excision in the inguinal canal or in transinguinal hysteropexy surgery (Fig. 6.12).

Inferior Epigastric Artery

Anatomical Landmarks 5

Origin: External iliac artery.

Origin: In the external iliac artery, a few millimeters above the inguinal ligament. It is the second branch of the external iliac artery.

Path: Runs horizontally and superiorly to the transverse fascia and follows anteriorly to the arched line, between the rectus abdominis muscle and the posterior layer of its sheath. Then, the inferior epigastric artery anastomoses with the superior epigastric artery.

Branches: It provides branches to the spermatic cord, a suprapubic branch, and an anastomotic branch to the obturator artery.

Irrigation: Abdominal muscles and peritoneum.

Anastomosis: Anastomoses with the superior epigastric artery, a branch of the internal thoracic artery.

Tips and Tricks 5

The inferior epigastric artery and the inguinal ligament divide the inguinal region into three main areas:

- The first area is the so-called Hesselbach's triangle, whose lower boundary is the inguinal ligament, the medial boundary is the lateral approach to the rectus abdominis muscle, and the upper boundary is the inferior epigastric artery.
- The second area is the region lateral to the inferior epigastric artery, just above the inguinal ligament.
- The third area is the femoral region, inferior to the inguinal ligament and lateral to the femoral vein.

Surgical importance in inguinal hernia corrections: during laparoscopy, there should be concern with the inferior epigastric artery during the performance of the accessory punctures in the right and left iliac fossae. It is necessary to proceed to the transillumination of the wall, as well as the correct marking of the point of performance (2 cm above the superior iliac crest and medially), avoiding the risk of injury during the accessory punctures (Figs. 6.13, 6.14, and 6.15).

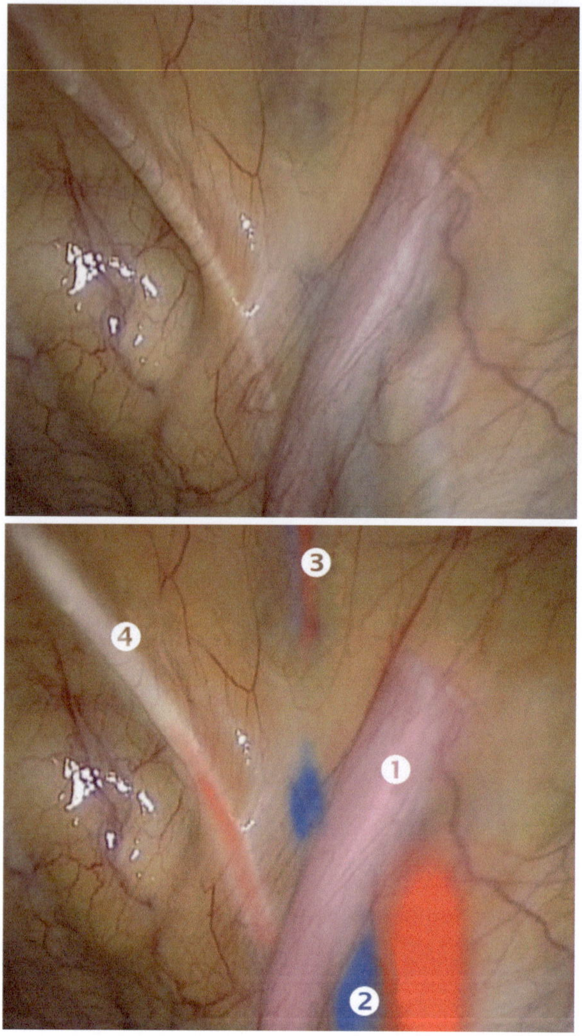

Fig. 6.13 Pelvic wall transparency of the right iliac fossa. (1) Right round ligament, (2) right external iliac vessels, (3) right inferior epigastric vessels, (4) right obliterated umbilical artery

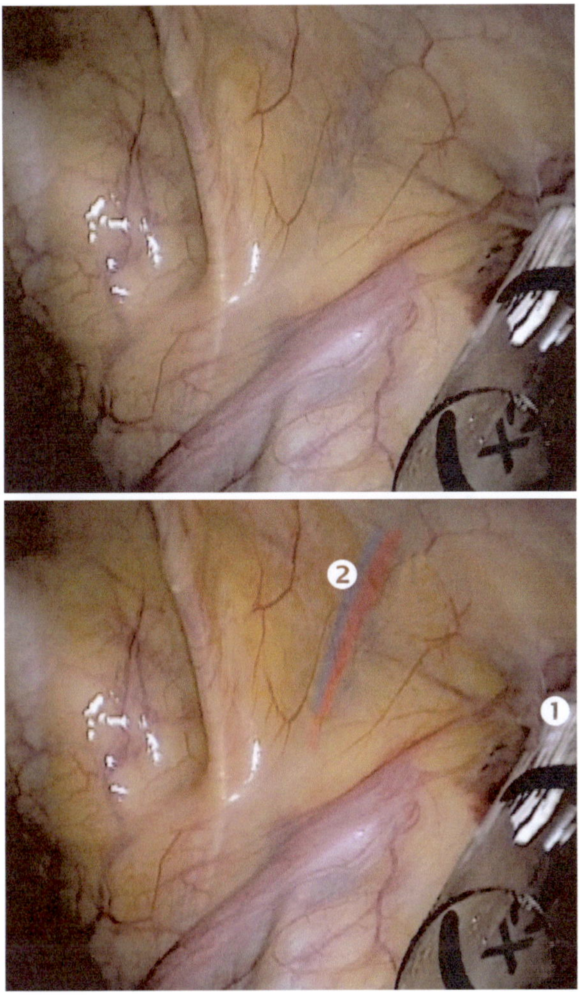

Fig. 6.14 In the right hemipelvis, you can see the positioning of the trocar of the accessory puncture, during laparoscopy, laterally to the inferior epigastric vessels. (1) Trocar, (2) lower epigastric vessels to the right

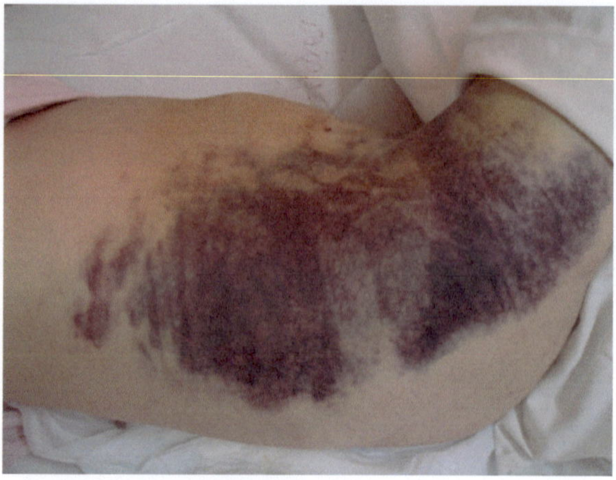

Fig. 6.15 Ecchymosis on right flank and thigh, after injury to the lower epigastric vessels during accessory puncture in laparoscopy

Femoral Artery

Anatomical Landmarks 6

Origin: External iliac artery.

Origin: The external iliac artery passes under the inguinal ligament and reaches the lower limb, when it is called the femoral artery.

Branch: Terminal branch of the external iliac artery.

Irrigation: It is the main source of irrigation of the lower limb.

Tips and Tricks 6

It has no application for laparoscopic pelvic surgery. Knowledge of the anatomy of the inguinal region is essential before performing vulvectomy and/or inguinal lymphadenectomy. The lymphatics of the vulva drain to the superficial inguinal and femoral lymph nodes, as well as to the external iliac lymph nodes (Figs. 6.16 and 6.17).

Internal Iliac Arteries

Anatomical Landmarks 7

They are the most important arteries of the pelvis, responsible for much of the irrigation of the pelvic viscera and skeletal muscle structures of the pelvic wall, gluteal region, medial regions of the thigh, and perineum.

Origin: Common iliac artery.

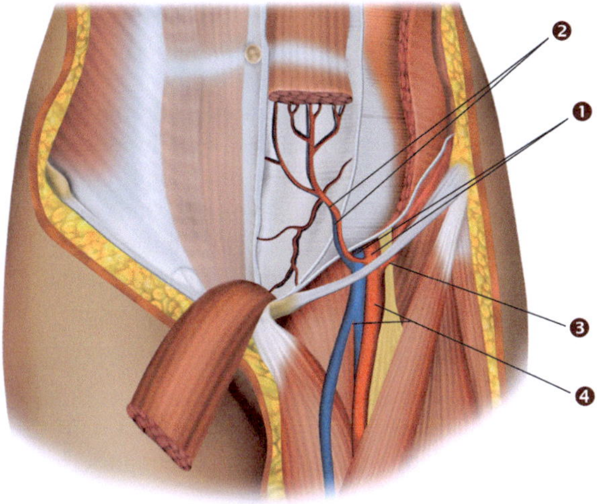

Fig. 6.16 Epigastric vessels. On the left side, the external iliac vessels and their branches are identified. (1) External iliac vessels, (2) inferior epigastric vessels, (3) deep circumflex iliac artery, and (4) femoral vessels

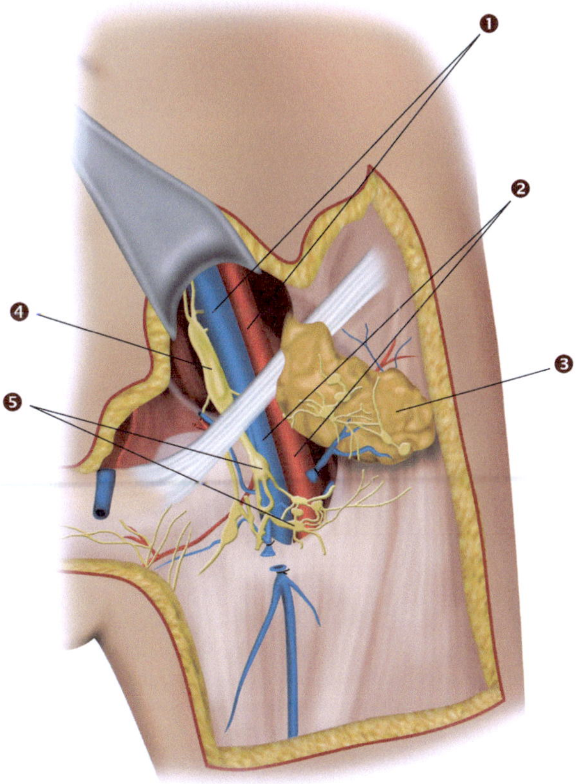

Fig. 6.17 External iliac artery. On the left side, we identify (1) external iliac vessels, (2) femoral vessels and their relations with the (3) subinguinal ganglia, (4) Cloquet's ganglion, and (5) deep inguinal lymph nodes, important anatomical landmarks in inguinal lymphadenectomy

Origin: From the bifurcation of the common iliac arteries along the wing of the sacrum anterior to the sacroiliac joint. Between the sacroiliac joint lie the internal iliac vein and the lumbosacral trunk.

Path: It descends in a posteromedial orientation to the beginning of the lesser pelvis, medial to the external iliac vein. In its medial portion, it is immediately covered by peritoneum. Its path is short, approximately 2–4 cm, when they bifurcate, giving rise to the anterior and posterior trunks.

Branches: Anterior and posterior trunks.

Irrigation: Main vascularization for pelvic organs, gluteal muscles, and perineum. They receive lymph from the internal iliac lymph nodes.

Tips and Tricks 7

The internal iliac artery represents the most cranial and medial landmark of the pelvic lymphadenectomy. Attention should be paid to its medial portion in close proximity to the ureter and its lateral and posterior portions near the bifurcation of the common iliac vein.

Difficult-to-control arterial pelvic bleeding is common in extensive obstetric and gynecological procedures, and clamping the internal iliac artery is a safe option that usually results in the cessation and control of bleeding. It is worth noting that it should be done not in the internal iliac artery, but in the anterior trunk, just after the bifurcation, avoiding interruption of blood to the posterior trunk and especially to the gluteal branches (Fig. 6.18).

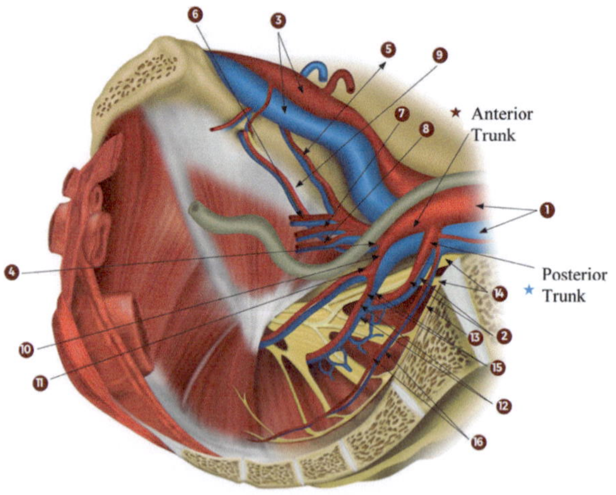

Fig. 6.18 Sagittal section of the pelvic structures on the right. The bifurcation of the (1) right common iliac vessels into (2) hypogastric and (3) external iliac vessels is identified. The internal iliac, or hypogastric, vessels supply the pelvic viscera through several branches and tributary veins. The internal iliac artery is divided into an anterior trunk (red star) and a posterior trunk (blue star). The anterior trunk is divided into anterior and posterior branches. The (4) anterior branches of the anterior trunk are (5) umbilical artery, (6) superior vesical artery, (7) uterine artery, (8) vaginal artery, and (9) obturator artery. And the (10) posterior branches of the anterior trunk are (11) rectus medius artery, (12) internal pudendal artery, and (13) inferior gluteal artery. From the posterior trunk of the internal iliac artery emanate the following branches: (14) iliolumbar artery, (15) superior gluteal artery, and (16) lateral sacral artery

Anterior Trunk of the Internal Iliac Artery

Anatomical Landmarks 8

Origin: Internal iliac artery (Fig. 6.19).

Origin: Division of the internal iliac artery into anterior and posterior at the level of the greater ischial foramen.

Branches: Mainly visceral, but include branches to the thigh and buttock. The arrangement of the branches is variable; these are:

- Anterior branches of the anterior trunk of the internal iliac artery:
  - Umbilical artery/upper vesical artery
  - Uterine artery
  - Obturator artery
  - Vaginal artery
- Posterior branches of the anterior trunk of the internal iliac artery:
  - Middle rectal artery
  - Internal pudendal artery
  - Inferior gluteal artery

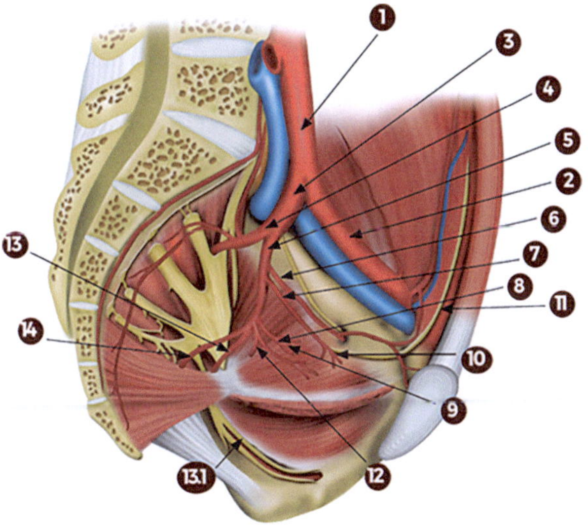

Fig. 6.19 Sagittal section of the left hemipelvis, (1) common iliac artery, and its branches: (2) external iliac artery and (3) internal iliac artery with its (4) posterior trunk and its (5) anterior trunk. From the anterior trunk emanate the following anterior branches: (6) obturator artery, (7) umbilical artery, (8) uterine artery, and (9) vaginal artery. The first branch of the umbilical artery is the (10) superior vesical artery, and its terminal branch is the (11) obliterated umbilical artery that will form the median umbilical ligament. The posterior branches of the anterior trunk of the internal iliac artery are (12) rectus medius artery, (13) internal pudendal artery, (13.1) internal pudendal artery within Alcock's canal, and (14) inferior gluteal artery

Anterior Branches of the Anterior Trunk of the Internal Iliac Artery

Umbilical Artery/Superior Vesical Artery

Anatomical Landmarks 9

Origin: Anterior trunk of the internal iliac artery (usually the first branch).

Origin: The superior vesical arteries are two to three in number, arising from the anterior trunk of the internal iliac artery.

Path: The vessels, usually two or three in number, branch from the anterior trunk of the internal iliac artery and follow the surface of the obturator internus muscle. The arteries then diverge from this course and descend to provide the main arterial supply to the bladder. The superior vesical artery forms the umbilical artery, an occluded remnant that is seen in the continuation of the course of the artery, from the obturator internus to the umbilicus, as the median umbilical ligament. This ligament elevates the fold of peritoneum, called the median umbilical fold, on the deep side of the anterior wall of the abdomen.

Irrigation: Upper part of the bladder and ureter.

Anastomosis: Vaginal artery.

Tips and Tricks 8

From a surgical point of view, the most obvious and important portion of the superior umbilical/vesical artery is the obliterated one, which runs through the median umbilical ligament forming the median umbilical fold, easily seen on the pelvic wall. Since, in most cases, the superior umbilical/vesical artery is the first branch of the internal iliac artery, traction is performed on the median umbilical fold, for its correct identification at its origin, finding, in the sequence, the uterine artery (usually the second medial branch), without the need for dissection of the latter by a long route when the goal is the permanent or temporary ligation of the uterine arteries at their origin.

Special attention should be given to the differentiation of the umbilical artery and obturator nerve, especially during pelvic lymphadenectomy. The identification of the umbilical fold and the obliterated umbilical artery is also considered for the initiation of Retzius space dissection during laparoscopic Burch surgery (Figs. 6.20, 6.21, 6.22, and 6.23).

Uterine Artery

Anatomical Landmarks 10

Origin: Anterior trunk of the internal iliac artery.

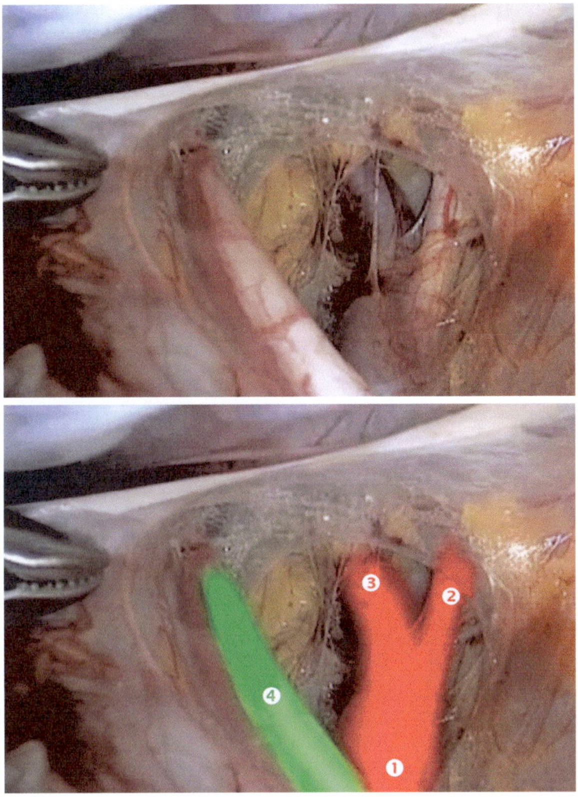

Fig. 6.20 Retroperitoneal opening in the right hemipelvis. (1) Right internal iliac artery, (2) right umbilical artery, (3) right uterine artery, (4) right ureter

Origin: Direct branch of the anterior trunk of the internal iliac artery. It may originate from the superior umbilical/vesical artery.

- The origin of the uterine artery has four types described (Figs. 6.24, 6.25, 6.26, and 6.27):

Path: The uterine artery runs medial to the levator ani muscle towards the cervix. Immediately before reaching the cervix, the artery sends a branch to the ureter, crossing it superiorly and anteriorly to reach the uterus. Arriving at the cervix, it gives the vaginal branch (descending and minor), and the ascending portion follows in the broad ligament, bordering and irrigating the uterine lateral wall up to the junction of the uterine tube and uterus. Near the cornual region, it issues the ovarian and tubal branches.

Branches:

- Vaginal branch: descending and minor (irrigates cervix and vagina)
- Ovarian branch: anastomoses with the ovarian branches of the ovarian artery (irrigates the ovary)
- Tubal branch: anastomoses with the tubal branches of the ovarian artery, forming the irrigation of the mesosalpinx (irrigates the uterine tube)

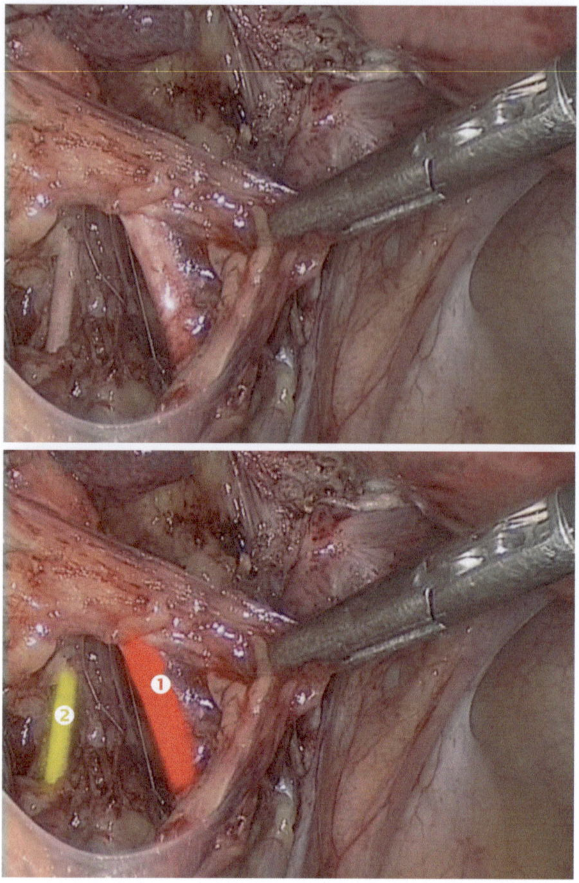

Fig. 6.21 Retroperitoneal opening in the left hemipelvis. (1) Left umbilical artery, (2) left obturator nerve

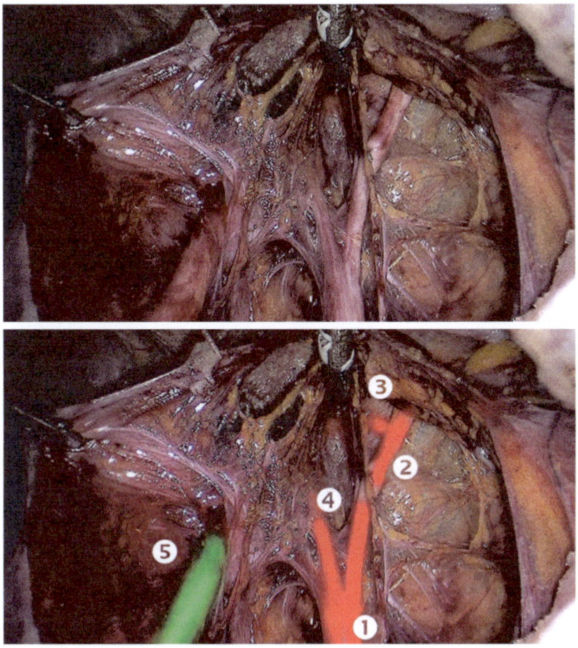

Fig. 6.22 Dissection of the right ovarian fossa. (1) Right internal iliac artery, (2) right umbilical artery, (3) right superior vesical artery, (4) right uterine artery, (5) right ureter

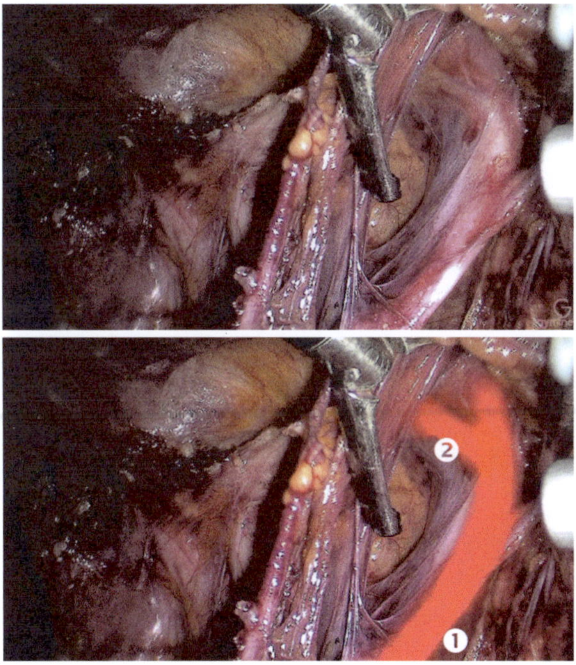

Fig. 6.23 Close-up view of the previous image. (1) Right umbilical artery, (2) right superior vesical artery

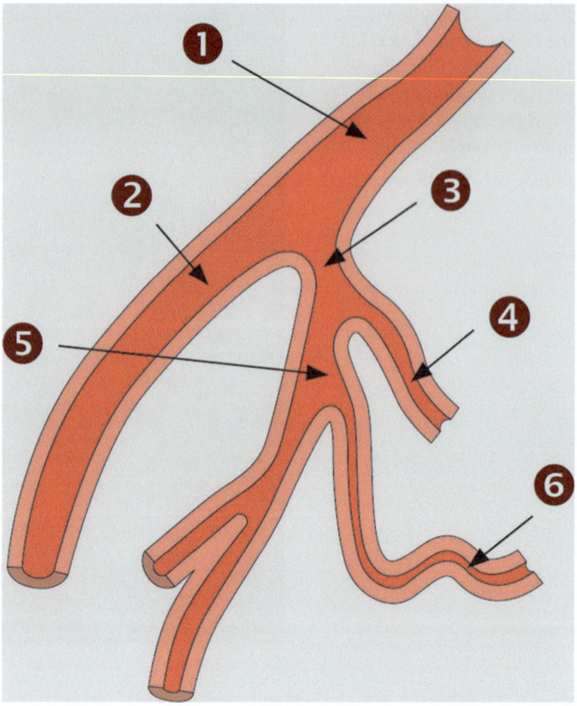

Fig. 6.24 Type I: in 45% of the cases, the uterine artery is a branch of the inferior gluteal artery. (1) Common iliac artery, (2) external iliac artery, (3) internal iliac artery, (4) superior gluteal artery, (5) inferior gluteal artery, (6) uterine artery

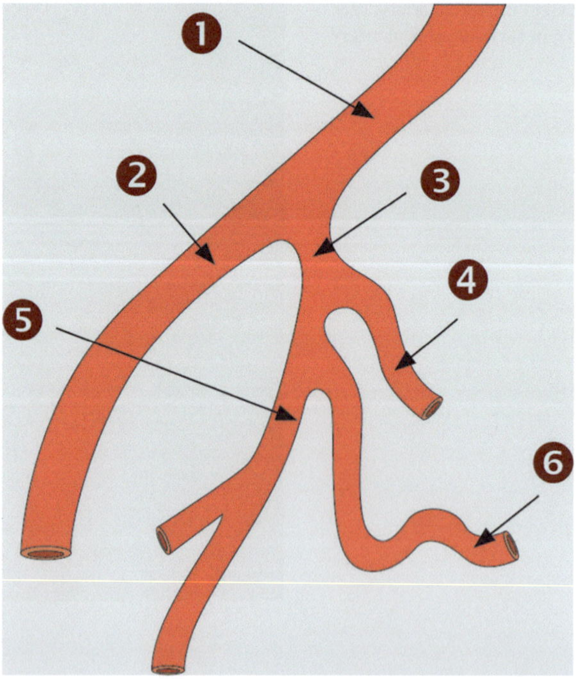

Fig. 6.25 Type II: in 6% of the cases, the uterine artery originates from the bifurcation with the inferior gluteal artery. (1) Common iliac artery, (2) external iliac artery, (3) internal iliac artery, (4) superior gluteal artery, (5) inferior gluteal artery, (6) uterine artery

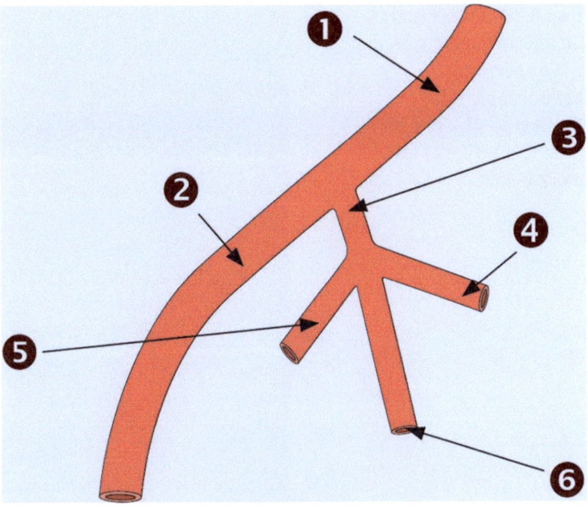

Fig. 6.26 Type III: in 43% of the cases, the uterine artery originates from the common trifurcation with the inferior superior gluteal arteries. (1) Common iliac artery, (2) external iliac artery, (3) internal iliac artery, (4) superior gluteal artery, (5) inferior gluteal artery, (6) uterine artery

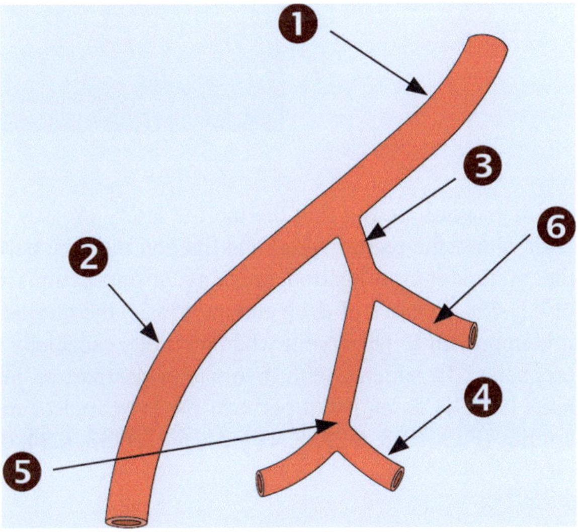

Fig. 6.27 Type IV: in 6% of the cases, the uterine artery is close to where the gluteal arteries originate. (1) Common iliac artery, (2) external iliac artery, (3) internal iliac artery, (4) uterine artery, (5) inferior gluteal artery, (6) superior gluteal artery

Irrigation: Uterus, ligaments of the uterus, medial parts of the uterine tubes and ovaries, and upper part of the vagina.

Anastomosis: Vaginal artery (by the vaginal branch) and ovarian artery (by the tubal and ovarian branches).

Tips and Tricks 9

The anatomical knowledge of the uterine artery is extremely important for gynecologists, because this artery is mainly responsible for uterine irrigation. To perform the hysterectomy, either laparotomic or laparoscopic, it is necessary to proceed to the ligation of the uterine arteries in its entry into the uterus, in the isthmic region,

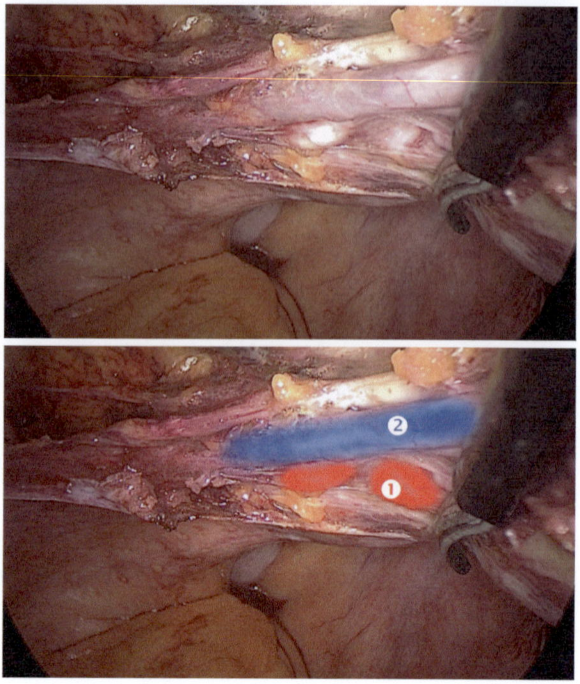

Fig. 6.28 Dissection of the uterine vessels on the left to perform laparoscopic total hysterectomy. (1) Left uterine artery; (2) left uterine vein

and it is worth noting that the uterine artery crosses the ureter (anteriorly), about 2 cm above the region where the ligation must be performed. It is at this moment that ureteral injury (ligation, crushing, or transection) may occur, with an incidence of 0.5–1%. In cases of deep endometriosis, the uterine artery may be affected, and it is important to preserve it when possible, especially for women with a desire for pregnancy. In patients with myomas or postpartum uterine atony, this anatomical knowledge is essential to perform the proximal or distal ligations of the uterine arteries (Figs. 6.28, 6.29, 6.30, 6.31, 6.32, 6.33, 6.34, 6.35, and 6.36).

Obturator Artery

Anatomical Landmarks 11

Origin: Anterior trunk of the internal iliac artery.

Origin: Variable; in general, it arises near where the superior vesical/umbilical artery originates, when it is crossed by the ureter.

Path: It follows anteroinferiorly over the obturator fascia on the lateral wall of the pelvis and passes between the obturator nerve and the obturator vein.

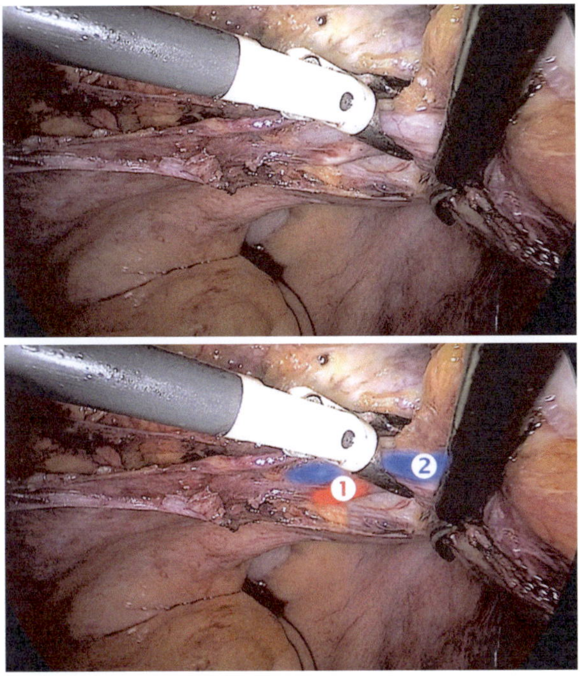

Fig. 6.29 Coagulation of the left uterine vessels, in the isthmo-cervical region and at the height of the insertion of the uterosacral ligaments, during laparoscopic total hysterectomy using the intrafascial technique. (1) Left uterine artery; (2) left uterine vein

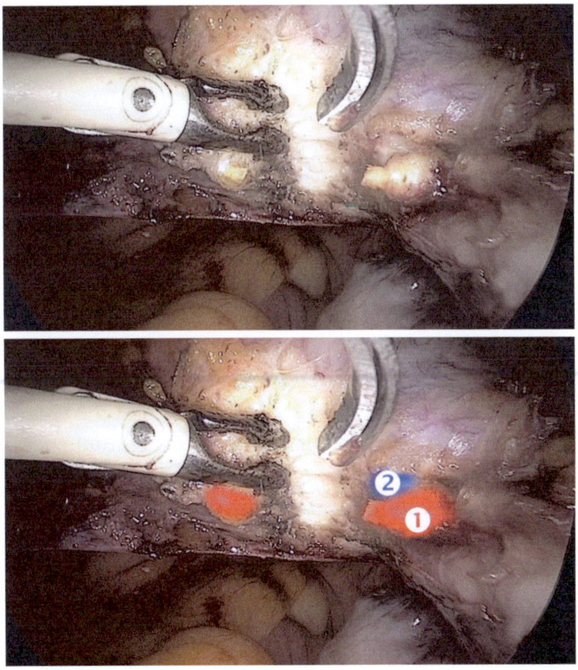

Fig. 6.30 Bipolar coagulation and section with scissors of the left uterine vessels in total hysterectomy. (1) Left uterine artery; (2) left uterine vein

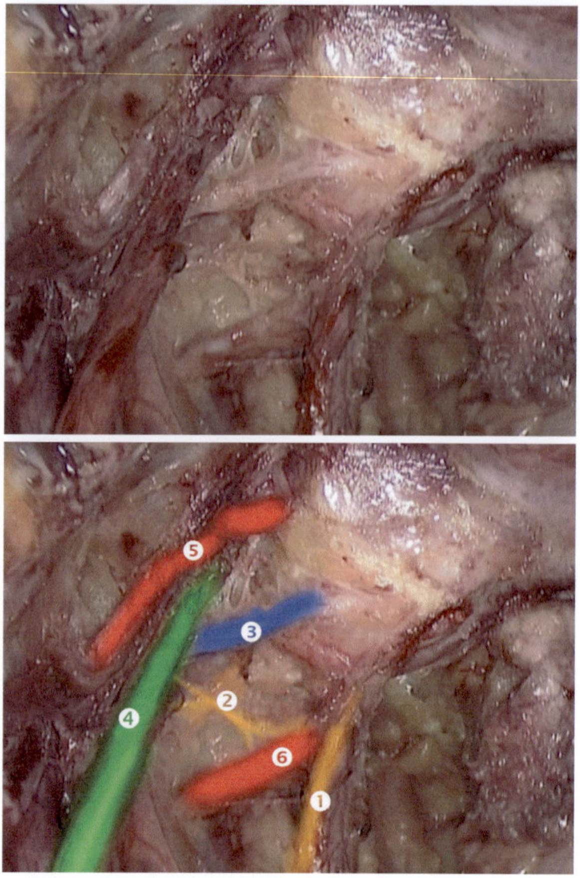

Fig. 6.31 Left hemipelvis after resection of deep endometriosis with identification of the main anatomical landmarks used in this procedure. (1) Left inferior hypogastric plexus; (2) branch of the left inferior hypogastric plexus; (3) left deep uterine vein; (4) left ureter; (5) left uterine artery crossing the left ureter, (6) left middle rectal artery

Branches: In the pelvis, it gives off muscular branches, an artery to the ilium, and a pubic branch. The pubic branch originates just before the obturator artery leaves the pelvis; it ascends on the pelvic side of the pubis to anastomose with the same contralateral branch and with the pubic branch of the inferior epigastric artery (branch of the external iliac artery).

Variation: In 20% of cases, an aberrant or accessory obturator artery originates from the inferior epigastric artery (branch of the external iliac artery) and descends into the pelvis along the usual pubic branch route.

Irrigation: The pelvic muscles, the ilium, the head of the femur, and the muscles of the medial compartment of the thigh.

Anastomosis: Inferior epigastric artery (via the pubic branch) and umbilical artery.

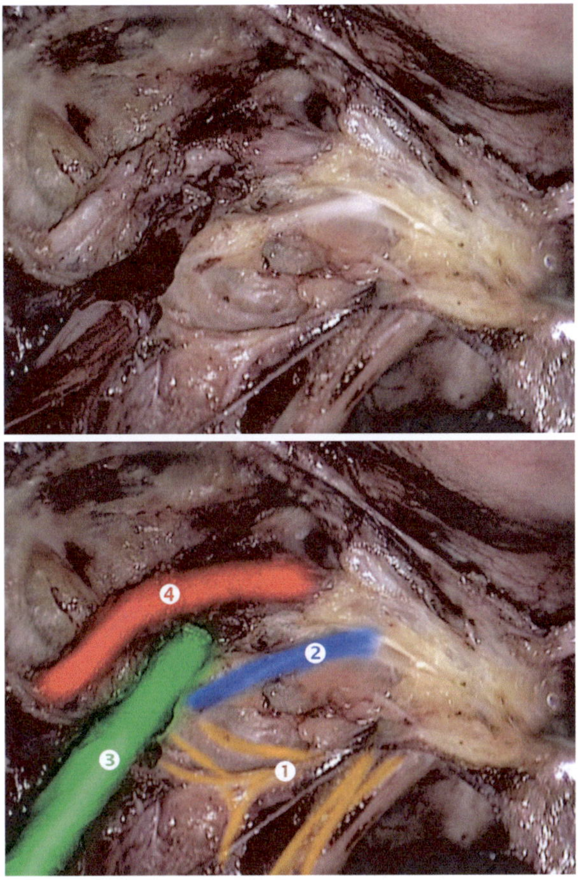

Fig. 6.32 Close-up view of the previous image. (1) Inferior hypogastric plexus with its branches, (2) deep uterine vein, (3) ureter, (4) uterine artery crossing the ureter

Tips and Tricks 10

The recommended surgery for both staging and treatment of endometrial cancer consists of exploration of the peritoneal cavity, peritoneal lavage, hysterectomy, bilateral salpingo-oophorectomy, and bilateral pelvic and para-aortic lymph node dissection. Complications from pelvic lymphadenectomy are usually few, such as acute hemorrhage, postoperative lymphocysts, and obturator vessels and nerve damage.

In Burch surgery, this artery should be studied, as there is a risk of injury to the obturator vessels during surgery, as well as corona mortis.

In surgery for deep infiltrative endometriosis affecting the obturator fossa, dissection of the spaces and identification of obturator vessels and nerve should be performed to preserve them (Figs. 6.37, 6.38, and 6.39).

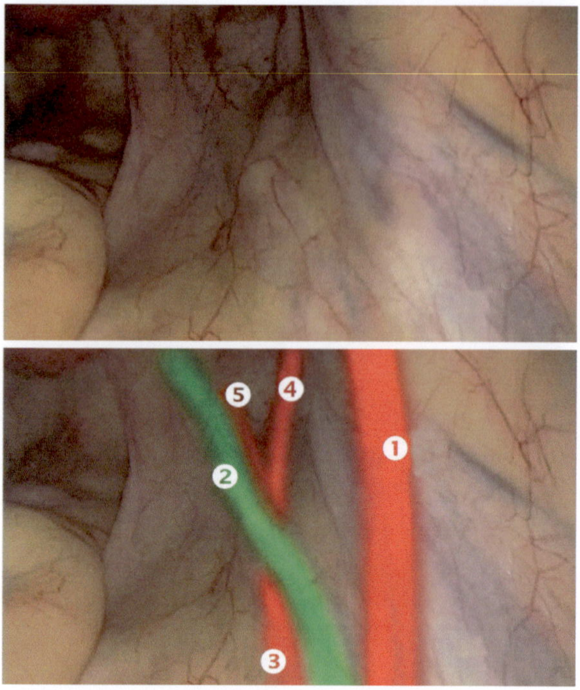

Fig. 6.33 Anatomical inventory before performing temporary ligation of the right uterine artery for myomectomy. (1) External iliac artery, (2) ureter, (3) internal iliac artery, (4) umbilical artery, (5) uterine artery

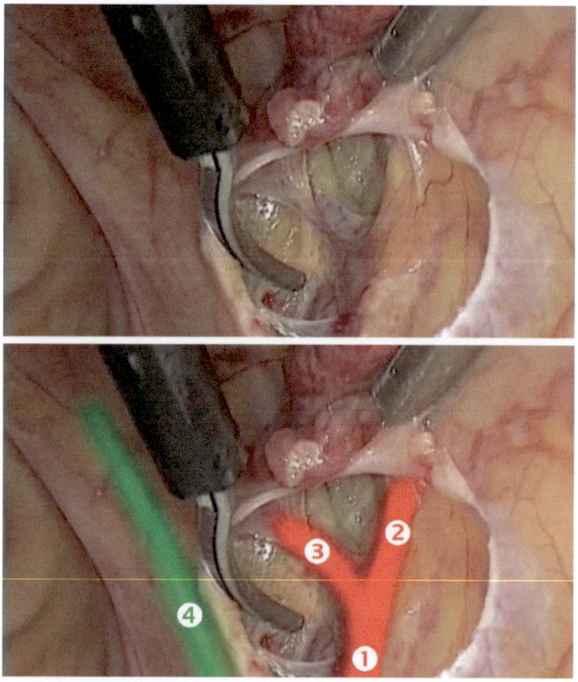

Fig. 6.34 The peritoneum is opened at the site where the internal iliac artery crosses the ureter. (1) Right internal iliac artery, (2) right umbilical artery, (3) right uterine artery, (4) right ureter (through transparency)

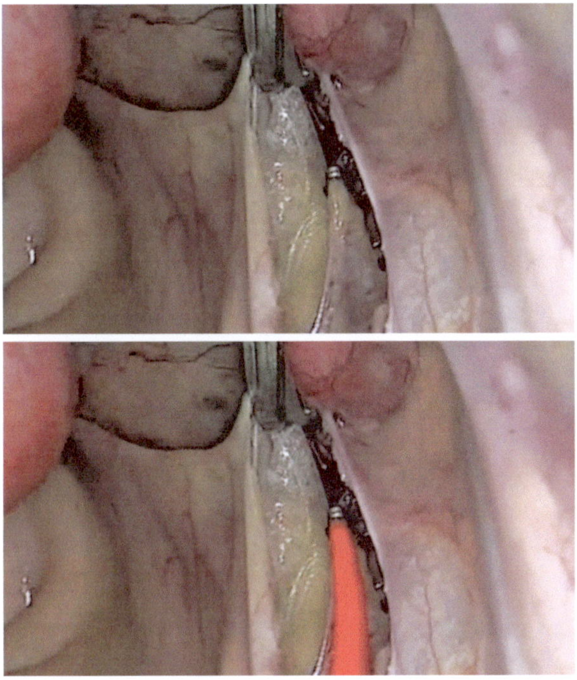

Fig. 6.35 Temporary ligation of the right uterine artery (in red) with a metal clip

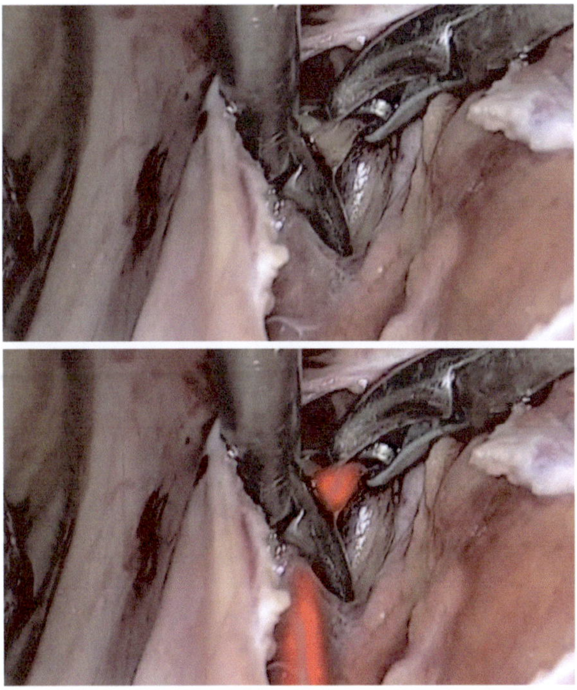

Fig. 6.36 Right uterine artery clip removal (in red)

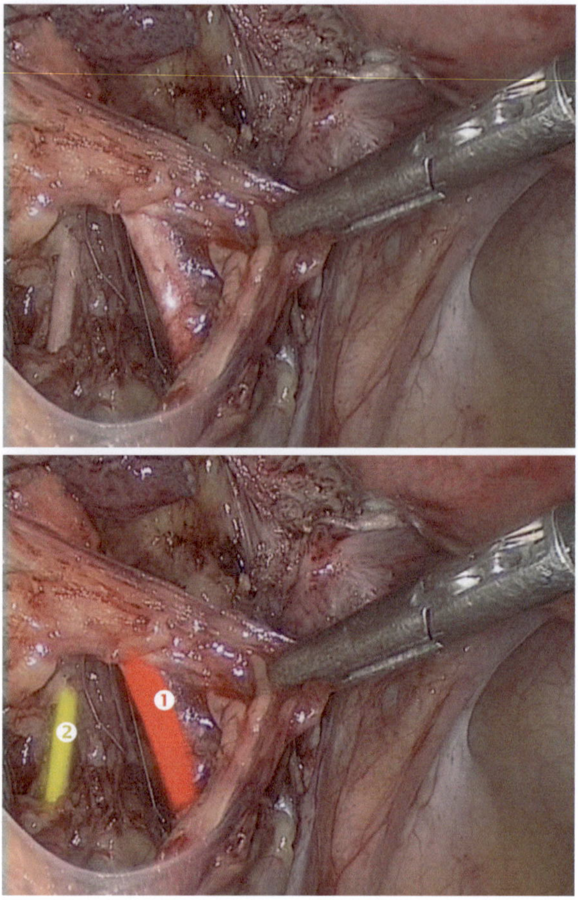

Fig. 6.37 Retroperitoneal opening in the left hemipelvis identifying the obturator fossa with umbilical artery, obturator vessels, and nerves. (1) Umbilical artery, (2) obturator nerve

Vaginal Artery

Anatomical Landmarks 12

Origin: In the anterior division of the internal iliac artery (or it may originate from the uterine artery).

Pathway: The artery usually divides into two branches: vaginal and inferior vesical. The vaginal branch descends over the vagina, supplying the mucosa, and then joins branches of the uterine artery to form the azygos arteries of the vagina.

Branches: Vaginal, inferior vesical, and azygos arteries of the vagina.

Irrigation: The vaginal branch irrigates the vagina, the bulb of the vestibule, and the adjacent rectum. The inferior vesical branch irrigates the fundus of the bladder.

Anastomosis: Vaginal branch of the uterine artery (azygos arteries of the vagina) and superior vesical artery.

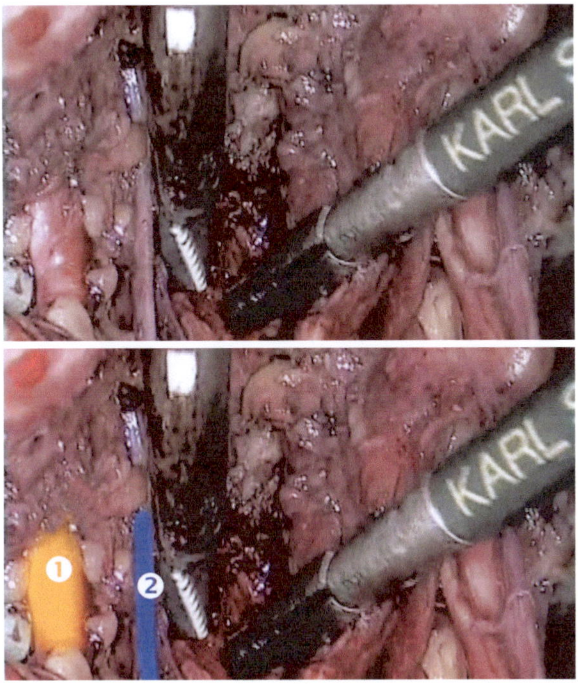

Fig. 6.38 Left hemipelvis during dissection for resection of a deep endometriosis nodule. Obturator nerve and vein are identified. (1) Left obturator nerve, (2) left obturator vein

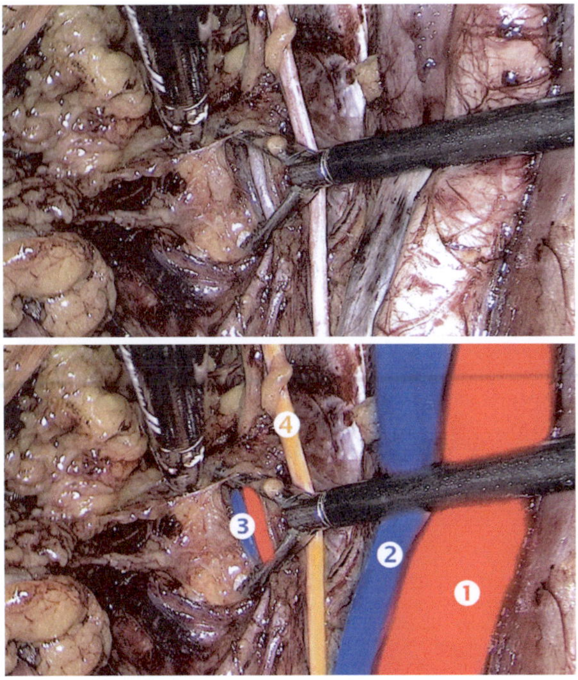

Fig. 6.39 Right hemipelvis during pelvic lymphadenectomy. (1) Right external iliac artery, (2) right external iliac vein, (3) right obturator vessels, (4) right obturator nerve

Tips and Tricks 11

In total hysterectomy, laparotomy, or laparoscopy, injury to the vaginal artery can occur during colpectomy, requiring repair that can be with coagulating energy or sealant or suture with thread. It is important to emphasize care with the use of energy at the edge of the vagina that will be sutured to avoid dehiscence of the vaginal dome.

In surgery for deep infiltrative endometriosis affecting the vaginal fornix, dissection of the pararectal and rectovaginal spaces should be performed for isolation and resection of the nodule, with preservation of the vaginal vessels when possible (Figs. 6.40 and 6.41).

Posterior Branches of the Anterior Trunk of the Internal Iliac Artery

Middle Rectal Artery

Anatomical Landmarks 13

Origin: May be in the anterior division of the internal iliac artery or in the internal pudendal artery.

Path: It descends in the pelvis to the lower part of the rectum, through the lateral ligaments of the rectum, to supply the muscle tissue of the lower rectum and anastomoses with the superior and inferior rectal arteries.

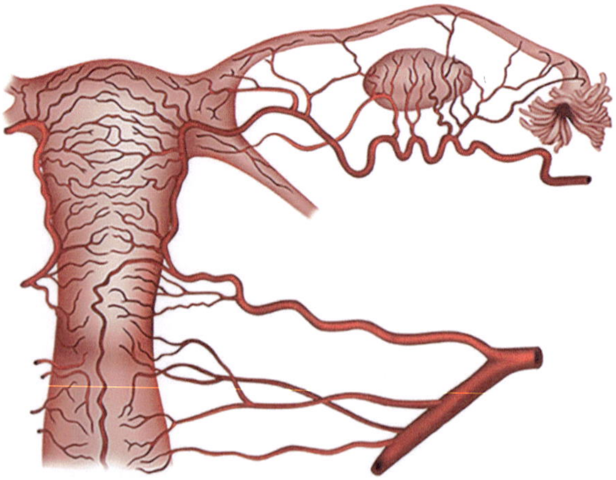

Fig. 6.40 Irrigation of the uterus, vagina, fallopian tubes, and ovaries

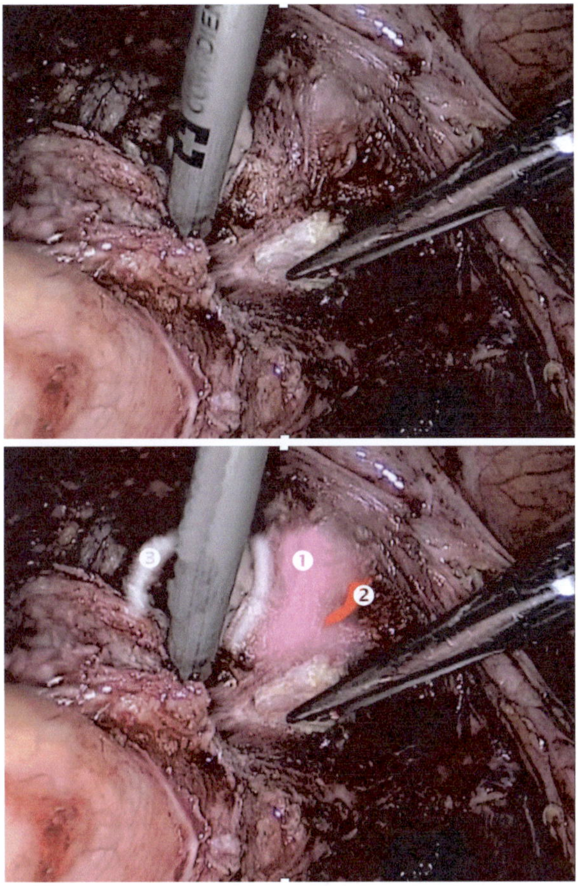

Fig. 6.41 Resection of a vaginal endometriosis nodule. (1) Vagina, (2) right vaginal artery, (3) colpectomy (open vagina)

Irrigation: Lower portion of the rectum and vagina.
Anastomosis: Superior and inferior rectal arteries.

Tips and Tricks 12

In colposacrofixation surgery, dissection of the Okabayashi space is performed until the identification of the puborectal bundle of the levator ani muscle, and, in this space, it is possible to identify the middle rectal artery that must be preserved on this occasion. In surgery for deep infiltrative endometriosis affecting the pararectal fossa, with obliteration of the "pouch of Douglas" and rectovaginal fossae, affecting or not the rectosigmoid with low and extensive lesions, the Okabayashi space dissection can identify the middle rectal artery for its preservation or for coagulation and sectioning, when necessary, due to the extension of the disease, thus preventing unwanted bleeding and intraoperative bleeding (Figs. 6.42, 6.43, and 6.44).

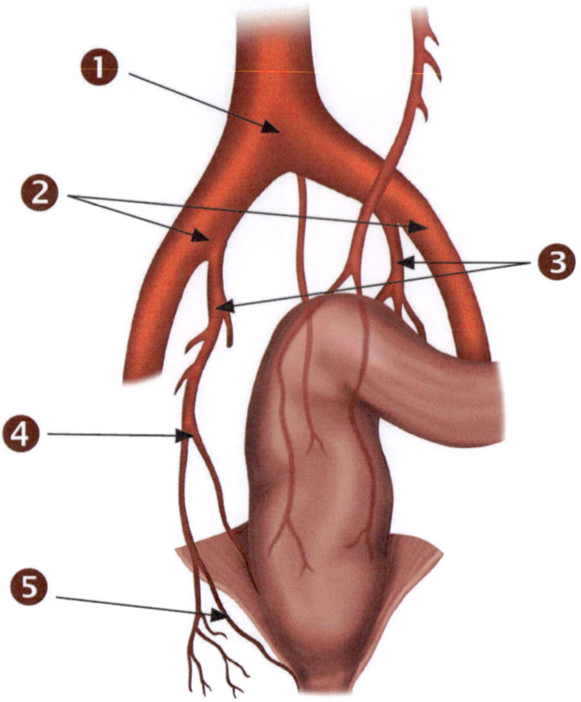

Fig. 6.42 Irrigation of the rectum. (1) Common iliac arteries, (2) external iliac arteries, (3) internal iliac arteries, (4) middle rectal artery, (5) internal rectal artery

Internal Pudendal Artery

Anatomical Landmarks 14

Origin: Branch of the anterior division of the internal iliac artery at the ischium.

Path: The internal pudendal artery descends anteriorly to the sacral plexus to the bottom of the greater ischial foramen, entering the gluteal region, and then passes through the lesser ischial foramen to enter the perineum. From there, with the internal pudendal veins and the pudendal nerve, it continues through the pudendal canal (Alcock's canal) to the urogenital region. Medially to the ischial tubercle, the internal pudendal artery divides into terminal branches.

Branches: Deep artery of the clitoris and dorsal artery of the clitoris.

Irrigation: Main artery of the perineum, irrigates muscles and skin of the anal and urogenital regions.

Anastomosis: Superior umbilical/vesical artery.

Tips and Tricks 13

It is important to be aware of the internal pudendal artery in cases of endometriosis surgery that affects Alcock's canal, immediately medial to the ischial tuberosity (Figs. 6.45 and 6.46).

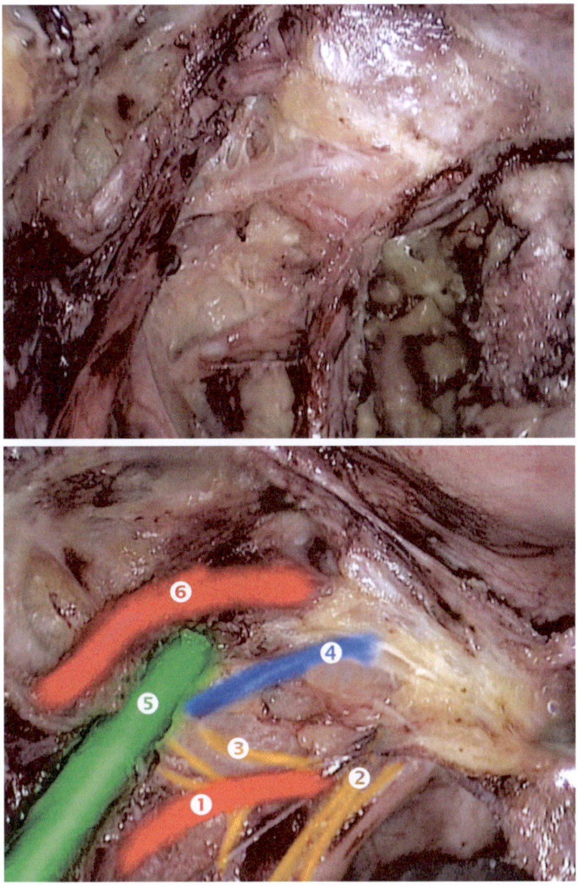

Fig. 6.43 Left hemipelvis, during dissection of the pararectal space for resection of deep endometriosis. (1) Left middle rectal artery, (2) left hypogastric nerve, (3) left inferior hypogastric plexus, (4) left deep uterine vein, (5) left ureter, (6) uterine artery crossing the left ureter

Inferior Gluteal Artery

Anatomical Landmarks 15

Origin: Anterior trunk of the internal iliac artery.

Origin: Terminal branch of the anterior trunk of the internal iliac artery, but may originate from the posterior trunk.

Path: Follows posteriorly between the S2 and S3 sacral nerves and leaves the pelvis through the lower part of the greater ischial foramen, inferiorly to the piriformis muscle.

Irrigation: It irrigates the diaphragm of the pelvis (ischiococcygeus and levator ani muscle), piriformis and quadratus femoris muscles, upper portion of the ischiotibial muscles, gluteus maximus muscle, and ischial nerve.

Anastomosis: Deep femoral artery through the medial and lateral circumflex femoral arteries.

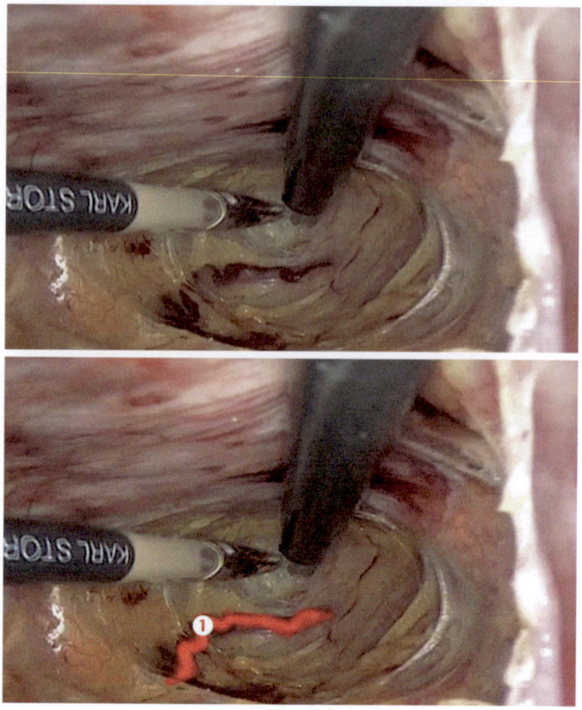

Fig. 6.44 Dissection of the left Okabayashi space, to perform colposacrofixation. (1) Middle rectal artery

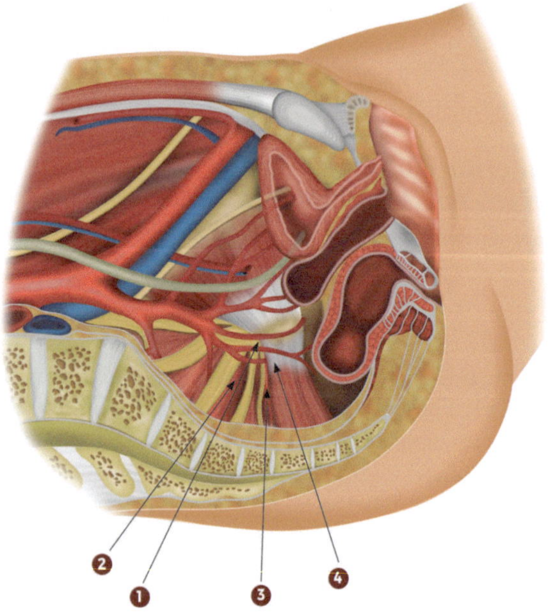

Fig. 6.45 Sagittal section of the pelvic anatomy, identifying: (1) internal pudendal artery and its relationship to the (2) piriformis muscle, (3) sacrospinal ligament, and (4) ischial spine

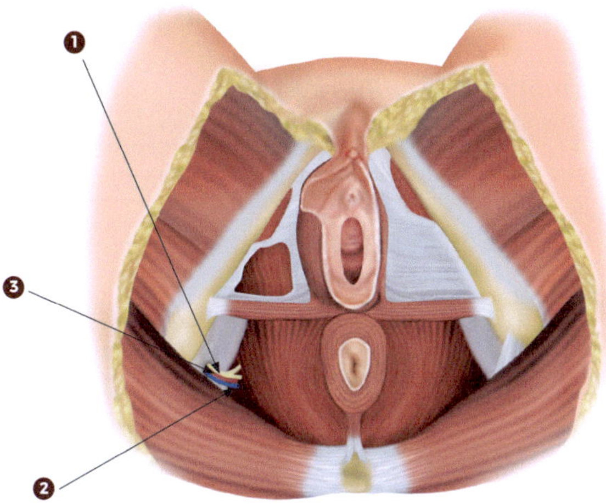

Fig. 6.46 Pudendal vessels and nerve: (1) internal pudendal nerves and (2) vessels emerge from (3) Alcock's canal, immediately medial to the ischial tuberosity. Their branches pierce the fascia covering the muscles and can be found in the perineal fat

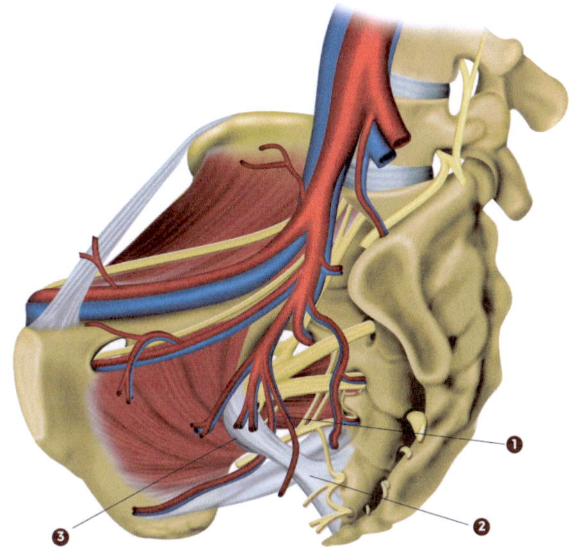

Fig. 6.47 In the sagittal section of the pelvis on the right, we identify (1) inferior gluteal artery and its relationship to the (2) sacrospinous ligament and the (3) ischial spine

Tips and Tricks 14

The relationship of the sacrospinous and sacrotuberous ligaments to the major pelvic vessels and nerves is of important clinical value, because surgery performed in this area, such as colposacrofixation or excision of pelvic floor endometriosis, must be precise in order to avoid injury to these vital structures such as the gluteal vessels (superior, inferior, or both) as well as the sciatic nerve (Fig. 6.47).

Posterior Trunk of the Internal Iliac Artery

Anatomical Landmarks 16

Origin: Division of the internal iliac artery into anterior and posterior at the height of the greater ischial foramen.

Branches: There are three parietal branches (Figs. 6.48 and 6.49):

- Iliolumbar artery
- Lateral sacral artery
- Superior gluteal artery

Iliolumbar Artery

Anatomical Landmarks 17

Origin: Posterior trunk of the internal iliac artery

Origin: First branch of the posterior trunk of the internal iliac artery.

Path: Ascends anteriorly to the sacroiliac joint and posteriorly to the common iliac vessels and the psoas major muscle; when it enters the iliac fossa, it splits into two branches.

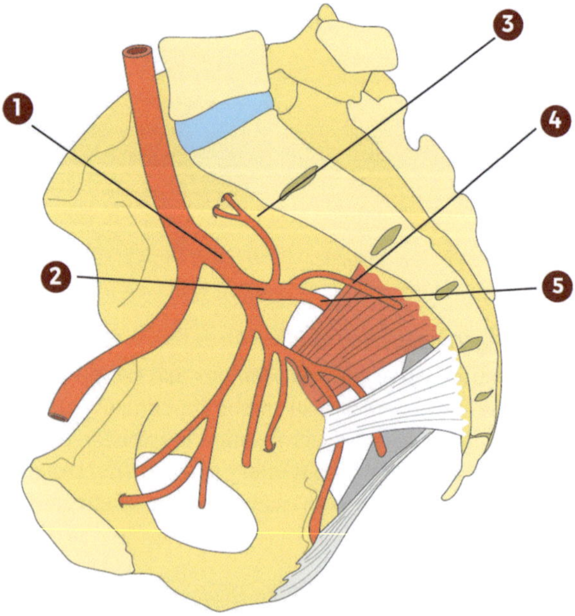

Fig. 6.48 Sagittal section of the right hemipelvis. (1) Internal iliac artery and its (2) posterior trunk, from which the following branches emanate: (3) iliolumbar artery, (4) lateral sacral artery, and (5) superior gluteal artery

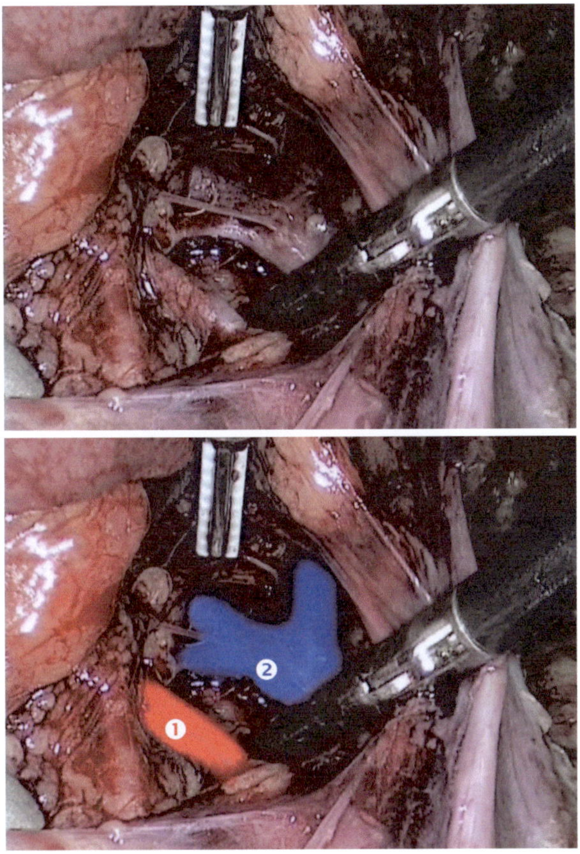

Fig. 6.49 Identification of the posterior trunk of the left internal iliac artery after deep dissection. (1) Posterior trunk of the left internal iliac artery, (2) posterior trunk of the left internal iliac vein

Branches: Iliac branch, which supplies the iliac and iliacus muscles, and lumbar branch, which supplies the psoas major and quadratus lumborum muscles.

Irrigation: Psoas major muscle, quadratus lumborum muscle, iliacus muscle, and ilium.

Anastomosis: Deep circumflex iliac artery and fourth lumbar artery.

Tips and Tricks 15

The iliolumbar artery assumes a deep and difficult-to-reach position. It is rarely identified in dissections during gynecological pelvic surgery (Fig. 6.50).

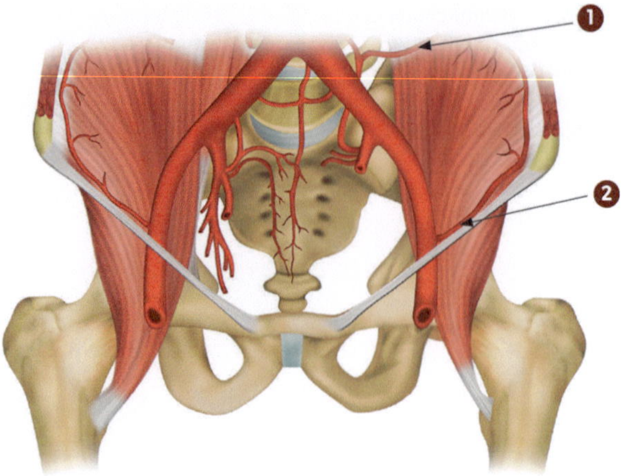

Fig. 6.50 In coronal section of the female pelvis: (1) iliolumbar artery, a branch of the posterior trunk of the internal iliac artery, ascends anterior to the sacroiliac joint and anastomoses with the (2) deep circumflex iliac artery

Lateral Sacral Arteries

Anatomical Landmarks 18

There are two lateral sacral arteries: the superior and the inferior.

Origin: Posterior trunk of the internal iliac artery.

Origin: Second branch of the posterior trunk of the internal iliac artery, may originate from a single trunk or from independent trunks.

Path: They follow the anteromedial face of the piriformis muscle, sending branches to the sacral foramen.

Branches: Spinal branches that cross anterior sacral foramen and irrigate the vertebral meninges; other branches follow the posterior sacral foramen and irrigate the erector spinae muscle and the skin over the sacrum.

Irrigation: Piriformis muscle, structures of the sacral canal, erector spinae muscle, and overlying skin.

Anastomosis: Median sacral artery.

Tips and Tricks 16

The lateral sacral arteries run closely to the sacrum bone. Separation of the sacroiliac joints or posterior iliac wing fractures that extend to the iliac gutter can cause trauma to these arteries, and they are therefore vessels of most interest to orthopedic surgeons (Fig. 6.51).

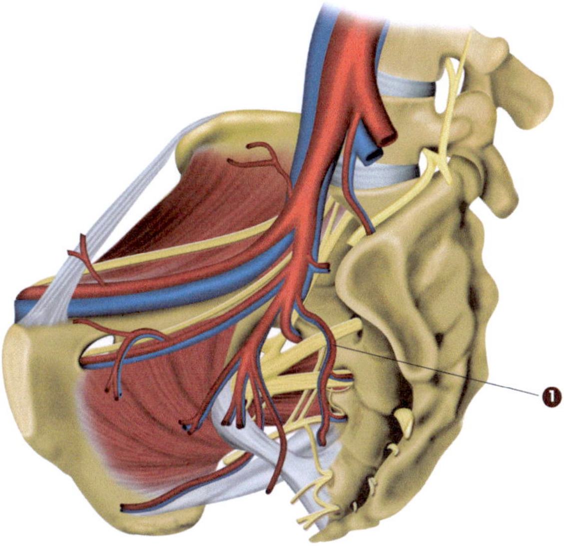

Fig. 6.51 Sagittal section of the female pelvis, in which the (1) lateral sacral artery can be seen sending branches to the sacral foramen

Superior Gluteal Artery

Anatomical Landmarks 19

Origin: Posterior trunk of the internal iliac artery.

Origin: Largest branch of the posterior trunk of the internal iliac artery.

Path: Runs between the lumbosacral trunk and the anterior branch of the S1 spinal nerve and exits the pelvis through the supra-piriform part of the greater ischial foramen.

Irrigation: Piriformis muscle, the three gluteal muscles, and the tensor fascia lata muscle.

Anastomosis: Lateral sacral, inferior gluteal, internal pudendal, deep circumflex femoral, and lateral circumflex femoral arteries.

Tips and Tricks 17

The relationship of the sacrospinous and sacrotuberous ligaments to the major pelvic vessels and nerves is of important clinical value because surgery performed in this area, such as colposacrofixation or excision of pelvic floor endometriosis, must be precise to avoid injury to these vital structures. An inadequate suture could injure the gluteal vessels (superior, inferior, or both) as well as the sciatic nerve (Fig. 6.52).

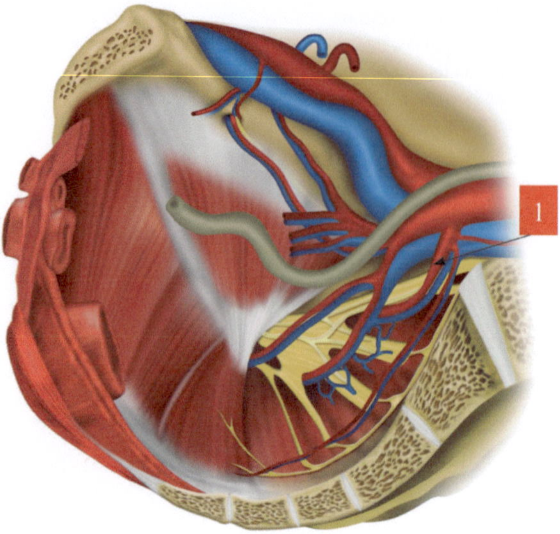

Fig. 6.52 The superior gluteal artery: (1) superior gluteal artery, the largest branch of the posterior trunk of the internal iliac artery, is identified

Ovarian Artery

Anatomical Landmarks 20

Origin: Aorta.

Origin: In 80% of individuals, the two ovarian arteries originate separately from the aorta, equidistant from the renal arteries and the inferior mesenteric artery.

Path: Both have a retroperitoneal path accompanying the psoas major muscle, crossing in front of the ureter and the external iliac vessels. In the lesser pelvis, the ovarian arteries assume a medial orientation, between the two layers of the ligament towards the ovaries and the uterine tubes. They continue through the broad ligament towards the side of the uterus, where they anastomose with the ascending portion of the uterine artery.

Branches: Ovarian branch and tubal branch.

Irrigation: Uterus, ovary, ureter, skin of the labia, and inguinal region. Receives lymph from the lumbar lymph nodes.

Anastomosis: Tubal and ovarian branches of the uterine artery.

Tips and Tricks 18

Anatomically, the ovarian vessels constitute the medial portion of the so-called posterior wide ligament triangle, formed by round ligament and external iliac vessels. Knowledge of the arrangement of the ovarian vessels (infundibulopelvic) is important for the procedures of adnexectomy and total hysterectomy with adnexectomy. For some authors, the removal of the ovarian vessels from their origin in the aorta is essential to decrease the chances of metastasis in cases of ovarian cancer (Figs. 6.53 and 6.54).

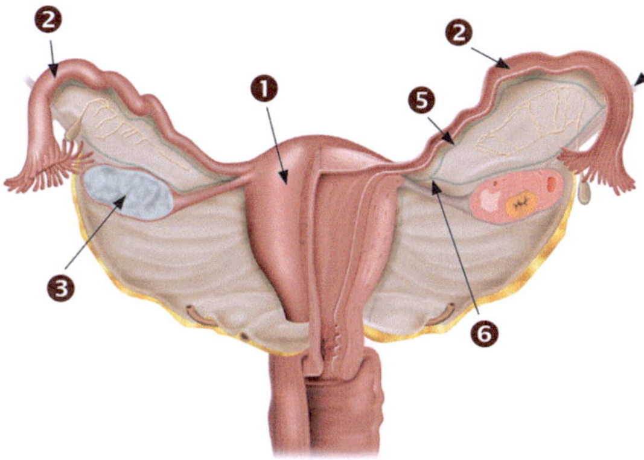

Fig. 6.53 Uterus and adnexa: (1) the uterus, uterine tubes, ovaries, ovarian artery, tubal branch of the ovarian artery, and ovarian branch of the ovarian artery are identified

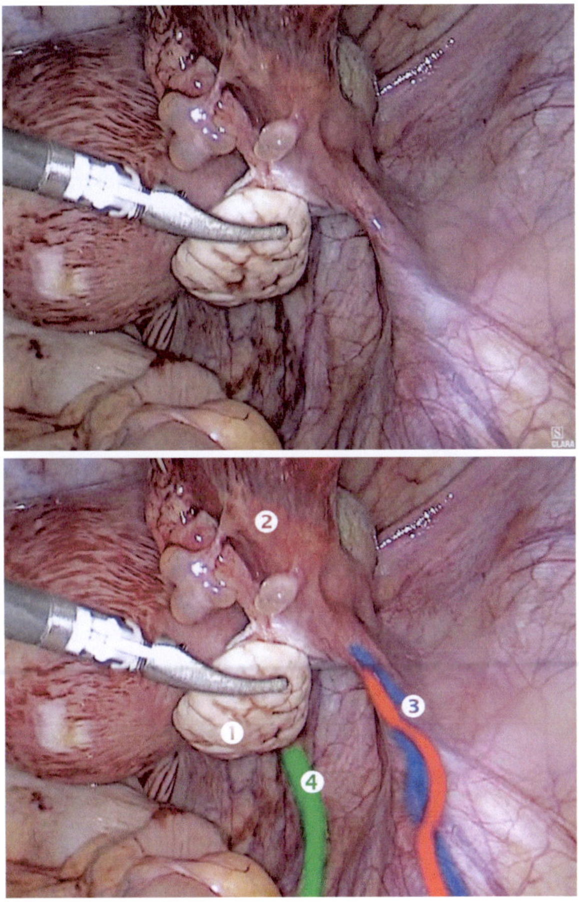

Fig. 6.54 Panoramic view of the pelvis with identification of the ovarian vessels and the infundibulopelvic ligament. (1) Right ovary, (2) right tube, (3) right infundibulopelvic ligament with right ovarian artery and vein, (4) right ureter

Median Sacral Artery

Anatomical Landmarks 21

It is a small odd artery, located in the promontory region.

Origin: Bifurcation of the aorta into common iliac arteries.

Origin: Posterior face of the abdominal part of the aorta, at the bifurcation of the aorta into common iliac arteries.

Path: It descends near the midline over the L4 and L5 vertebrae and over the sacrum and coccyx.

Branches: Two small branches that irrigate the L5 vertebrae bilaterally, before the median sacral artery enters the lesser pelvis; lateral sacral branches when descending over the sacrum; visceral branches to the posterior part of the rectum, passing through anastomosis with the superior and middle rectal arteries.

Irrigation: Lower lumbar vertebrae, sacrum, and coccyx.

Anastomosis: Sacral branches of the lateral sacral artery.

Tips and Tricks 19

In some cases, during the colposacrofixation or colposacropexy procedure, the median sacral vessels can be found slightly lateralized at the point of fixation of the mesh. The region should be dissected and the vessels retracted to reduce the risk of bleeding (Figs. 6.55, 6.56, 6.57, and 6.58).

Superior Rectal Artery

Anatomical Landmarks 22

Origin: Inferior mesenteric artery.

Origin: It is the direct continuation of the inferior mesenteric artery.

Path: It crosses the left common iliac vessels and descends into the sigmoid mesocolon to the lesser pelvis.

Branches: At the S3 level, it divides into two branches that irrigate the rectum up to the internal anus sphincter muscle.

Irrigation: Upper part of the rectum and internal sphincter muscle of the anus.

Anastomosis: Middle and inferior rectal arteries and internal pudendal artery.

Tips and Tricks 20

Rectosigmoidectomy for adenocarcinoma of the rectosigmoid should be associated with removal of the mesosigmoid with the inclusion of the superior rectal artery. In cases of rectosigmoidectomy for endometriosis, economic resection in the wall of the intestinal loop ensures better blood support, among other aspects, preserving the superior rectal artery and its branches (Fig. 6.59).

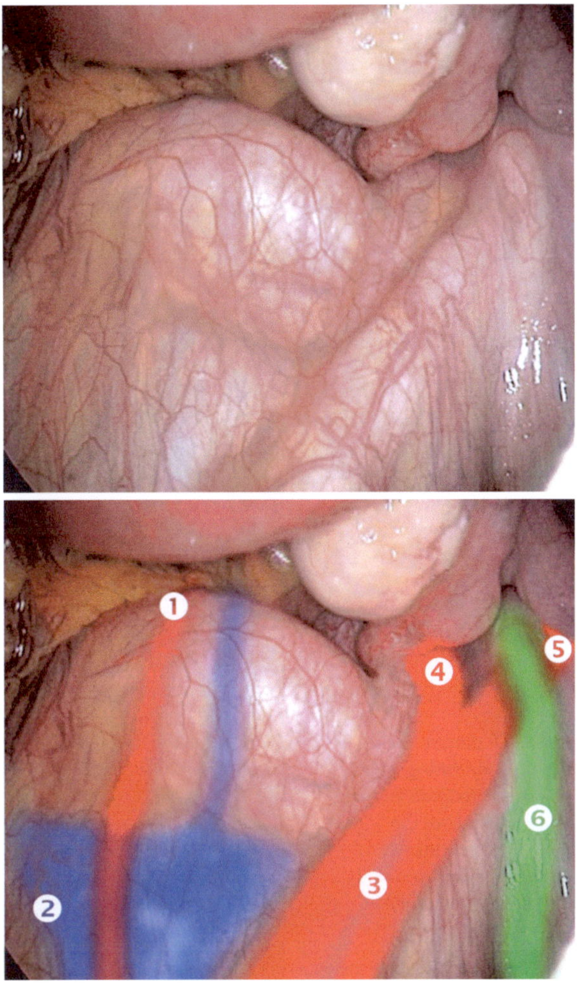

Fig. 6.55 Transparency view of the promontory. (1) Median sacral vessels, (2) left common iliac vein, (3) right common iliac artery, (4) right internal iliac artery, (5) right external iliac artery, (6) right ureter

Pelvic Veins

The venous system of pelvic drainage has a complex distribution, making its dissection more difficult. While the larger caliber veins have a distribution similar to that of the arterial system, the branches and venous endings present frequent anatomical variations, confluences, and large plexuses.

From the point of view of surgical importance, five veins are emphasized: deep uterine vein, median sacral vein, middle rectus vein, left common iliac vein, and corona mortis.

Some veins must be well known by gynecologic surgeons, because they are “treacherous” and have more delicate walls, with a middle layer smaller than the adventitia, leading to non-sealing of the vein if little energy is used or to rupture (explosion) of its wall if excessive energy is used (Figs. 6.60 and 6.61).

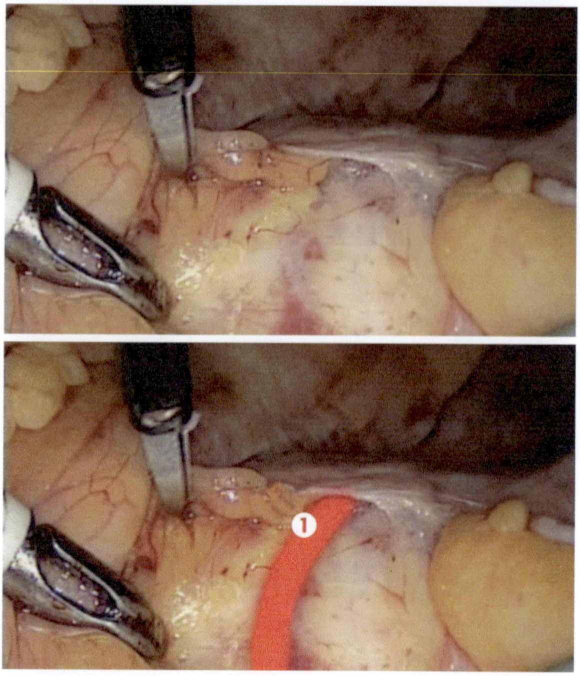

Fig. 6.56 Identification of the median sacral artery, after opening the retroperitoneum. (1) Median sacral artery

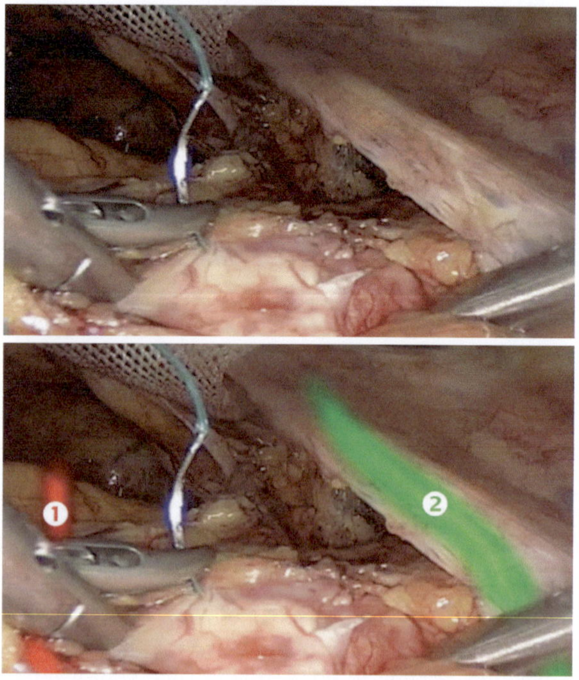

Fig. 6.57 Suture at the promontory during colposacrofixation and the relationship with the median sacral artery and ureter. (1) Median sacral artery, (2) right ureter

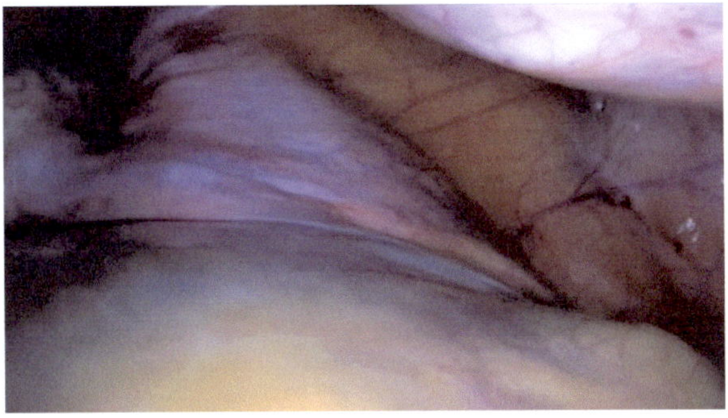

Fig. 6.58 Hematoma due to injury of the median sacral vessels due to a first-puncture accident with a Veress needle

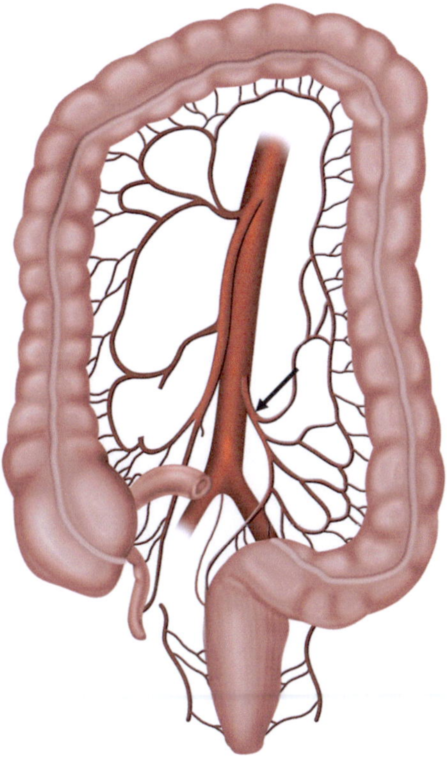

Fig. 6.59 Inferior mesenteric artery (black arrow) and its branches

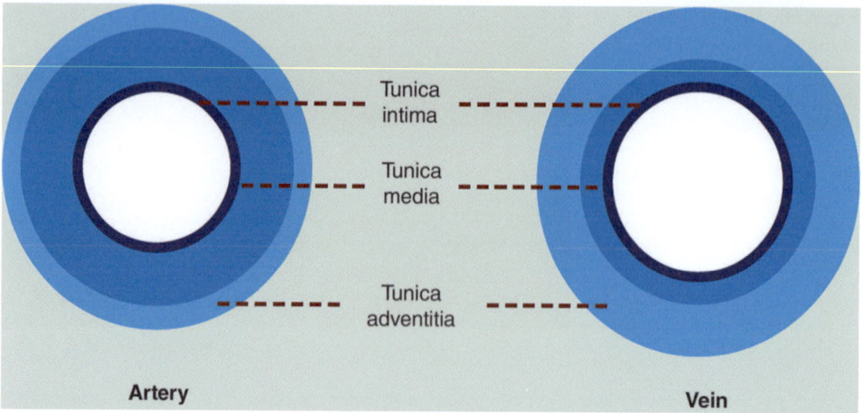

Fig. 6.60 Structural differences between arteries and veins

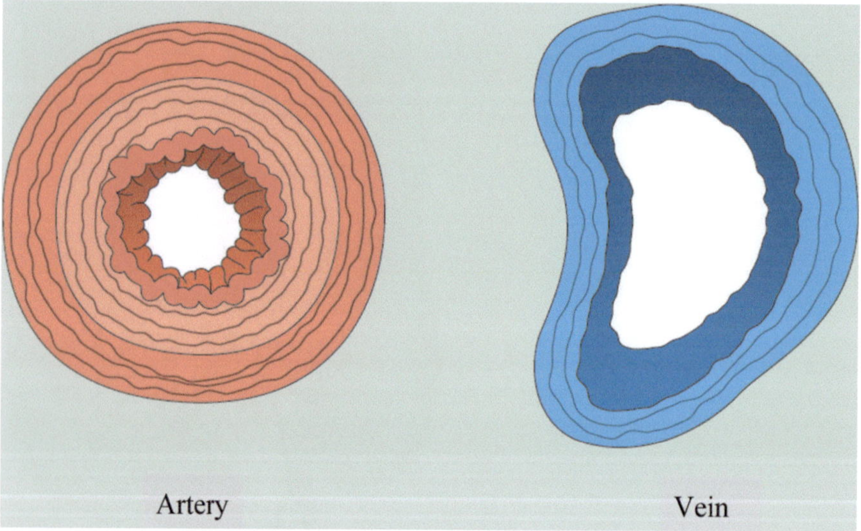

Fig. 6.61 Structural differences between arteries and veins

Deep Uterine Vein

Anatomical Landmarks 23

Located in the paracervical space, just below the ureter.

Origin: Parauterine branches (in the paracervical space, below the ureter).

Origin: From the confluence of the parauterine branches coming from the cervix and the uterine body.

Pathway: Lateral orientation below the ureter and just above the inferior hypogastric plexus towards the internal iliac vein.

Drainage: Uterine body, cervix, and upper vagina.

Tips and Tricks 21

The deep uterine vein is an anatomical landmark of great importance for performing radical hysterectomies in cases of cervical cancer. In the most recent classification by Querleu and Morrow, revised by Cibulla, radical hysterectomies limited to the depth of the deep uterine vein are classified as C1, also called neuropreservative. Those resections that consider the structures below the deep uterine vein are classified as C2 and non-neuropreservative. The latter include the removal of the inferior hypogastric plexus, presenting a high risk of functional damage to the pelvic organs, especially the bladder and rectum (Figs. 6.62 and 6.63).

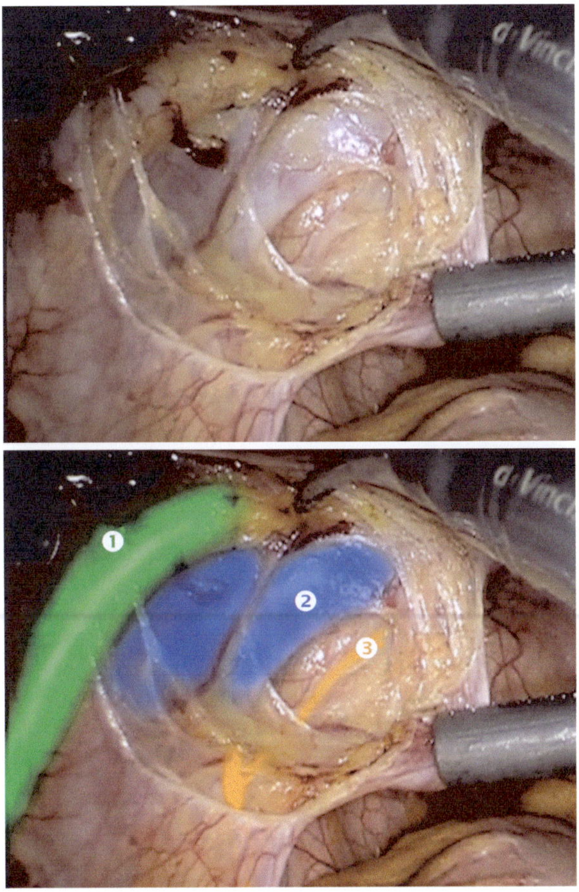

Fig. 6.62 Laparoscopic view of the left paracervical region. (1) Left ureter, (2) left deep uterine vein, (3) left hypogastric nerve

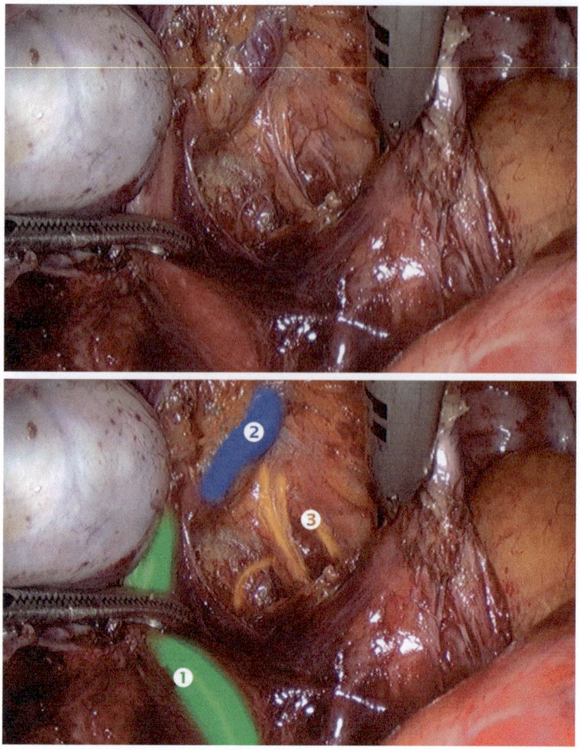

Fig. 6.63 Identification of the structures of the left Okabayashi space during excision of infiltrating deep endometriosis. (1) Left ureter, (2) left deep uterine vein, (3) left inferior hypogastric plexus

Median Sacral Vein

Anatomical Landmarks 24

Origin: Sacral vessels (with drainage into the left common iliac vein).

Origin: Sacral vessels.

Path: Accompanies the median sacral artery on the right side, ascending near the midline over the L4 and L5 vertebrae, sacrum, and coccyx.

Drainage: To the regions of the sacrum, coccyx, and rectum.

Tips and Tricks 22

The median sacral vein is clinically important due to the risk of first-puncture accident, since it is in the region of the sacrum, with a 9% rate of injury during abdominal access. During colposacrofixation and sacropexy, the path of this vein must be known in order to avoid both arterial and venous injury when suturing the mesh to the sacrum (Fig. 6.64).

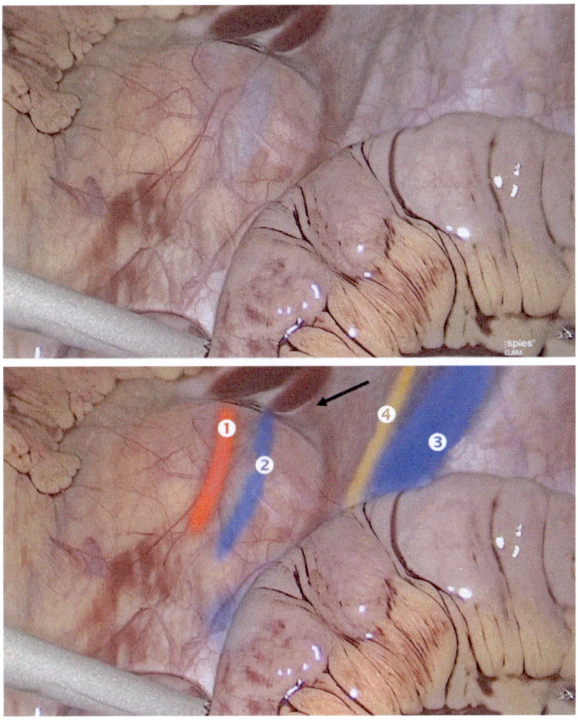

Fig. 6.64 Evaluation, by transparency, of the promontory region. The arrow shows the right hypogastric nerve. (1) Median sacral artery, (2) median sacral vein, (3) right common iliac vein, (4) right ureter

Middle Rectal Vein

Anatomical Landmarks 25

Origin: They originate from the confluence of the arcuate veins of the mesorectum.

Origin: Arched veins of the mesorectum.

Path: Towards the internal iliac vein, crossing the medial pararectal space.

Drainage: From part of the mesorectum.

Tips and Tricks 23

Anatomical knowledge of the middle rectal vein and its identification are fundamental during the dissection of the pararectal spaces in deep endometriosis surgery, as well as when performing rectosigmoidectomy (Fig. 6.65).

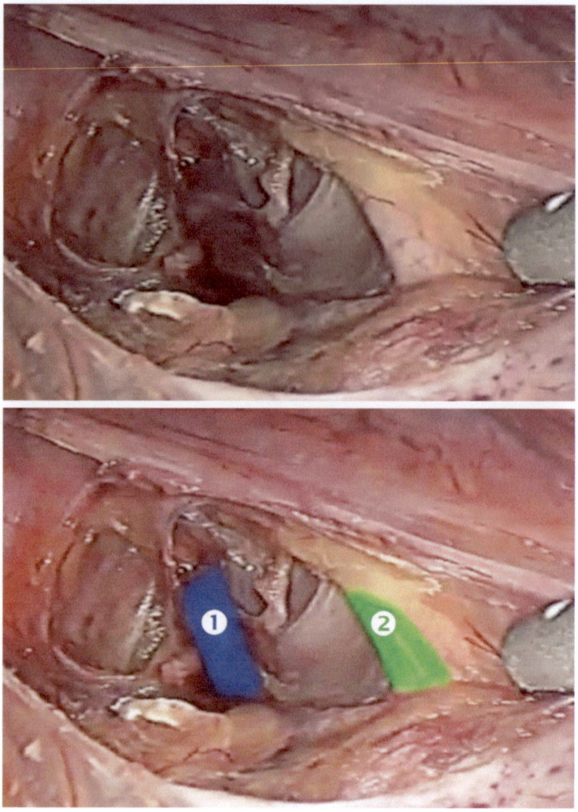

Fig. 6.65 Dissection of the right pararectal space and its structures. (1) Right middle rectal vein, (2) right ureter (lateral to the vein)

Left Common Iliac Vein

Anatomical Landmarks 26

Origin: Confluence of the external and internal iliac veins.

Origin: From the confluence of the left iliac veins (external and internal), anteriorly to the left sacroiliac synostosis.

Path: Towards the vena cava, passing through the posterior aspect of both common iliac arteries. It is located anteriorly to the L5 vertebra and, in its central portion, is covered by lymph nodes and the parietal peritoneum.

Drainage: From the left hemipelvis and left leg.

Tips and Tricks 24

The left common iliac vein is directly linked to vascular complications of first puncture in laparoscopy. Its position, anterior to L4 and L5, is in the same orientation as the umbilical scar (Figs. 6.66 and 6.67).

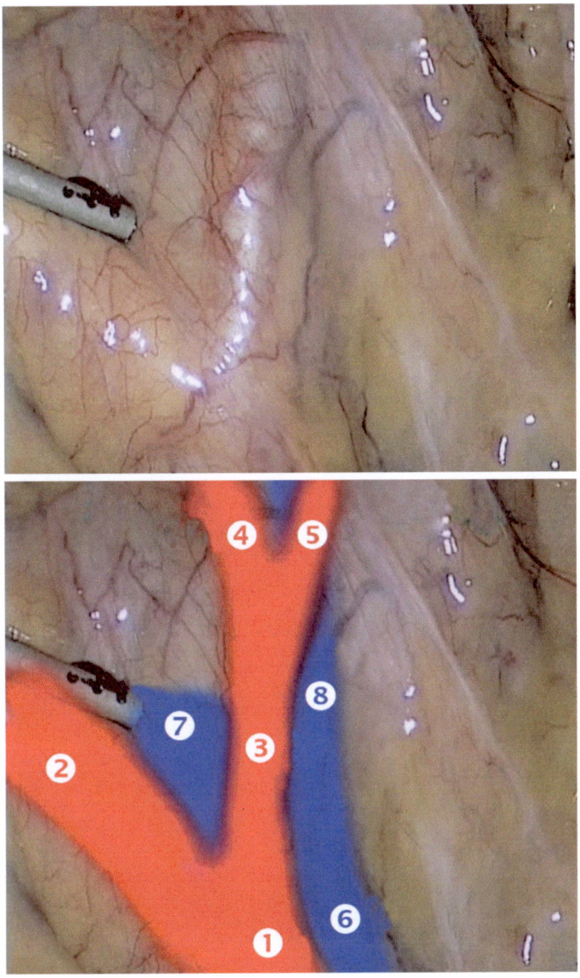

Fig. 6.66 Transparency evaluation of the large retroperitoneal vessels in the anatomical plane corresponding to the umbilical scar. (1) Aorta, (2) left common iliac artery, (3) right common iliac artery, (4) right internal iliac artery, (5) right external iliac artery, (6) vena cava, (7) left common iliac vein, (8) right common iliac vein

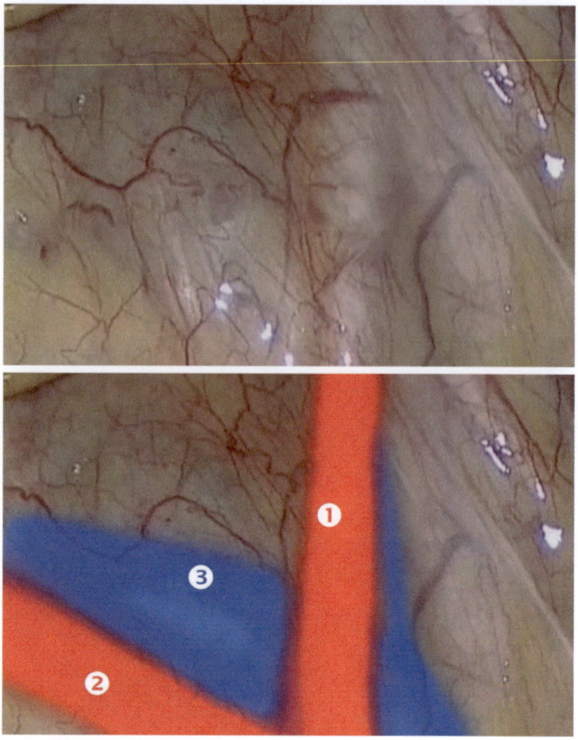

Fig. 6.67 Through transparency, the risk area for first-puncture accidents is identified, in a triangle delimited between the left and right common iliac arteries, and over the left common iliac vein. (1) Right common iliac artery, (2) left common iliac artery, (3) left common iliac vein

Corona Mortis

Anatomical Landmarks 27

The corona mortis, or crown of death, is widely known as the communication between the internal and external iliac vascular systems, more specifically between the external iliac vessels and the obturator artery. It is also described, by some authors, as the crown formed by the obturator vessels, internal iliac artery, external iliac vessels, plus the communication itself. It can be a communication between veins (the most common), between arteries, or between both, and also a shunt between vein and artery.

Origin: Anastomosis between external iliac vessels and obturator vessels.

Origin: Communication between the internal and external iliac vascular systems, more specifically between external iliac vessels and obturator vessels.

Path: Near the obturator foramen and the terminal part of the external iliac vessels over the pectineal ligament.

Drainage/support: Structures of the leg, due to its relationship with the external iliac and femoral vessels, and structures of the acetabulum, due to the obturator vessels.

Tips and Tricks 25

The anastomosis known as corona mortis is important in lymphadenectomy and in urinary incontinence surgeries, more specifically in the passage of transobturator bands. In the former, it represents the deep anterior limit for lymph node removal. If it is necessary to sacrifice it during the procedure, it is recommended to do so far from the external iliac vessels. A lesion of this vessel near the origin of the external iliac vessels would, in practice, represent a lesion of the external iliac vein itself (Figs. 6.68 and 6.69).

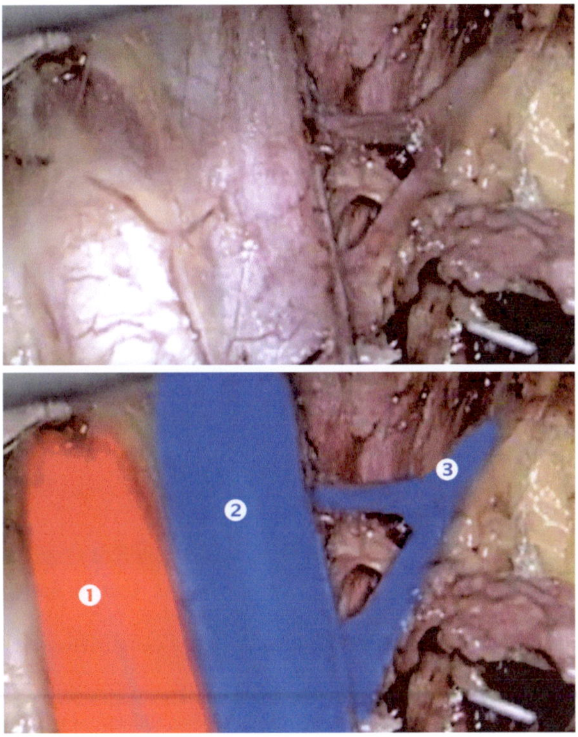

Fig. 6.68 Identification of corona mortis, after lymphadenectomy. (1) Left external iliac artery, (2) left external iliac vein, (3) corona mortis

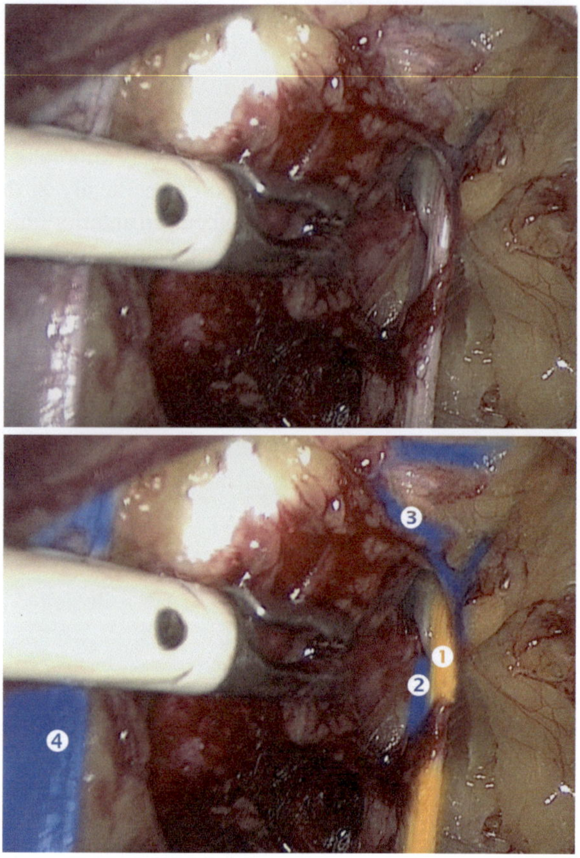

Fig. 6.69 Identification of the corona mortis, and other structures of the left lateral paravesical space, after lymphadenectomy. (1) Left obturator nerve, (2) left obturator vein (below the nerve), (3) left corona mortis, (4) left external iliac vein

Bibliography

1. Albulescu D, Constantin C, Constantin C. Uterine artery emerging variants: angiographic aspects. Curr Health Sci J. 2014;40(3):214–6.
2. Baggish MS, Karram MM. Atlas de anatomia pélvica e cirurgia ginecológica. 4th ed. São Paulo: Elsevier; 2017.
3. Cibula D, Abu-Rustum NR, Benedetti-Panici P, Köhler C, Raspagliesi F, Querleu D, et al. New classification system of radical hysterectomy: emphasis on a three-dimensional anatomic template for parametrial resection. Gynecol Oncol. 2011;122(2):264–8.
4. Giraudet G, Protat A, Cosson M. The anatomy of the sacral promontory: how to avoid complications of the sacrocolpopexy procedure. Am J Obstet Gynecol. 2018;218:457.e1–3.
5. Good MM, Abele TA, Balgobin S, Montoya TI, McIntire D, Corton MM. Vascular and ureteral anatomy relative to the midsacral promontory. Am J Obstet Gynecol. 2013;208:486.e1–7.
6. Hoffman BL, Schorge JO, Bradshaw KD, Halvorson LM, Schaffer JI, Corton MM. Williams gynecology. 3rd ed. New York: McGraw Hill Education; 2016.
7. Leite TFO, Pires LAS, Goke K, Silva JG, Chagas CAA. Corona mortis: descrição anatômica e cirúrgica em 60 hemipelves cadavéricas. Rev Col Bras Cir. 2017;44(6):553–9.
8. Magrina JF. Complications of laparoscopic surgery. Clin Obstet Gynecol. 2002;45(2):469–80.

9. Mamatha H, Hemalatha B, Vinodini P, Souza AS, Suhani S. Anatomical study on the variations in the branching pattern of internal iliac artery. Indian J Surg. 2015;77(2):248–52.
10. Moore KL, Dalley AF, Agur AMR. Anatomia orientada para a clínica. 8th ed. Rio de Janeiro: Guanabara Koogan; 2019.
11. Nayak SB, Shetty SD, Sirasanagandla SR, Vasanthakumar P, Jetti R. Multiple variations in the pelvic vasculature: a case report. J Clin Diagn Res. 2015;9(2):AD01-2.
12. Papadia A, Remorgida V, Salom EM, Ragni N. Laparoscopic pelvic and paraaortic lymphadenectomy in gynecologic oncology. J Am Assoc Gynecol Laparosc. 2004;11:297.
13. Roach MK, Andreotti RF. The normal female pelvis. Clin Obstet Gynecol. 2017;60(1):3–10.
14. Rock JA, Jones HW. Te Linde's operative gynecology. 10th ed. Philadelphia: Wolters Kluwer, Lippincott Williams & Wilkins; 2008.
15. Rusu MC, Cergan R, Motoc AG, Folescu R, Pop E. Anatomical considerations on the corona mortis. Surg Radiol Anat. 2010;32(1):17–24.
16. Stavropoulou-Deli A, Anagnostopoulou S. Corona mortis: anatomical data and clinical considerations. Aust N Z J Obstet Gynaecol. 2013;53(3):283–6.
17. Tajra JBM, Lima CF, Pires FR, Sales L, Junqueira D, Mauro E. Variability of the obturator artery with its surgical implications. J Morphol Sci. 2016;33(2):96–8.

Chapter 7
Pelvic Innervation

Augusta Morgado, Guilherme Karam Corrêa Leite, Gustavo Leme Fernandes, Nucélio Barros Moreira Lemos, and Paulo Ayroza Ribeiro

Supplementary Information The online version contains supplementary material available at https://doi.org/10.1007/978-3-031-63520-5_7.

A. Morgado
Brazilian Federation of Associations of Gynecology and Obstetrics (FEBRASGO), São Paulo, Brazil

Pelvic Neuropsychiatric Outpatient Clinic of the Urogynecology Section of the Gynecology Department of the Federal University of São Paulo, São Paulo, Brazil
e-mail: augusta.morgado@increasing.com.br

G. K. C. Leite
Brazilian Federation of Associations of Gynecology and Obstetrics (FEBRASGO), São Paulo, Brazil

Faculdade de Ciências Médicas da Universidade Metropolitana de Santos (UNIMES), Santos, Brazil

Faculty of Medical Sciences, Santa Casa de Misericórdia de São Paulo (SCMSP), São Paulo, Brazil

Hospital Ana Costa de Santos/United Health Group (UHG), Santos, Brazil

G. L. Fernandes
Faculty of Medical Sciences, Santa Casa de Misericórdia de São Paulo (SCMSP), São Paulo, Brazil

Santa Casa de São Paulo School of Medical Sciences, São Paulo, Brazil

Department of Obstetrics and Gynaecology, Faculty of Medicine, University of Toronto, Toronto, ON, Canada

Department of Gynecology, Paulista School of Medicine, Federal University of São Paulo (EPM/UNIFESP), São Paulo, Brazil

N. B. M. Lemos
Department of Obstetrics and Gynaecology, Faculty of Medicine, University of Toronto, Toronto, ON, Canada

Department of Gynecology, Paulista School of Medicine, Federal University of São Paulo (EPM/UNIFESP), São Paulo, Brazil
e-mail: nucelio.lemos@utoronto.ca

H. Salomão Ayroza, P. Ayroza Ribeiro (eds.), *Atlas of Laparoscopic Gynecological Anatomy*, https://doi.org/10.1007/978-3-031-63520-5_7

P. Ayroza Ribeiro (✉)
Brazilian Federation of Associations of Gynecology and Obstetrics (FEBRASGO), São Paulo, Brazil

Department of Obstetrics and Gynecology, Santa Casa de São Paulo School of Medical Sciences, São Paulo, Brazil

Overview

The peripheral nervous system can be divided into two parts: the somatic nervous system (SNS) and the autonomic nervous system (ANS). The SNS is composed of sensory nerves (afferent) and motor nerves (efferent) that are responsible for conscious perception and regulate the voluntary motor processes of skeletal muscles. The ANS, on the other hand, performs the internal control and regulation of the viscera in an unconscious manner.

The knowledge of pelvic neuroanatomy is fundamental for the successful treatment of intrapelvic nerve entrapment and, mainly, to avoid functional complications in reconstructive pelvic surgeries, in the radical treatment of pelvic infiltrative endometriosis, and in oncologic surgeries. Technological advances in recent decades, provided by laparoscopy, allowed a better anatomical recognition of nerve fibers and the consequent development of nerve preservation techniques [1].

The access to the nerves of the retroperitoneum can be obtained in a reproducible and safe way in several points. However, it is necessary to recognize the avascular anatomical spaces (Chap. 6), as well as the use of dissection techniques that allow adequate exposure of the deeper nervous structures of the pelvis without damaging them. The most relevant anatomical spaces for the identification of nerve bundles of the pelvis are the presacral space, the iliolumbar fossa, and the obturator space.

Pelvic Visceral Innervation

In the pelvis, the ANS is composed of superior hypogastric plexus (SHP), hypogastric nerves (HNs), pelvic splanchnic nerves (PSNs), and inferior hypogastric plexus (IHP).

Surgical Anatomy of the Pelvic Autonomic Plexuses

The SHP (or presacral nerve) is formed by nerve fibers that descend from the para-aortic sympathetic trunk, which converge at the level of the L5 vertebra, giving rise to a more or less rectangular web—generally of fenestrated or plexiform or, more

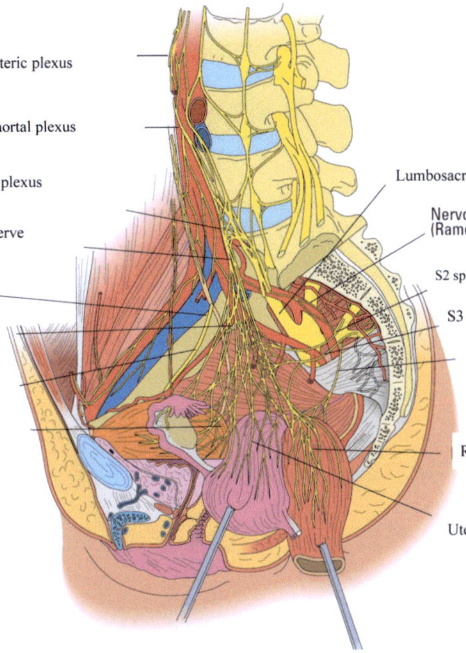

Fig. 7.1 Pelvic visceral innervation. In yellow, we can see the presacral nerve (SHP) dividing to form the hypogastric nerves (HNs) at the promontory. More inferiorly in the pelvis, the inferior hypogastric plexus (IHP) receives fibers from S2 and S3, through the pelvic splenic nerves (PSNs), inferiorly, and the left and right branches of the HNs, superiorly, connecting the nerve plexuses

rarely, cord-like appearance—that characterizes the plexus. The SHP is retroperitoneal, embedded in a sheet of fatty connective tissue—which follows distally, forming the presacral fascia—just below the peritoneum between the two common iliac arteries, usually lying a little to the left. These fibers converge at the distal angles of the plexus, giving rise to the right and left NHs at the height of the sacral promontory. The HNs and the SHP are formed primarily by efferent sympathetic fibers and afferent visceral fibers (Figs. 7.1 and 7.2).

Tips and Tricks 1

To access the SHP, the sigmoid is pulled back to the left, with gentle anterior traction, in order to incise the peritoneum and expose the presacral space. A delicate dissection is performed, with development of the space between the peritoneum and the presacral fascia and identification of the left common iliac vein, the left ureter, and the inferior mesenteric vessels. Dissection in the progression of the space must be cautious, avoiding injury to the median sacral vessels, located posteriorly to the most distal portion of the SHP, between the origins of the HNs, at the promontory. In presacral neurectomy (now proscribed), the objective was to identify and isolate the SHP and the proximal portion of the HNs in order to proceed to the transection of these nerves. Today, this dissection has its main applications in level II pelvic

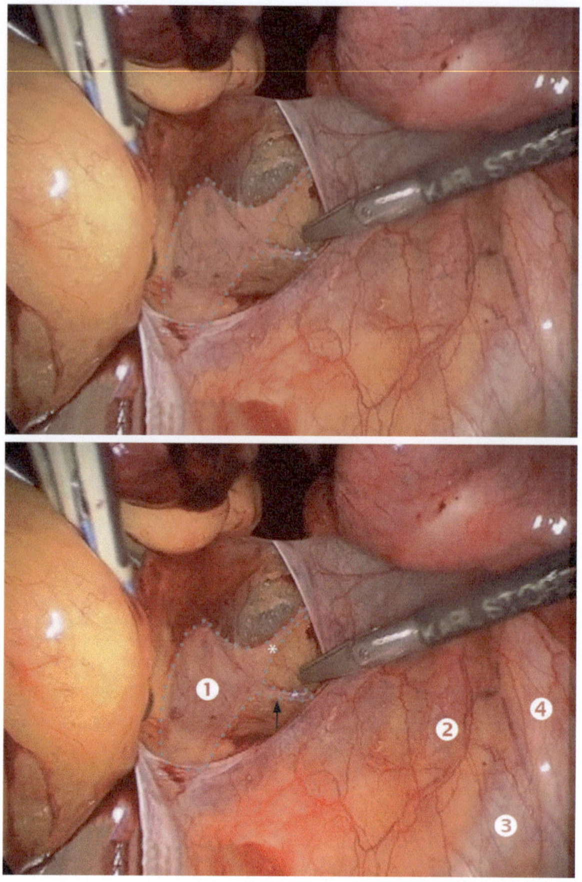

Fig. 7.2 Dissection at the level of L5–S1 demonstrating the superior hypogastric plexus (SHP) giving rise to the right hypogastric nerve (*) and the right ureter (black arrow). (1) Superior hypogastric plexus, (2) right internal iliac artery, (3) right external iliac artery, (4) right ureter

lymphadenectomy and in sacropromontofixations of uterovaginal or rectal prolapses, with the goal of avoiding transection or contact of the nerve fibers with the synthetic mesh [2, 3].

Formed at the bifurcation of the SHP, the HNs follow a course in a caudal and lateral direction, anteriorly to the presacral fascia, medially to the hypogastric fascia, and laterally to the fascia propria of the rectum; they follow in this direction in a posteromedial situation to the ureters (8 mm apart on the left and 14 mm apart on the right) [4], until they join the pelvic splanchnic nerves (PSNs—parasympathetic) to form the inferior hypogastric plexus (IHP), which is a mixed autonomic nervous plexus, sympathetic and parasympathetic, the latter being divided into three bundles: vesical, uterine, and rectal. In this tract, the HNs vary between 4 and 7 mm in thickness, and there may be asymmetry in the density of nerve fibers between the sides. Duplicity of HNs is seen in less than 20% of pelvis [3] (Figs. 7.3, 7.4, and 7.5).

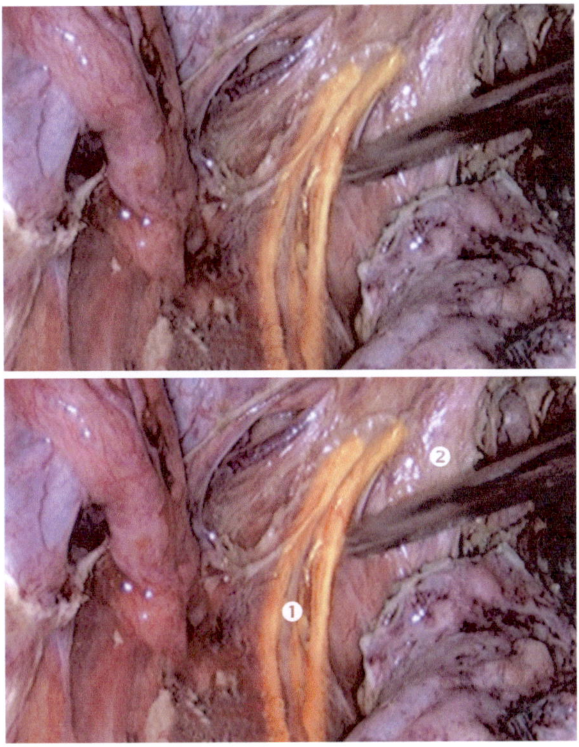

Fig. 7.3 Left hypogastric nerve and inferior hypogastric plexus. (1) Left hypogastric nerve, (2) inferior hypogastric plexus

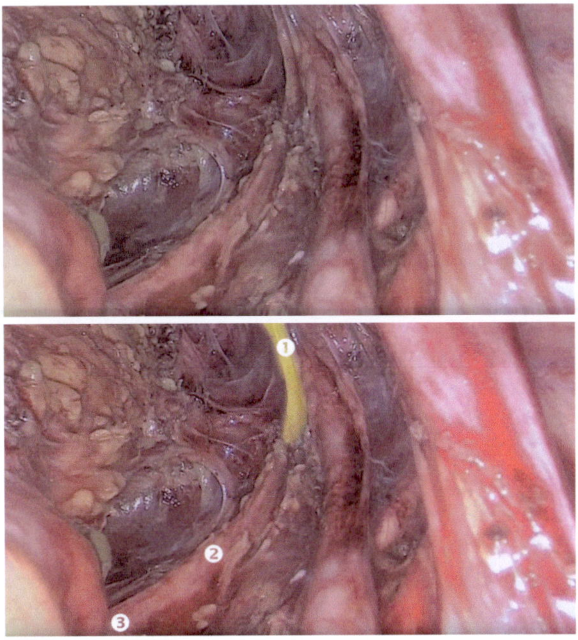

Fig. 7.4 Right hypogastric nerve and right inferior hypogastric plexus dissected during a nerve-preserving sacrocolpopexy. (1) Right inferior hypogastric plexus, (2) right hypogastric nerve, (3) superior hypogastric plexus

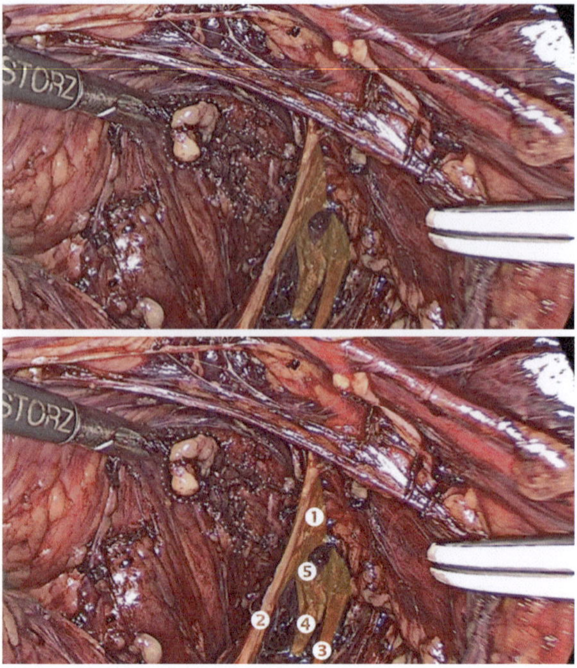

Fig. 7.5 Surgical image demonstrating deep endometriosis nodule in the right uterosacral ligament just after release, with neuropreservation, of the inferior hypogastric plexus. (1) Inferior hypogastric plexus, (2) right hypogastric nerve, (3) sacral root S2, (4) sacral root S3, (5) pelvic splanchnic nerves

Tips and Tricks 2
Surgical resection of endometriosis of the uterosacral ligaments and/or the recto-vaginal septum may injure nerve fibers of the HNs and the IHP; such injury may cause urinary retention, loss of bladder sensitivity and/or urinary incontinence, constipation, loss of rectal sensitivity, and/or anal incontinence. In this context, the nerve-sparing surgical technique consists of isolating the nerve bundles. For this, the surgeon performs the dissection in the craniocaudal direction, laterally to the mesorectum and medially to the mesoureter, aided by the cranial traction of the rectosigmoid by the assistant surgeon. Following the dissection steps described above, the HNs are dissected, and the endometriosis is resected with cold scissors, or other energy source, in parallel to the nerve fibers, with a technique similar to that used in tunneling the ureters. In the case of bilaterality, the possibility of leaving residual disease is considered in order to avoid too much denervation [5–7].

The PHI (or pelvic plexus) is formed primarily by the sympathetic fibers of the HNs described above and by the PSNs—parasympathetic—originating from the roots S2, S3, and S4. Besides these, contributions of fibers from the sacral sympathetic trunk are observed. This confluence of fibers occurs in the height of the medial portion of the uterosacral ligaments (hypogastric fascia), where the distal portion of the ipsilateral HNs opens in a triangular blade of nervous tissue and fuses with the PSNs, forming the IHP, in the height of the middle rectal vein. Thus, IHPs are described as triangular nerve networks, located in the pararectal fossae, whose proximal angle follows the ipsilateral HN, while the distal lateral angle forms the vesical

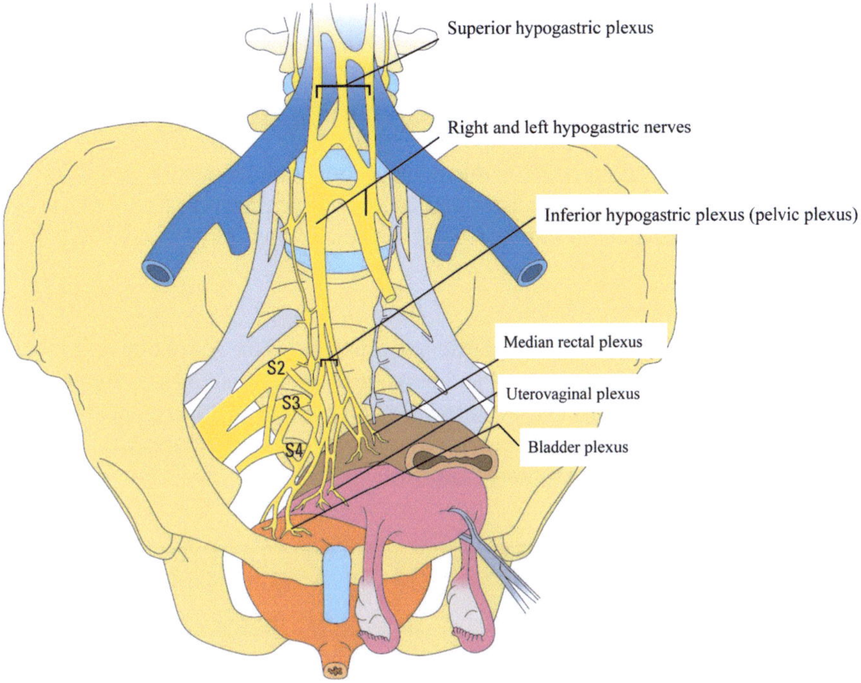

Fig. 7.6 Schematic illustration of the autonomic innervation of the pelvic organs: showing the nerve fibers of the superior hypogastric plexus (SHP), the hypogastric nerves (HNs), the fibers originating from the sympathetic trunk in close contact with the fibers of the sacral plexus (S2, S3, S4), forming the pelvic splanchnic nerves and, in sequence, the inferior hypogastric plexus (IHP) and its three branches: rectal, uterovaginal, and vesical

plexus—which follows the posterolateral margin of the ureter after crossing the deep uterine vein to its entry into the bladder—and the distal medial angle forms the middle rectal plexus—which follows the levator ani muscle and enters the anal canal between the external and internal sphincters of the anus, continuing with the myenteric plexus [3, 7] (Fig. 7.6).

Tips and Tricks 3

In resection of infiltrative pelvic endometriosis of the posterior compartment, the PSNs, as thin nerves, may be confused with retroperitoneal connective trabeculae and suffer injury by transection. Therefore, some authors advocate the identification of these nerves in their dorsal origin from the sacral nerve roots near the sacral foramen (LANN technique—laparoscopic neuronavigation) to reduce postoperative functional morbidity [6, 8, 9].

Tips and Tricks 4

In resection of intestinal endometriosis, conservative techniques, such as nodulectomy of the anterior wall of the rectosigmoid, with linear stapling or discoid resection, should be preferred over segmental resection whenever possible to avoid bladder dysfunctional complications (urinary retention), as they have better preservation of the bowel function. The better functional outcomes are due to less need for manipulation of the pararectal fossae and, therefore, the lower risk of injury to the IHP [5, 6, 10].

To facilitate the understanding and mastery of pelvic neuroanatomy and, in particular, the surgical application of this complex topographic anatomy, we present below a sequence of surgical images and cadaveric specimen dissections that will certainly allow the reader to sediment these concepts (Figs. 7.7, 7.8, 7.9, 7.10, 7.11, and 7.12).

Tips and Tricks 5

Watch the didactic video on the laparoscopic anatomy of the Autonomous Nervous System (ANS) nerves of the pelvis and nerve preservation techniques in the treatment of deep endometriosis at http://fertstertforum.com/lemosn-laparoscopic-neuroanatomy/ [in English; accessed Apr 15, 2019]. http://fertstertforum.com/lemosn-laparoscopic-neuroanatomy

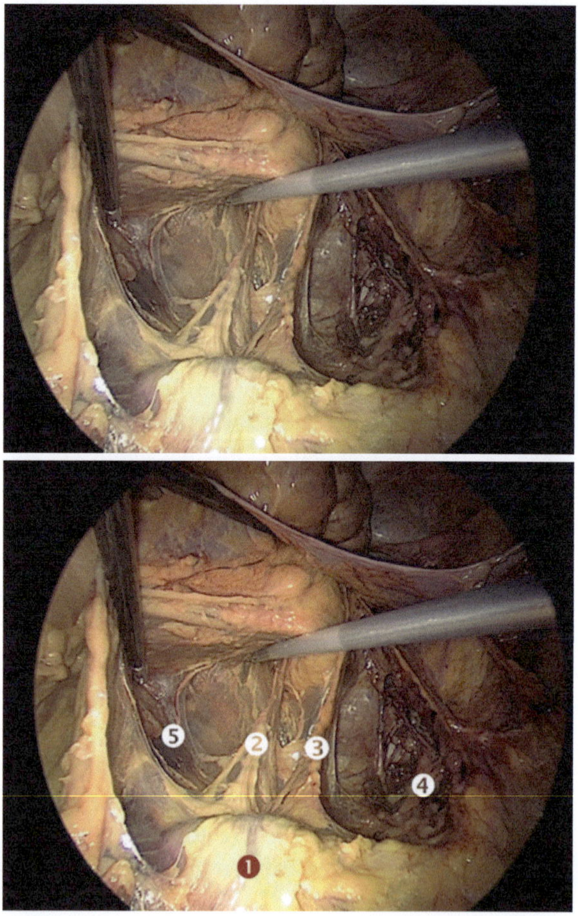

Fig. 7.7 Cadaveric dissection with image demonstrating the HNs (hypogastric nerve bilaterally) and the formation of the inferior hypogastric plexus (IHP) from fibers of the pelvic splanchnic nerves. (1) Superior hypogastric plexus, (2) left hypogastric nerve, (3) right hypogastric nerve, (4) right pararectal space, (5) left pararectal space. (Courtesy of Dr. Nucelio Lemos)

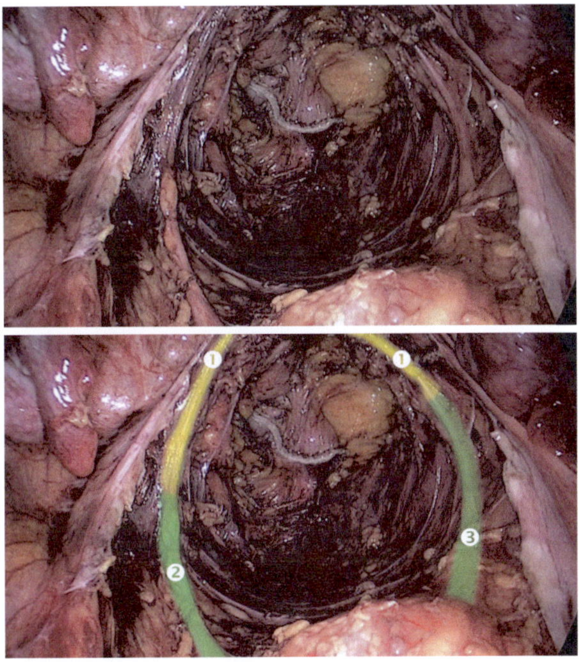

Fig. 7.8 Surgical image demonstrating the HNs bilaterally and the formation of the inferior hypogastric plexus (IHP). (1) Inferior hypogastric plexus bilaterally, (2) left hypogastric nerve, (3) right hypogastric nerve

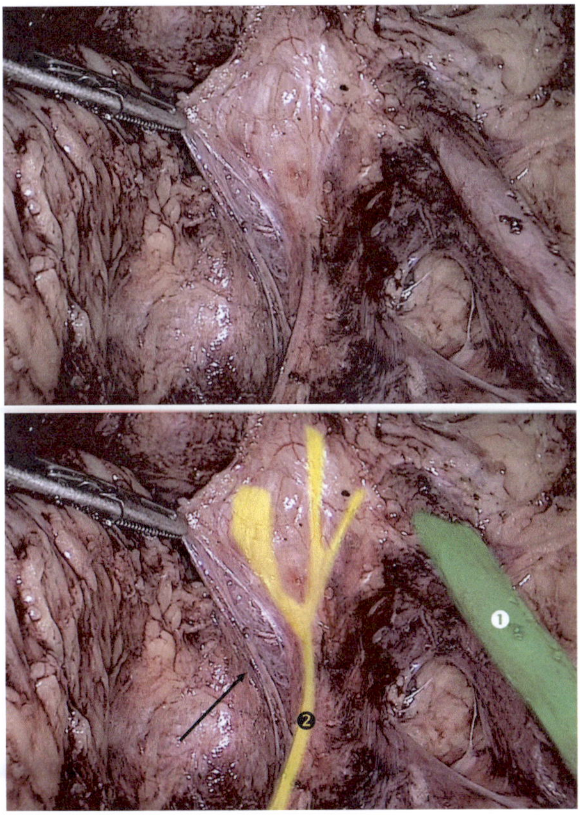

Fig. 7.9 Surgical image demonstrating the uterosacral ligament with the inferior hypogastric plexus, and its branches, painted and some fibers of the PSNs (black arrow). (1) Right ureter, (2) right hypogastric nerve, and right inferior hypogastric plexus

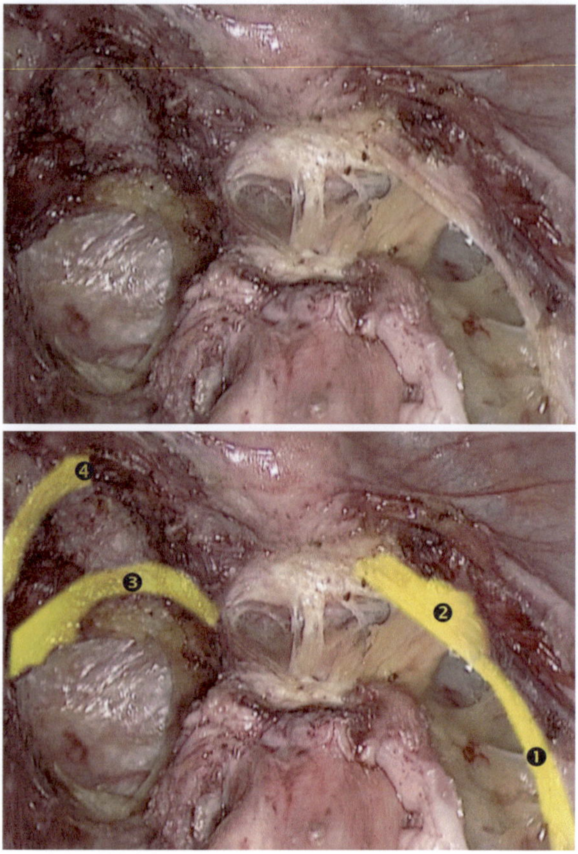

Fig. 7.10 Surgical image showing, on the right side, the HN and IHP preserved and on the left side, after removal of an endometriotic nodule, the vaginal branch of the IHP not visible, with the RVe (vesical) and RR (rectal) branches identified. (1) Right hypogastric nerve, (2) right inferior hypogastric plexus, (3) rectal branch of the left inferior hypogastric plexus, (4) vesical branch of the left inferior hypogastric plexus

Collateral Branches

More laterally in the pelvis, the PHI sends out branches that form, together with the direct branches of the PHS, the lower part of the ovarian plexus. The upper part of the ovarian plexus, on the other hand, is formed by the renal and aortic plexuses. Three main nerve trunks converge from the aortic plexus and follow the ovarian vessels to the ovary. At the point where the ovarian vessels cross the ureter, the ovarian plexus merges with the ureteral plexus. These nerves are responsible for the innervation of the ovary and the uterine tube.

The ureteric plexus has its fibers coming from several plexuses along its path. In its proximal portion, the ureter is supplied by a plexus of nerves from the renal, mesenteric, and aortic plexuses and, in its pelvic portion, by the superior and inferior hypogastric plexuses. The urinary tract is intimately connected through these nerve plexuses with all the other abdominal viscera. The plexus increases in thickness when it reaches the bladder.

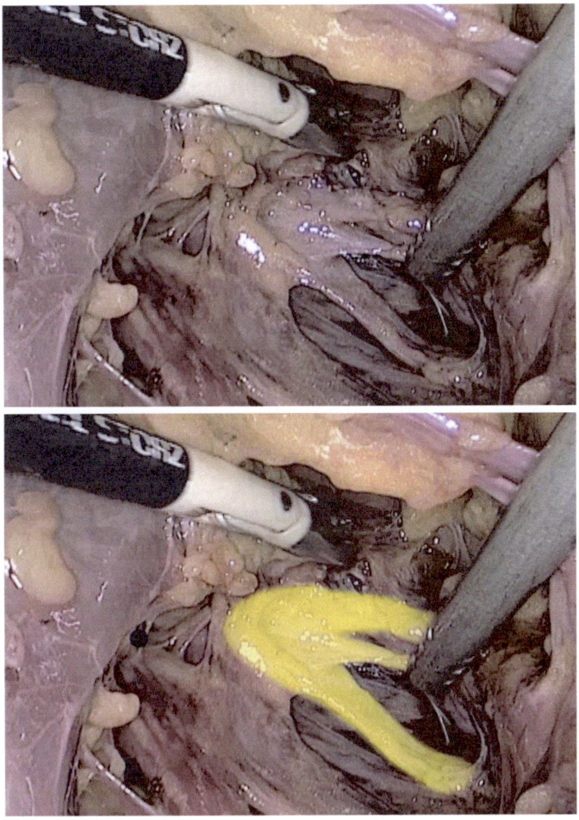

Fig. 7.11 Cadaveric dissection image showing the sacral roots of S2, S3, and S4 in yellow

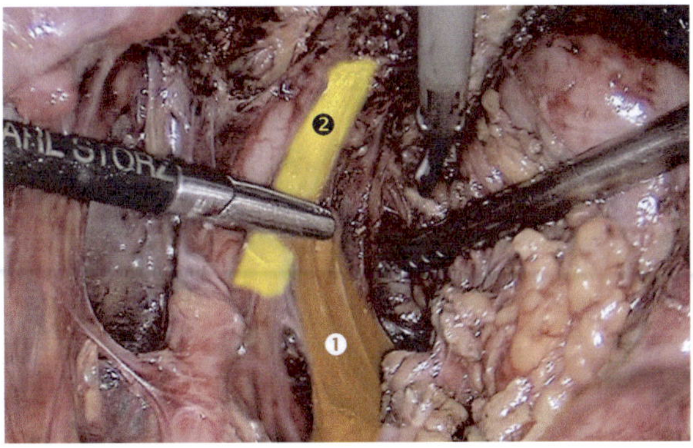

Fig. 7.12 Surgical image showing the left pelvic splanchnic nerves (PSNs) and the formation of the inferior hypogastric plexus. (1) Pelvic splanchnic nerves, (2) inferior hypogastric plexus

Somatic Innervation

Nerves of the Anterior Abdominal Wall

Iliohypogastric, ilioinguinal, genitofemoral, and femoral nerves.

These are sensitive branches of the lumbosacral plexus that enter the retroperitoneal space, emerging from the lateral or anterior border of the psoas muscle and following anteriorly and distally to leave the abdomen through the femoral and inguinal canals. Fibrotic incarceration of these branches is related to postsurgical inguinal pain (herniorrhaphy, cesarean delivery, or transverse pelvic incision surgeries) (Fig. 7.13).

Iliohypogastric Nerve

The iliohypogastric nerve emerges from the first lumbar nerve (L1) in the superolateral portion of the psoas major muscle and crosses obliquely the anterior aspect of the quadratus muscle towards the iliac crest, when it pierces the posterior aspect of

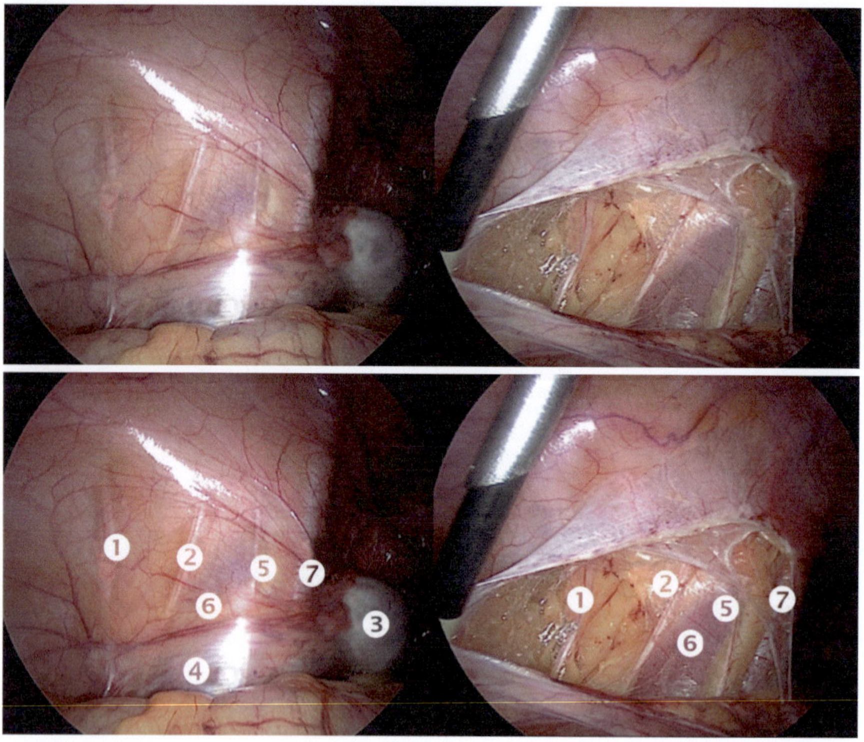

Fig. 7.13 Somatic nerves visible on the left lateral wall of the pelvis. (1) Iliohypogastric nerve, (2) ilioinguinal nerve, (3) left ovary, (4) left ovary suspensor ligament, (5) genitofemoral nerve, (6) psoas muscle, (7) external iliac artery

the transverse abdominis muscle and branches to innervate the skin over the iliac wing and meso-hypogastric region.

Tips and Tricks 6
The iliohypogastric and ilioinguinal nerves can be injured during the passage of lateral trocars or in larger transverse incisions. To avoid injury to these nerves, one should position the trocars as close as possible to the lateral borders of the rectus abdominis muscles, taking care not to injure the epigastric vessels. Photo 7.12 shows the 95% path of the iliohypogastric and ilioinguinal nerves.

Ilioinguinal Nerve

Smaller than the anterior one, it emerges with it from L1, on the lateral aspect of the psoas major muscle, just below the iliohypogastric nerve, traveling the same path until it leaves the abdominal cavity through the inguinal canal.

Genitofemoral Nerve

Formed by fibers from L1 and L2, it emerges in the anterior edge of the psoas major muscle, close to the spine, and follows obliquely and divides into a genital branch, which leaves the abdominal cavity through the inguinal canal, and a femoral branch, which crosses the wall through the femoral canal.

Femoral Nerve

It originates from the dorsal divisions of roots L2, L3, and L4 and has the largest motor and sensory portion of the lumbar plexus. The femoral nerve enters the abdomen through the lateral fibers of the psoas major muscle in its inferior portion and continues distally between it and the iliac muscle, under the fascia of the latter, leaving the cavity through the femoral canal to innervate the quadriceps femoris muscle and the skin that covers the anterior surface of the thigh (Fig. 7.14).

Nerves of the Obturator Space

The obturator space can be developed by the opening of the parietal peritoneum, between the external iliac vessels and the psoas major muscle. Besides being crossed by the obturator nerve, the space houses deeper the confluence of the lumbosacral trunk with the roots S1–S4, forming the main nerve trunks of the sacral plexus—sciatic nerve, pudendal nerve, anus levator nerves, superior gluteal nerve, inferior gluteal nerve, and, in some cases, posterior femoral cutaneous nerve (in most cases, the

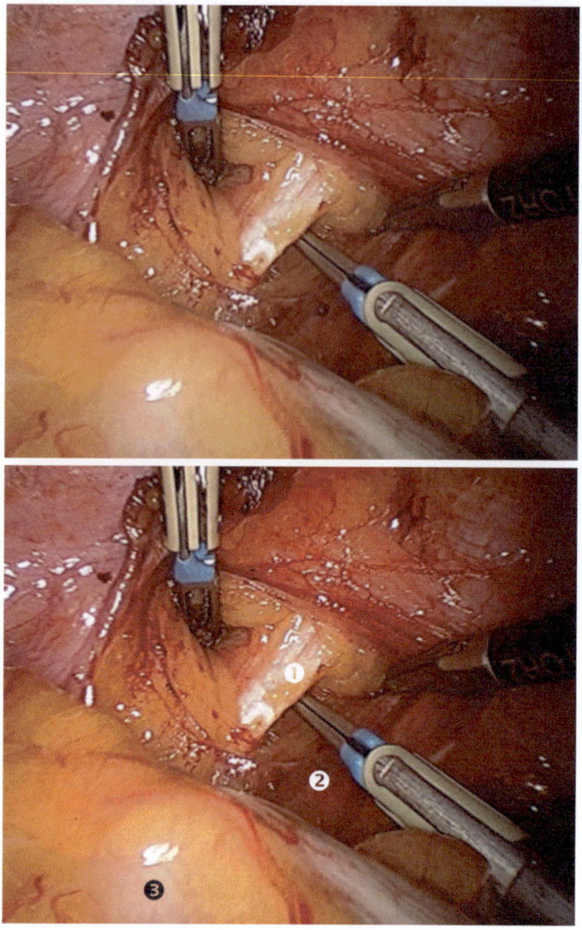

Fig. 7.14 Left femoral nerve (FN) dissected at the lateral border of the psoas muscle (PM). (1) Left femoral nerve, (2) lateral border of the left psoas muscle, (3) left colon. (Courtesy of Dr. Nucelio Lemos)

posterior femoral cutaneous nerve is an extrapelvic branch of the sciatic nerve, originating after the latter passes through the greater ischial foramen) (Fig. 7.15).

Obturator Nerve

The obturator nerve emerges from the ventral branches of L2, L3, and L4, at the medial border of the psoas major muscle, just proximal to the iliopectineal eminence. It follows distally and passes posteriorly to the common iliac vessels and laterally to the internal iliac vessels, which separate it from the ureter. It walks on the lateral wall of the lesser pelvis, anteriorly to the obturator vessels, up to the obturator canal, through which it leaves the pelvis issuing branches that sensitively innervate the medial skin of the thigh and motorly the adductor muscles of the hip.

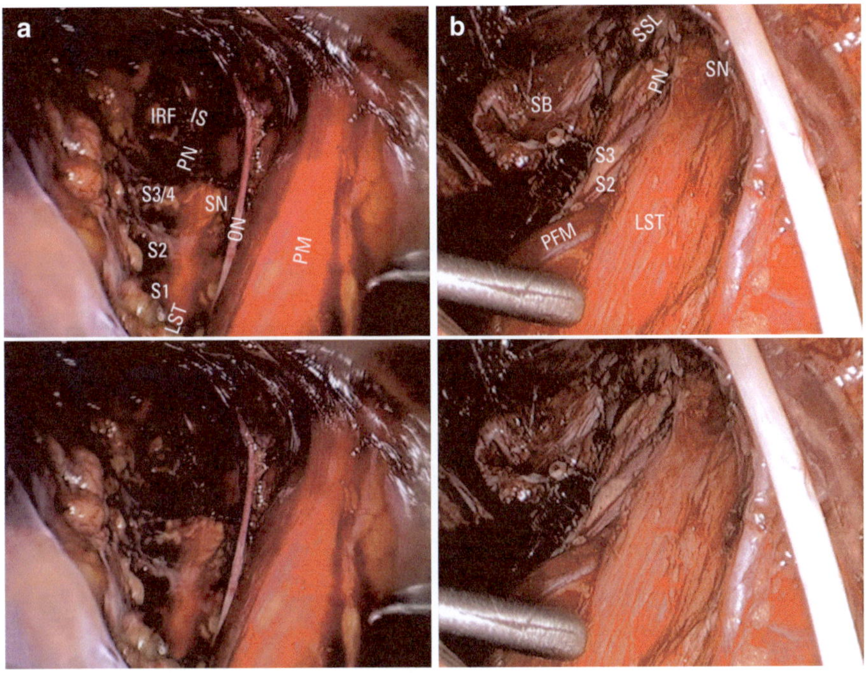

Fig. 7.15 Nerves of the obturator space at right. (**a**) On left, pudendal nerve dissection with transection of the sacral spinal ligament, exposing the ischiorectal fossa (IRF). (**b**) On right, the sacral plexus after resection of an endometriotic nodule that required resection of the internal iliac vessels, connecting the presacral and obturator spaces. Obturator nerve (ON), lumbosacral trunk (LST), sciatic nerve (SN), pudendal nerve (PN), and S1, S2, S3, and S4 roots. Piriformis muscle (PFM), psoas muscle (PM), sacrum bone (SB), ischial spine (IS). (Courtesy of Dr. Nucelio Lemos)

Lumbosacral Trunk

The lumbosacral trunk is formed by branches from L4 and L5. It emerges medially from the psoas major muscle and follows distally over L5 and over the sacroiliac synostosis towards the obturator space, to join the distal portions of roots S1, S2, and S3, giving rise to the sciatic nerve (Figs. 7.16 and 7.17).

Sciatic Nerve

The sciatic nerve is the largest nerve in the body, and its proximal portion is 2 cm thick. It is formed by fibers from L4 and L5, coming from the lumbosacral trunk, and by fibers from S1, S2, and S3. It leaves the pelvis through the supra-piriform hiatus of the greater sciatic foramen, bounded anteriorly by the ischial incisure of the iliac bone and posteriorly by the piriformis muscle (Figs. 7.18 and 7.19).

The sciatic nerve sends sensory branches to the superior gluteal and posterolateral regions of the thigh, as well as to the leg, ankle, and foot, and motor branches

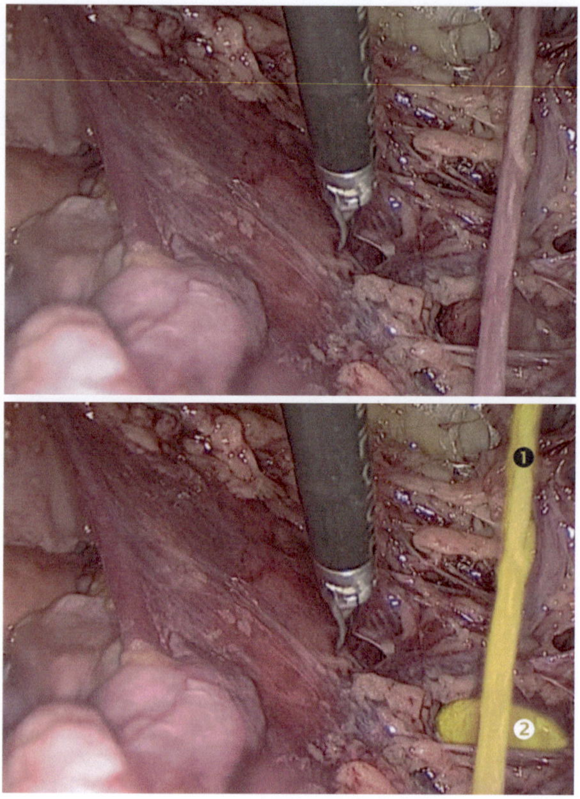

Fig. 7.16 Anatomical relationship of the lumbosacral trunk and obturator nerve. (1) Obturator nerve, (2) lumbosacral trunk

to the hip extensor, abductor, and rotator muscles, knee flexors, and all ankle and foot muscles. In some people, the gluteal, posterior femoral cutaneous, and lateral femoral cutaneous nerves emerge before the sciatic nerve exits the pelvis.

Pudendal Nerve

The pudendal nerve originates in the ventral branches of S2, S3, and S4 and travels between the piriformis and coccygeal muscles, crossing between the sacrospinal and sacrotuberous ligaments, to enter the Alcock's canal (pudendal canal), through which it leaves the pelvis towards the perineum.

The pudendal nerve sends sensory branches to the lower gluteal region and the skin of the perineal region and sends motor branches to the perineal muscles,

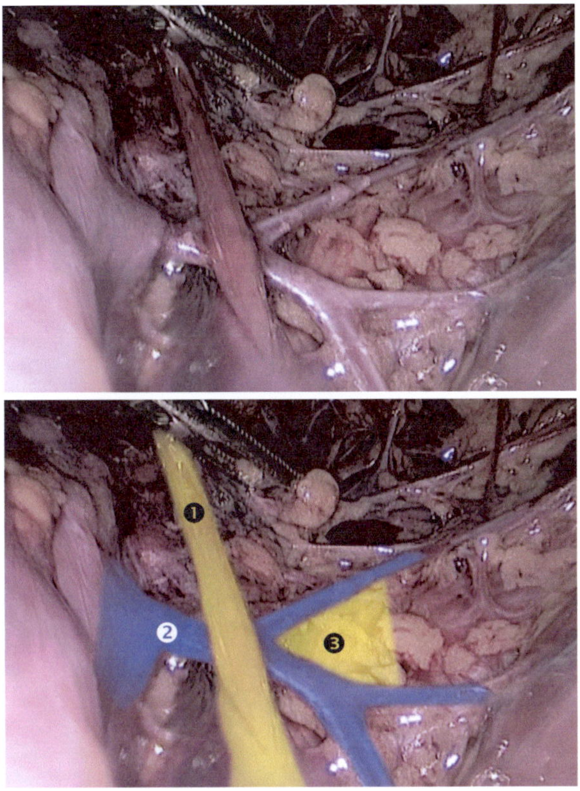

Fig. 7.17 Anatomical relationship of the lumbosacral trunk and vessels of the posterior trunk of the internal iliac vessels. (1) Obturator nerve, (2) posterior trunk of the internal iliac vessels and its branches, (3) lumbosacral trunk

including the external sphincters of the urethra and anus, and the anterior fibers of the levator ani muscle. The posterior fibers of the levator ani muscle are innervated by the levator ani muscle nerve, formed by motor and sensory branches of the S3 and S4 roots (Figs. 7.20 and 7.21).

Tips and Tricks 7

Traditionally, during the teaching of pelvic surgery, much attention is paid to the preservation of the ureter and great vessels; however, the fact that the pelvic walls are lined by nerves is often neglected. Injury to nerves of the lumbosacral plexus can have very serious consequences, such as lower limb motor changes (impairing gait) and chronic neuropathic pain. For more details, watch the video at https://youtu.be/Tm0qTeyzMHY [in English; accessed Apr. 16, 2019.

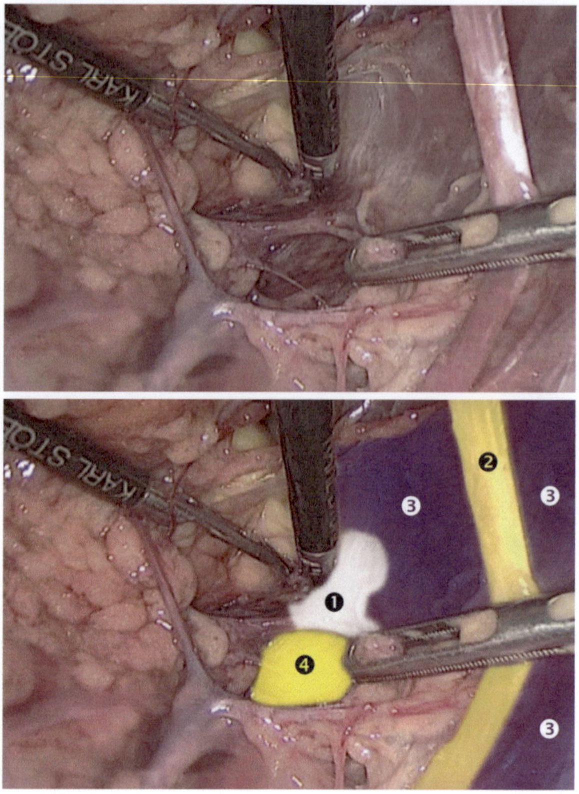

Fig. 7.18 Anatomical relationship of the lumbosacral trunk with the pudendal nerve, the sciatic spine, the obturator nerve, and the obturator muscle. (1) Sciatic spine, (2) obturator nerve, (3) obturator muscle, (4) lumbosacral trunk

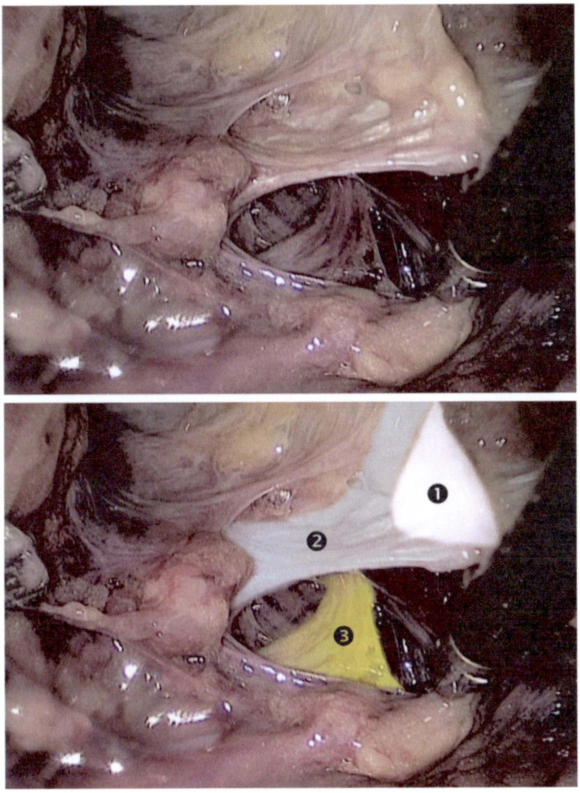

Fig. 7.19 Anatomical relationship of the pudendal nerve to the sciatic spine and sacrospinous ligament. (1) Sciatic spine, (2) sacrospinal ligament, (3) pudendal nerve

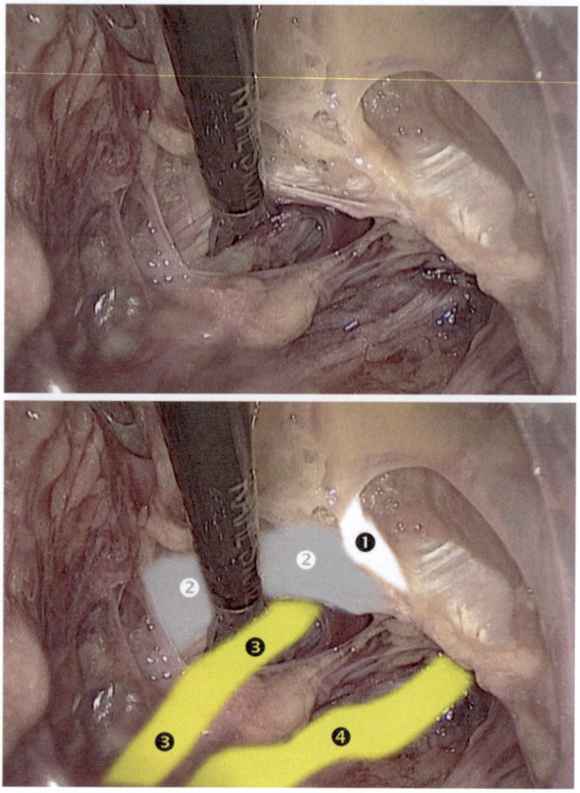

Fig. 7.20 Cadaveric dissection image demonstrating the relationship of the pudendal nerve to the sciatic nerve. (1) Sciatic spine, (2) sacrospinous ligament, (3) pudendal nerve, (4) sciatic nerve

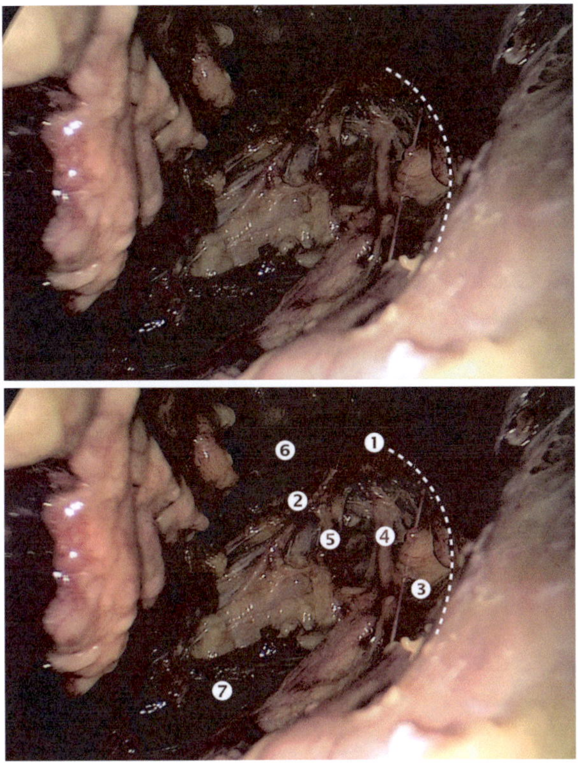

Fig. 7.21 Surgical image showing the pudendal nerve, the sciatic nerve, the piriformis muscle, and the levator ani muscle. (1) Sciatic spine, (2) sacrospinous ligament, (3) sciatic nerve, (4) pudendal nerve, (5) levator ani nerve, (6) levator ani muscle, (7) piriformis muscle. (Courtesy of Dr. Nucelio Lemos)

References

1. Lemos N, Souza C, Marques RM, Kamergorodsky G, Schor E, Girão MJ. Laparoscopic anatomy of the autonomic nerves of the pelvis and the concept of nerve-sparing surgery by direct visualization of autonomic nerve bundles. Fertil Steril. 2015;104(5):e11–2.
2. Baggish MS, Karram MM. Atlas de anatomia pélvica e cirurgia ginecológica. 4th ed. Rio de Janeiro: Revinter; 2012.
3. Ripperda CM, Jackson LA, Phelan JN, Carrick KS, Corton MM. Anatomic relationships of the pelvic autonomic nervous system in female cadavers: clinical applications to pelvic surgery. Am J Obstet Gynecol. 2017;216(4):388.e1–7.
4. Seracchioli R, Mabrouk M, Mastronardi M, Raimondo D, Arena A, Forno SD, et al. Anatomic cartography of the hypogastric nerves and surgical insights for autonomic preservation during radical pelvic procedures. J Minim Invasive Gynecol. 2019;S1553-4650(19):30054–8.
5. Ceccaroni M, Clarizia R, Bruni F, D'Urso E, Gagliardi ML, Roviglione G, et al. Nerve-sparing laparoscopic eradication of deep endometriosis with segmental rectal and parametrial resection: the Negrar method. A single-center, prospective, clinical trial. Surg Endosc. 2012;26(7):2029–45.
6. Lemos NLBM, Ribeiro R, Fernandes GL, Abrão MS, Moretti-Marques R. Nerve-sparing routes in radical pelvic surgery. In: Gomes-da-Silveira GG, da Silveira G, Pessini SA, editors. Minimally invasive gynecology. Cham: Springer; 2018. p. 61–75.

7. Kale A, Basol G, Usta T, Aytuluk HG. Laparoscopic evaluation of female pelvic neuroanatomy and autonomic plexuses in terms of gynecologic perspective. J Endometr Pelvic Pain Disord. 2018;10(4):216–21.
8. Volpi E, Ferrero A, Sismondi P. Laparoscopic identification of pelvic nerves in patients with deep infiltrating endometriosis. Surg Endosc. 2004;18(7):1109–12.
9. Possover M, Chiantera V, Baekelandt J. Anatomy of the sacral roots and the pelvic splanchnic nerves in women using the LANN technique. Surg Laparosc Endosc Percutan Tech. 2007;17(6):508–10.
10. Ceccaroni M, Clarizia R, Tebache L. Role and technique of nerve-sparing surgery in deep endometriosis. J Endometr Pelvic Pain Disord. 2016;8(4):141–51.
11. Ceccaroni M, Clarizia R, Roviglione G, Ruffo G. Neuro-anatomy of the posterior parametrium and surgical considerations for a nerve-sparing approach in radical pelvic surgery. Surg Endosc. 2013;27(11):4386–94.
12. Whiteside JL, Barber MD, Walters MD, Falcone T. Anatomy of ilioinguinal and iliohypogastric nerves in relation to trocar placement and low transverse incisions. Am J Obstet Gynecol. 2003;189(6):1574–8. discussion 1578

Chapter 8
Digestive System

Fabio Ohara, Francisco Cesar Rodrigues, Helizabet Salomão Ayroza, and Paulo Ayroza Ribeiro

Overview

In this chapter, the gastrointestinal organs of special interest to gynecologists will be discussed.

F. Ohara
Santa Casa de Misericórdia de São Paulo (SCMSP), São Paulo, Brazil

Brazilian Federation of Gynecology and Obstetrics Associations (FEBRASGO), São Paulo, Brazil

F. C. Rodrigues
Ob/Gyn Department, Santa Casa de Sao Paulo School of Medical Sciences, São Paulo, Brazil

H. Salomão Ayroza
Department of Obstetrics and Gynecology, Santa Casa de Sao Paulo School of Medical Sciences, São Paulo, Brazil

Gynecological Endoscopy and Endometriosis Division, Santa Casa de São Paulo Hospital, São Paulo, Brazil

P. Ayroza Ribeiro (✉)
Brazilian Federation of Gynecology and Obstetrics Associations (FEBRASGO), São Paulo, Brazil

Department of Obstetrics and Gynecology, Santa Casa de Sao Paulo School of Medical Sciences, São Paulo, Brazil

H. Salomão Ayroza, P. Ayroza Ribeiro (eds.), *Atlas of Laparoscopic Gynecological Anatomy*, https://doi.org/10.1007/978-3-031-63520-5_8

Large Intestine

The large intestine is responsible for the absorption of water from undigested waste, transforming it into semisolid feces, which are stored and accumulated until defecation occurs. It is composed of the cecum, appendix, colon (ascending, transverse, descending, and sigmoid), rectum, and anal canal.

Cecum

It measures approximately 7.5 cm in length and is situated in the right iliac fossa of the abdomen. It is usually attached to the lateral wall of the abdomen by one or more cecal folds of peritoneum. The terminal part of the ileum enters the cecum obliquely and partly invaginates into it.

Irrigation

Ileocolic Artery

Origin: Superior mesenteric artery.

Path: The superior mesenteric artery lies inferiorly to the celiac trunk at 1–2 cm posteriorly to the pancreas with a descending path, and the ileocolic artery is its most inferior branch. It follows along the root of the mesentery and divides into ileal and colic branches (Fig. 8.1a and b).

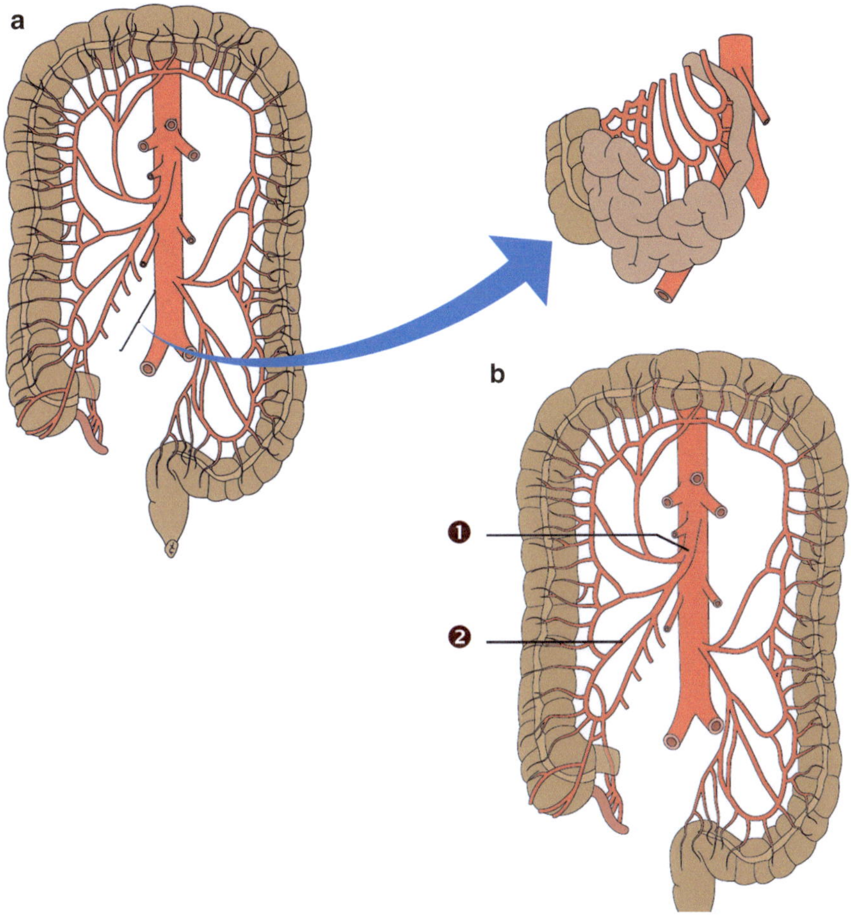

Fig. 8.1 (1) Superior mesenteric artery, (2) ileocolic artery

Ileocolic Vein

Drainage: Into the superior mesenteric vein.

Path: Accompanies the ileocolic artery (Fig. 8.2a and b).

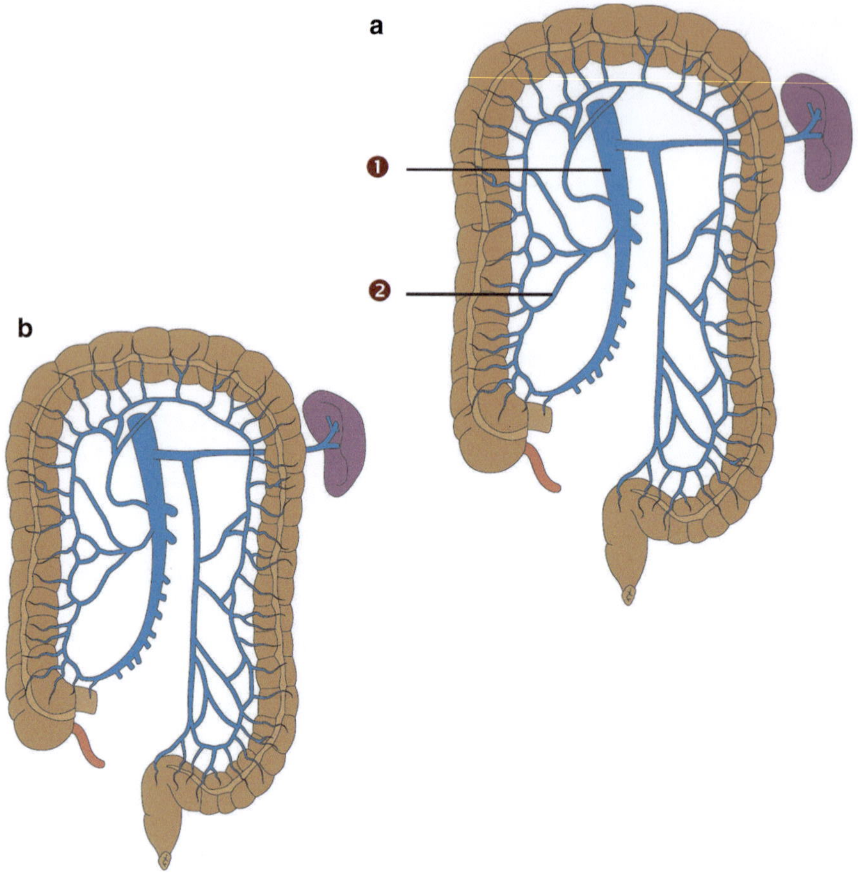

Fig. 8.2 (1) Inferior mesenteric vein, (2) ileocolic vein

Innervation

Sympathetic

The sympathetic innervation originates in the superior mesenteric plexus. The fibers originate from the lower thoracic (T8–T10).

Parasympathetic

The parasympathetic innervation originates from the superior mesenteric plexus. The fibers originate from the vagus nerves.

Appendix

It is an intestinal diverticulum that measures approximately 6–10 cm, containing lymphoid tissue, and originates on the medial side of the cecum, inferiorly to the ileocecal junction. It has a short mesentery, called the mesoappendix, which originates on the posterior surface of the mesentery of the terminal part of the ileum. The appendix is most often located retrocecally.

Irrigation

Appendicular Artery

Origin: Ileocolic artery.

Path: It is a retroileal artery, reaching the appendix through the mesoappendix (Fig. 8.3).

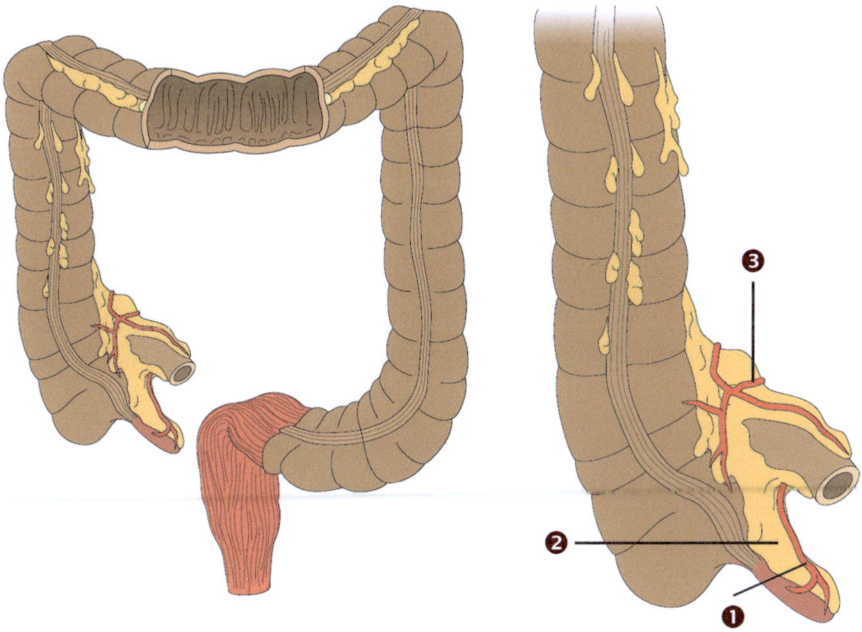

Fig. 8.3 (1) Appendicular artery, (2) mesoappendix, (3) ileocolic artery

Ileocolic Vein

Drainage: Superior mesenteric vein.

Path: Accompanies the ileocolic artery.

Tips and Tricks 1

Among all cases of deep endometriosis, the appendix has an incidence of 3–10%. In most situations, the finding is intraoperative because of the diagnostic difficulty prior to surgery for this pathology. The surgical technique consists of sectioning the mesoappendix at its base with linear stapling, ligation, or mechanic suturing (Figs. 8.4, 8.5, 8.6, and 8.7).

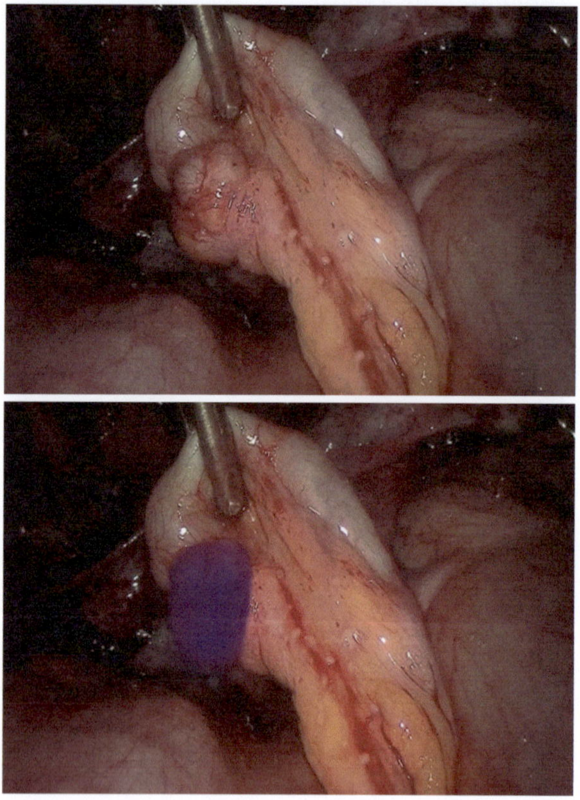

Fig. 8.4 Appendiceal endometriosis nodule

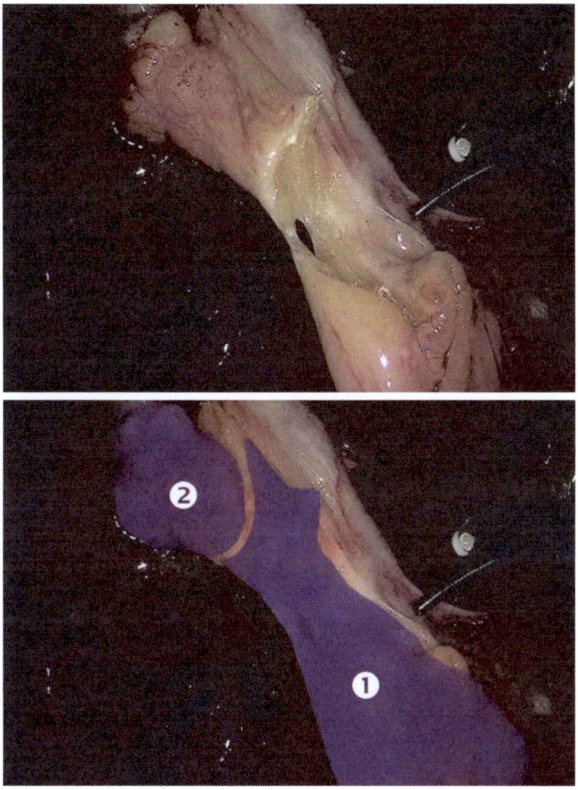

Fig. 8.5 Sectioning and coagulation of the mesoappendix. (1) Mesoappendix, (2) appendiceal endometriosis nodule

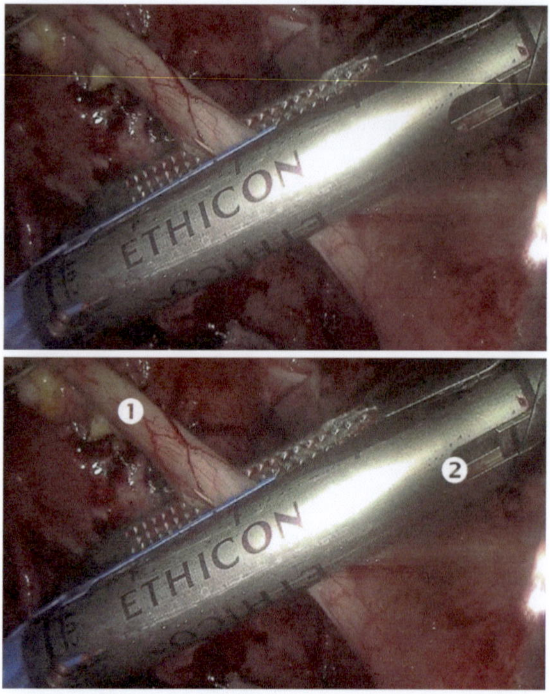

Fig. 8.6 Linear stapling at the base of the appendix. (1) Cecal appendix, (2) stapler

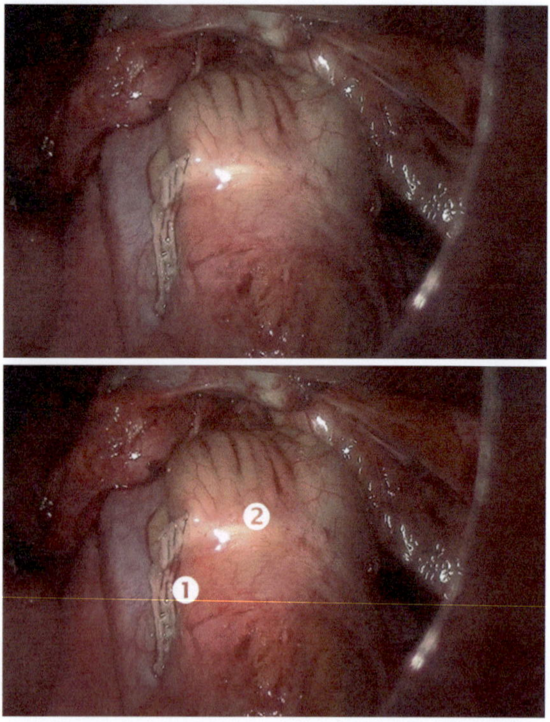

Fig. 8.7 Appendectomy with the linear stapling lines. (1) Staples line, (2) cecum

Colon

It is divided into four parts: ascending, transverse, descending, and sigmoid, forming an arch. The colon surrounds the small intestine as follows: the ascending colon to the right, the transverse colon superiorly and anteriorly, the descending colon to the left, and the sigmoid colon inferiorly.

Sigmoid Colon

It is characterized by its S-shaped shape of variable length (from 15 to 50 cm), joining the descending colon to the rectum. It extends from the iliac fossa to the third sacral segment (SIII), where it joins the rectum. The end-of-the-colon threads approximately 15 cm from the anal border indicate the rectosigmoid junction. In general, it has a long mesentery—the sigmoid mesocolon—which extends first medially and superiorly to the external iliac vessels, and then medially and inferiorly to the bifurcation of the common iliac vessels to the anterior face of the sacrum. The left ureter lies posterior to the apex of the root of the sigmoid mesocolon.

Tips and Tricks 2
The release of the physiological adherence of the sigmoid mesocolon known as Toldt's fascia is one of the initial steps in the treatment of deep endometriosis, allowing better mobilization of the rectosigmoid, besides allowing easy identification and access to the left ureter and lateral pelvic vessels, avoiding damage to them (Figs. 8.8 and 8.9).

Anatomical Landmarks 5

Arterial Irrigation

Origin: Sigmoid arteries (three to four), which are branches of the inferior mesenteric artery.

Path: The sigmoid arteries descend to the retroperitoneum to the left of the descending colon, dividing into ascending and descending branches. The superior branch of the superior sigmoid artery anastomoses with the descending branch of the left colic artery, forming a part of the marginal artery (Fig. 8.10).

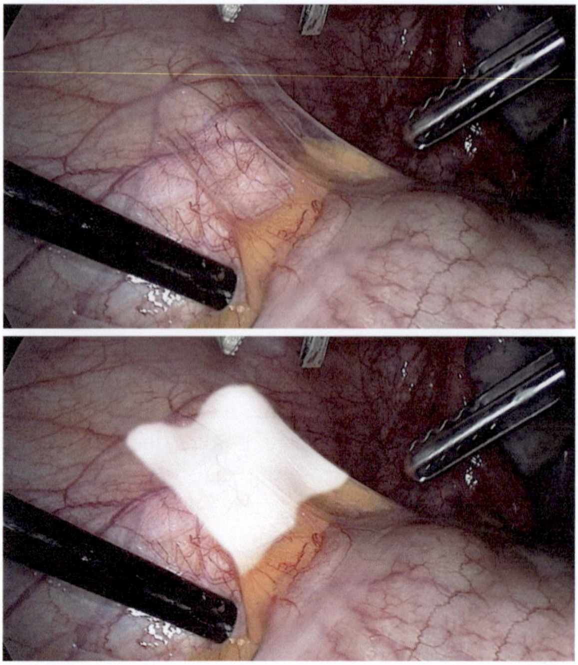

Fig. 8.8 Toldt's fascia

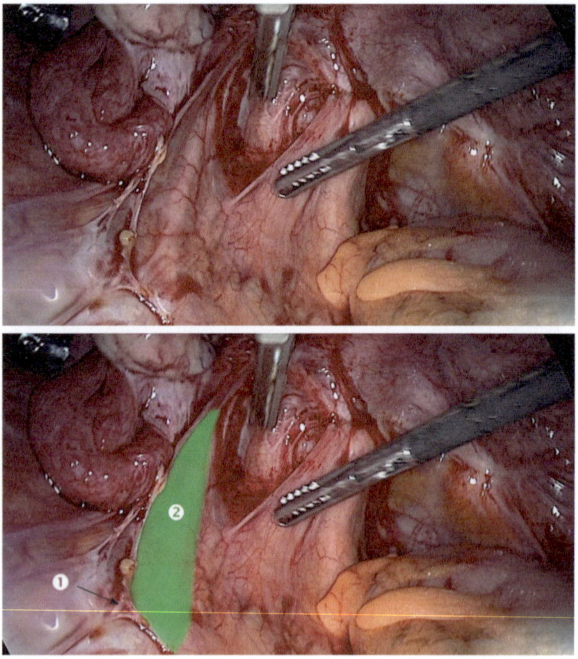

Fig. 8.9 Release of physiological adhesion from the mesocolon

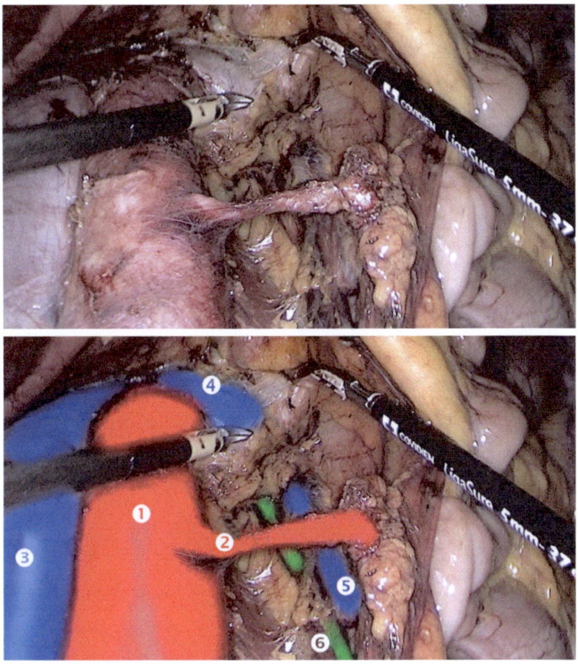

Fig. 8.10 Anatomical relations of the inferior mesenteric artery. (1) Aorta artery, (2) inferior mesenteric artery, (3) vena cava, (4) left renal vein, (5) left gonadal vein, (6) left ureter

Anatomical Landmarks 6

Venous Irrigation

Drainage: Venous drainage from the sigmoid vein is via the inferior mesenteric vein.

Path: The inferior mesenteric vein flows into the splenic vein and then into the portal vein on its way to the liver (Fig. 8.11).

Innervation

Anatomical Landmarks 7

Sympathetic

Origin: T10–L2 segment.

Pathway: Sympathetic innervation follows through the lumbar splanchnic nerves toward the nerves of the superior mesenteric plexus and those of the periarterial plexuses.

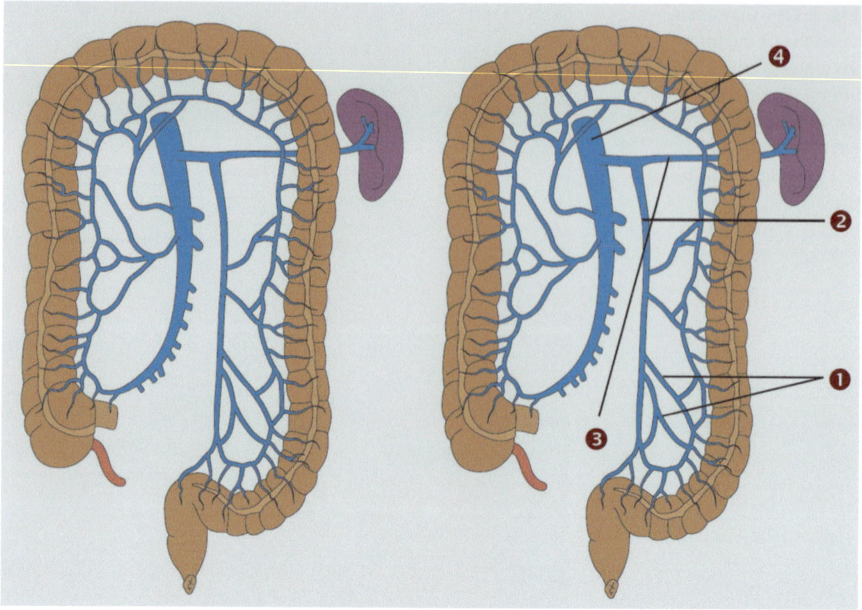

Fig. 8.11 Anatomical relationships of the inferior mesenteric vein. (1) Sigmoidal vein, (2) inferior mesenteric vein, (3) splenic vein, (4) portal vein

Anatomical Landmarks 8

Parasympathetic

Origin: Vertebrae S2–S4.

Pathway: Parasympathetic innervation follows through the pelvic splanchnic nerves, plexus, and inferior hypogastric nerves (Figs. 8.12, 8.13, 8.14, 8.15, 8.16, and 8.17).

Rectum

This is the terminal part of the large intestine, continuous with the sigmoid at the S3 vertebra and continuous inferiorly with the anal canal. The rectum follows the curve of the sacrum and coccyx, forming the sacral flexure of the rectum. The rectum terminates anteroinferior to the end of the coccyx, just before the anorectal flexure of the anal canal, the point at which the bowel pierces the diaphragm of the pelvis (levator anus muscle). The anorectal flexure is an important mechanism for fecal continence and is maintained by the tone of the puborectal muscle.

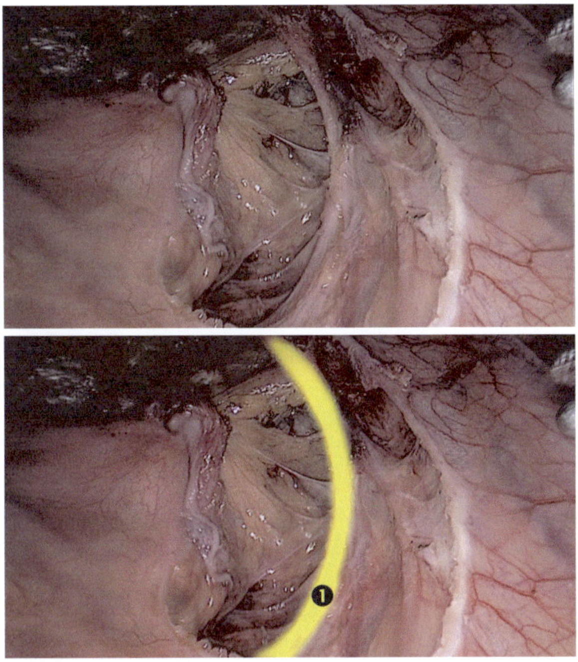

Fig. 8.12 Parasympathetic innervation of the rectum. (1) Right hypogastric nerve

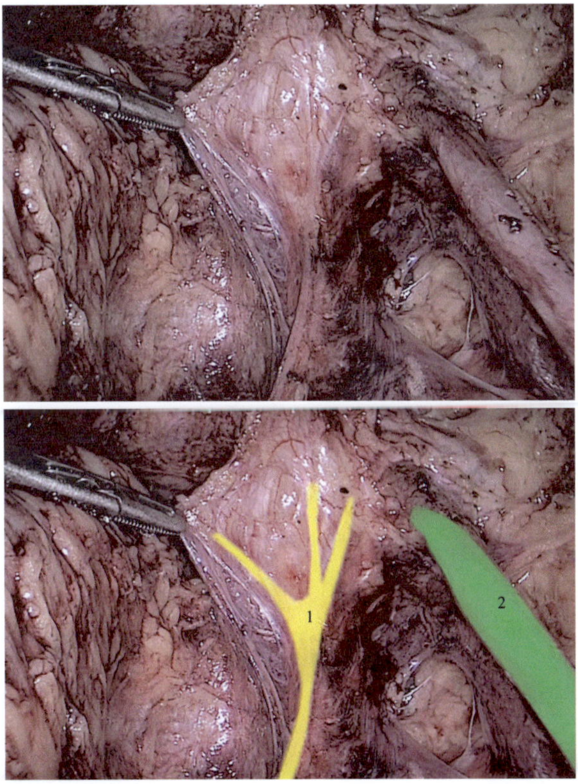

Fig. 8.13 Parasympathetic innervation of the rectum. (1) Right hypogastric nerve, (2) right ureter

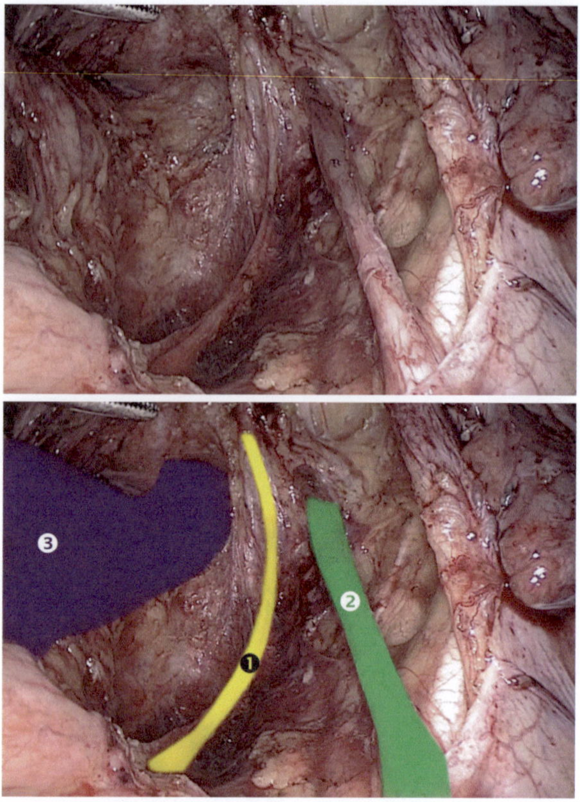

Fig. 8.14 Relations of the rectum and hypogastric nerve. (1) Right hypogastric nerve, (2) right ureter, (3) rectum

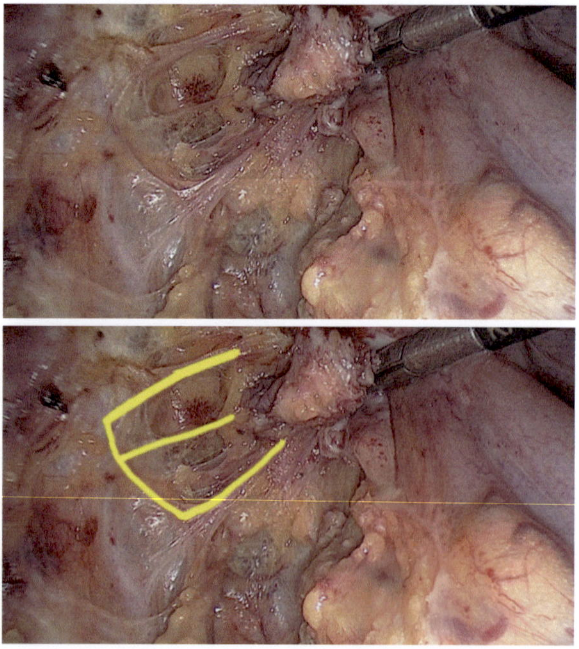

Fig. 8.15 Lower hypogastric plexus and pelvic splanchnic nerves (in yellow) and rectum medially. Surgery for deep endometriosis with involvement of rectum

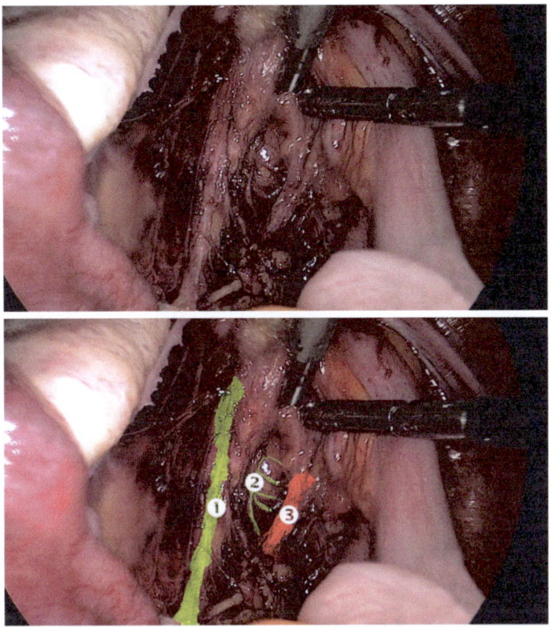

Fig. 8.16 Anatomical landmarks of rectal dissection in the treatment of deep endometriosis. (1) Left hypogastric nerve, (2) pelvic splanchnic nerves, (3) median rectal artery

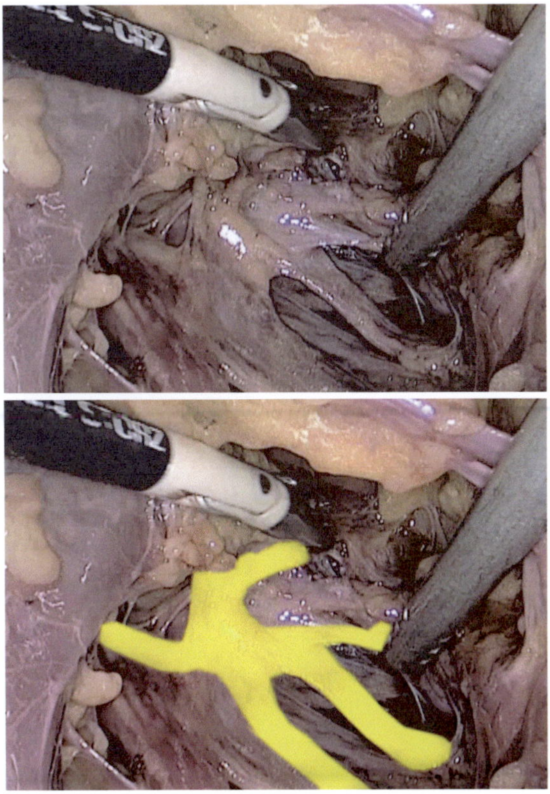

Fig. 8.17 Sacral roots (in yellow)

The dilated terminal part of the rectum, directly superior to the pelvic diaphragm, is known as the ampulla of the rectum, responsible for holding the fecal mass that accumulates until it is expelled during defecation. The peritoneum is flexed from the rectum to the posterior part of the fornix of the vagina, where it forms the floor of the rectouterine excavation; inferiorly to the excavation is the rectovaginal septum, and the lateral flexions of the peritoneum of the upper third of the rectum form the pararectal fossae. The rectovaginal septum separates the upper half of the posterior wall of the vagina from the rectum.

Tips and Tricks 3

In the surgery to treat deep intestinal endometriosis, dissection of the pararectal fossae is fundamental to better identify the anatomical landmarks (ureter and hypogastric nerve), also facilitating the dissection and identification of the rectovaginal septum, allowing the separation of the rectum from the retrocervical lesion.

It starts by identifying the pelvic excavation, with a longitudinal incision at the promontory, medially to the uterosacral ligament. With this dissection, an avascular space is found between the uterosacral ligament and the wall of the sigmoid, which is called the pararectal space (Figs. 8.18, 8.19, and 8.20).

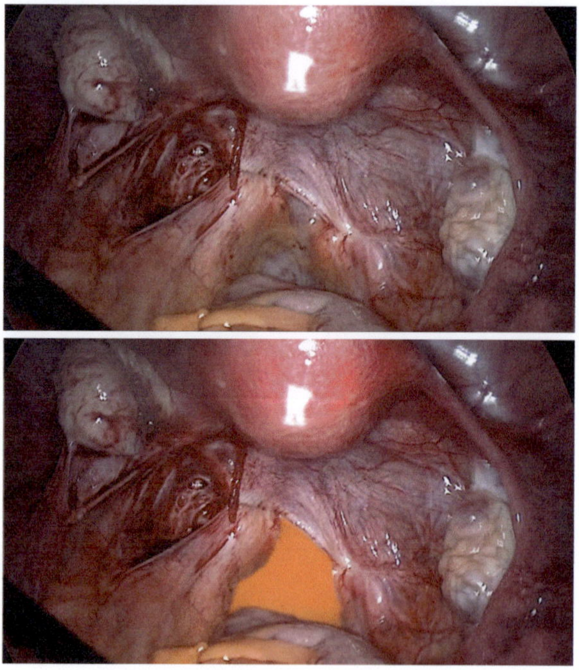

Fig. 8.18 Pelvic excavation (in orange), in a patient with deep retrocervical endometriosis with bilateral involvement of the uterosacral ligaments

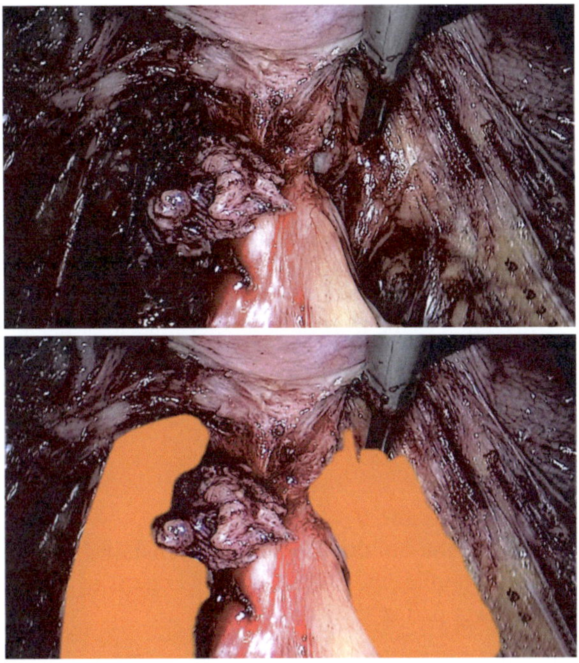

Fig. 8.19 Pararectal spaces (in orange) and rectal endometriosis nodule in the center

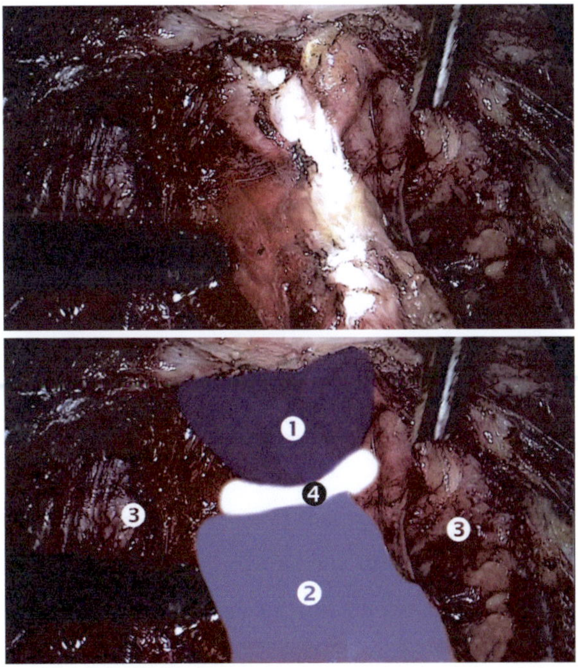

Fig. 8.20 Relations of the pararectal and rectovaginal spaces. (1) Vagina, (2) rectum, (3) pararectal spaces, (4) rectovaginal space

Arterial Irrigation

Anatomical Landmarks 9

Superior rectal artery.

Origin: Inferior mesenteric artery.

Path: It irrigates the upper part of the rectum, crosses the left common iliac vessels, and descends to the sigmoid mesocolon to the lesser pelvis. At the height of S3, it divides into two branches that descend on each side of the rectum and proceed to the irrigation to the internal sphincter muscle of the anus.

Anatomical Landmarks 10

Rectus medius artery.

Origin: Anterior division of the internal iliac arteries.

Path: Supplies the middle and lower parts of the rectum, going down the pelvis to the lower part of the rectum.

Tips and Tricks 4

The middle rectal artery is found at the dissection of the pararectal fossae and serves as an anatomical landmark for the pelvic splanchnic nerves that lie just below this structure (Figs. 8.21 and 8.22).

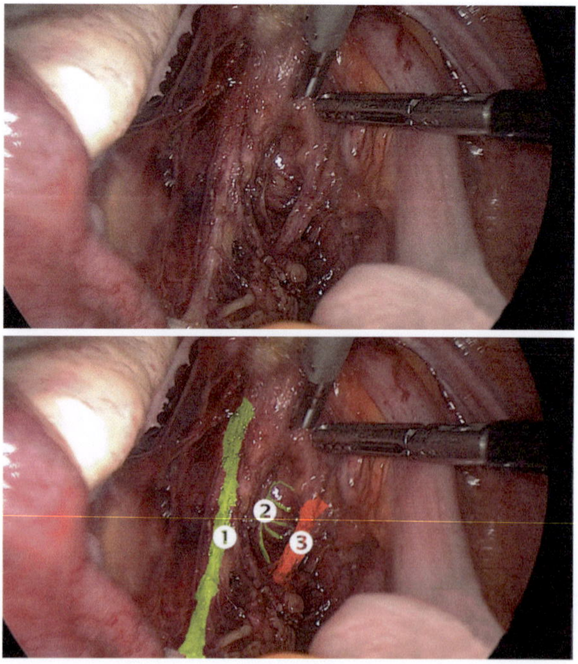

Fig. 8.21 Relevance of the middle rectal artery and splanchnic nerves in surgery for deep endometriosis of the rectosigmoid. (1) Left hypogastric nerve, (2) pelvic splanchnic nerves, (3) middle rectal artery

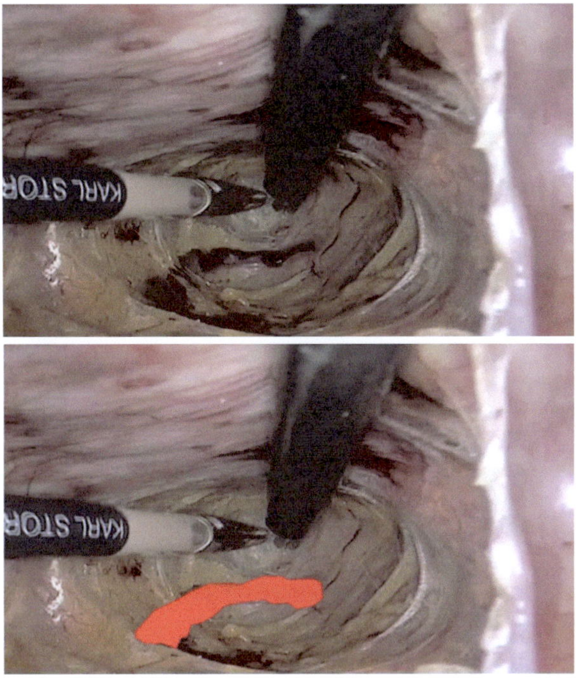

Fig. 8.22 Middle rectal artery (in red)

Anatomical Landmarks 11

Inferior Rectal Artery

Origin: Internal pudendal arteries.

Path: Supplies the anorectal junction and the anal canal (Fig. 8.23).

Anatomical Landmarks 12

Superior Rectal Vein

Drainage: To the portal venous system.

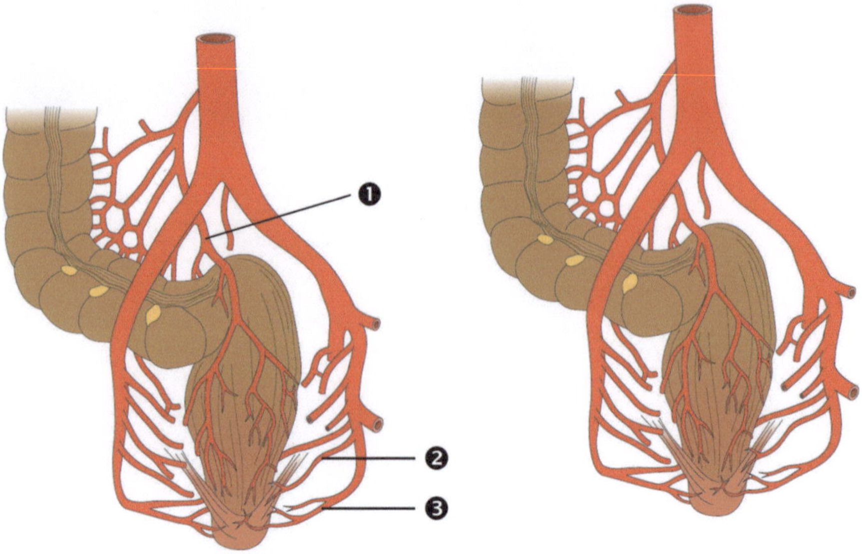

Fig. 8.23 Rectosigmoid irrigation. (1) Superior rectal artery, (2) right middle rectal artery, (3) right inferior rectal artery

Innervation

Anatomical Landmarks 14

Sympathetic

Origin: Vertebrae L1–L3.

Pathway: Conducted through the lumbar splanchnic nerves, the hypogastric plexus, and the periarterial plexus of the inferior mesenteric and superior rectal arteries, running with the arterial irrigation of the intestinal wall.

Parasympathetic

Origin: Vertebrae S2–S4.

Path: It follows through the pelvic splanchnic nerves and the right and left inferior hypogastric plexuses to the rectal (pelvic) plexus (Figs. 8.24 and 8.25).

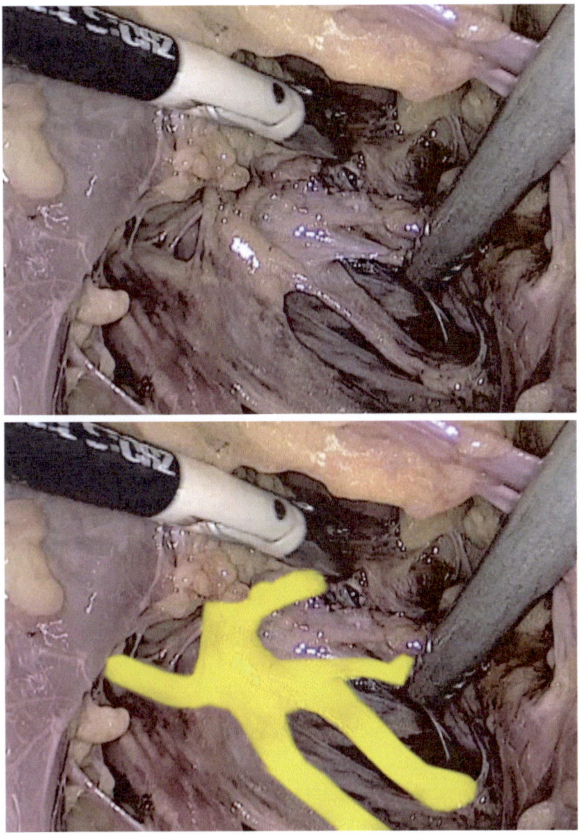

Fig. 8.24 Sacral roots

Anatomical Landmarks 15

Somatic

Origin: Vertebrae S2–S4.

Path: It follows through the pudendal nerves, passing through Alcock's canal, dividing into three branches: inferior rectal nerves, perineal nerves, and dorsal nerves of the clitoris.

Tips and Tricks 5

Dissection in deep intestinal endometriosis is always limited to the region of the lesion, and linear or discoid resection is preferred when possible, because this way we have less devascularization and less denervation of the intestinal segment since its irrigation and innervation run all the way to the mesocolon.

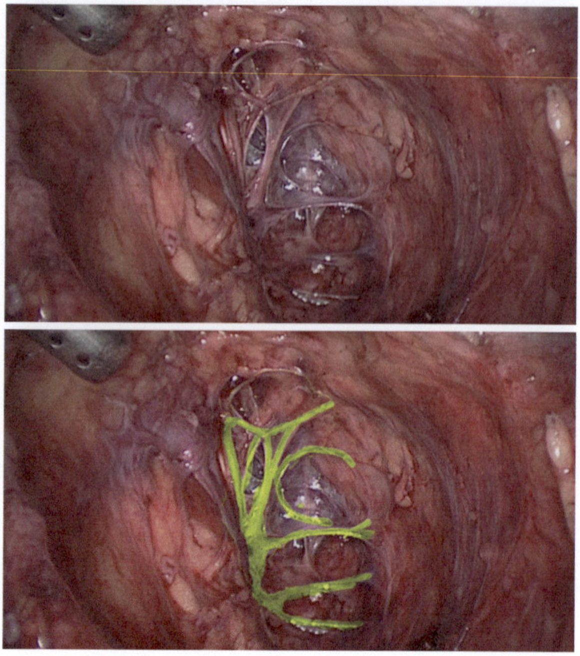

Fig. 8.25 Pelvic splanchnic nerves

Small Intestine

The small intestine consists of the duodenum, jejunum, and ileum. It is the main site for absorbing nutrients from the food ingested. It extends from the pylorus to the ileocecal junction.

In this chapter, we will discuss the ileum, which is of interest in addressing endometriosis.

The Ileum

This is the third part of the small intestine. Jejunum and ileum are approximately 6–7 m long; the ileum has about three-fifths of the intraperitoneal part of the small intestine. It is of importance for endometriosis because of its position in the right lower quadrant, with the terminal part being located in the pelvis (Fig. 8.26).

Arterial Irrigation

Superior mesenteric artery.

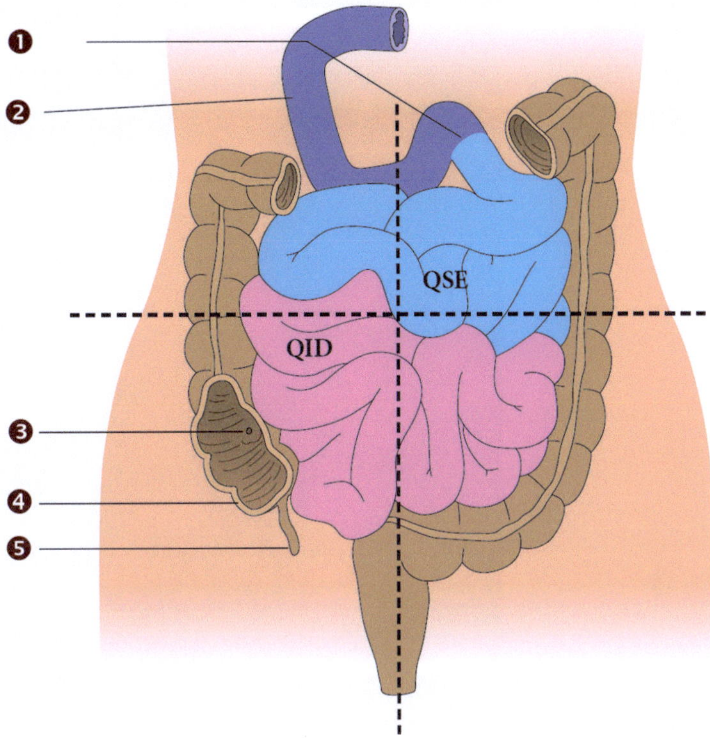

Fig. 8.26 Parts of the intestine. (1) Duodenojejunal flexure, (2) duodenum, (3) ileocecal junction, (4) cecum, (5) vermiform appendix

Anatomical Landmarks 16

Origin: Abdominal part of the aorta at L1.

Pathway: Follows between the layers of the mesentery, sending 15–18 branches to the jejunum and ileum. The arteries join to form the arterial arches (Fig. 8.27).

Anatomical Landmarks 17

Venous Irrigation

Drainage: Into the portal vein.

Path: Ends posteriorly to the pancreas, where it joins the splenic vein to form the portal vein.

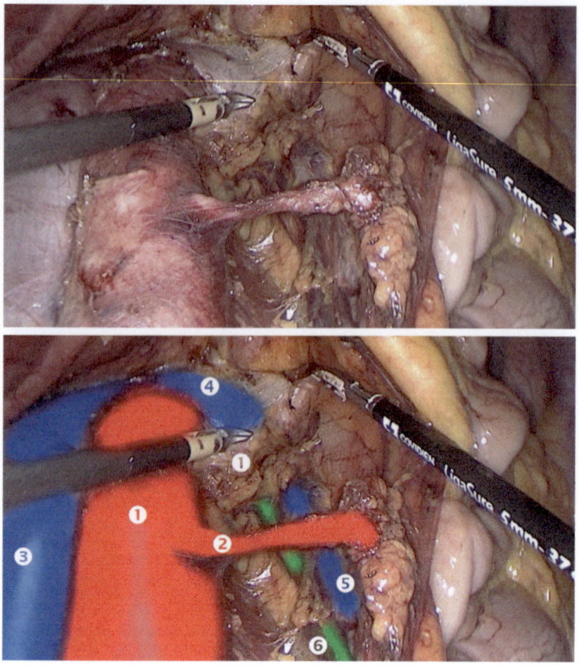

Fig. 8.27 Anatomical relations of the inferior mesenteric artery. (1) Aorta artery, (2) inferior mesenteric artery, (3) vena cava, (4) left renal vein, (5) left gonadal vein, (6) left ureter

Innervation

Anatomical Landmarks 18

Sympathetic

Origin: Vertebrae T8–T10.

Pathway: It reaches the superior mesenteric plexus through the sympathetic trunks and the thoracic abdominopelvic splanchnic nerves (major and minor).

Parasympathetic

Origin: Posterior vagal trunks.

Path: It reaches the superior mesenteric plexus through the sympathetic trunks and the abdominal pelvic thoracic splanchnic nerves (major, minor, and imo).

Bibliography

1. Abrão MS, Borelli GM, Clarizia R, Kho RM, Ceccaroni M. Strategies for management of colorectal endometriosis. Semin Reprod Med. 2017;35(1):65–71.
2. Baggish MS, Karram MM. Atlas de anatomia pélvica e cirurgia ginecológica. 4a ed. São Paulo: Elsevier; 2017.
3. De Cicco C, Corona R, Schonman R, Mailova K, Ussia A. Bowel resection for deep endometriosis: a systematic review. BJOG. 2011;118(3):285–91.
4. Kamina P. Anatomie clinique. 4a éd ed. Paris: Maloine; 2009.
5. Moore KL, Dalley AF, Agur AMR. Anatomia orientada para a clínica. 8a ed. Rio de Janeiro: Guanabara Koogan; 2011.
6. Possover M, Quakernack J, Chiantera V. The LANN technique to reduce postoperative functional morbidity in laparoscopic radical pelvic surgery. J Am Coll Surg. 2005;201(6):913–7.
7. Rock JA, Jones HW III. Te Linde's operative gynecology. 10th ed. Pennsylvania: Lippincott Williams & Wilkins; 2011.
8. Wattiez A, Puga M, Albornoz J, Faller E. Surgical strategy in endometriosis. Best Pract Res Clin Obstet Gynaecol. 2013;27(3):381–92.

Chapter 9
Urinary System

Beatriz Taliberti da Costa Porto, Deusdedit Cortez Vieira da Silva Neto, Fábio Sakae Kuteken, and Marina Miyuki Maekawa

Overview

Kidneys

Renal Anatomy

The kidneys are solid brownish-red parenchymatous organs with a lobulated surface (bean-like appearance), located bilaterally in the upper retroperitoneal space [1].

They measure approximately 10–12 cm vertically, 5–7 cm transversally, and 3 cm in the anteroposterior axis. They weigh about 130–150 g at home.

The left kidney lies between the body of the 12th thoracic vertebra and the top of the third lumbar vertebra, while the right kidney lies comparatively lower (due to

Supplementary Information The online version contains supplementary material available at https://doi.org/10.1007/978-3-031-63520-5_9.

B. T. da Costa Porto (✉) · M. M. Maekawa
Santa Casa São Paulo School of Medical Sciences (SCMSP), São Paulo, Brazil

Brazilian Federation of Gynecology and Obstetrics Associations (FEBRASGO), São Paulo, Brazil

D. C. V. da Silva Neto
Rede D'Or Sao Luiz, São Paulo, Brazil

F. S. Kuteken
Brazilian Federation of Gynecology and Obstetrics Associations (FEBRASGO), São Paulo, Brazil

Faculty of Medical Sciences, Santa Casa São Paulo School of Medical Sciences (SCMSP), São Paulo, Brazil

H. Salomão Ayroza, P. Ayroza Ribeiro (eds.), *Atlas of Laparoscopic Gynecological Anatomy*, https://doi.org/10.1007/978-3-031-63520-5_9

hepatic compression) between the first and third lumbar vertebrae. This positioning can change according to the degree of inspiration and the positioning of the patient.

Both kidneys have a spatial rotation, with the medial face rotated anteriorly in relation to the lateral face, at an angle of 30°. And the lower poles are arranged more laterally and anteriorly relative to the upper poles.

In the retroperitoneal space, the kidneys are surrounded by a fatty cushion and a fascia called the Gerota. It separates the kidneys and perirenal fat (internal to the Gerota) from adjacent structures and is an important anatomical barrier to the expansion of malignant tumors. This fascia is composed of an anterior and a posterior leaflet that meets and closes superiorly and laterally to the kidneys. The fusion of the two leaflets occurs laterally to the quadratus lumborum muscle; together they follow until they meet the transversalis fascia at Toldt's line (Fig. 9.1). This anatomy is important for access to the kidneys in transperitoneal laparoscopic surgeries (Figs. 9.2 and 9.3).

Toldt's line should be incised along its craniocaudal length into the parietocolic gutter on the side in question, and the colon and mesentery should be retracted medially to expose the kidney with the anterior leaflet of the Gerota still intact (Figs. 9.4 and 9.5). In their medial portion, the leaflets extend across the midline and do not meet, but the anterior leaflet has a loose adhesion with the connective tissue surrounding the aorta and vena cava, while the posterior leaflet has adhesions with the connective tissue anterior to the vertebrae. These adhesions are easily undone, and this is important for controlling the renal hilum even before access to the renal parenchyma and perirenal fat.

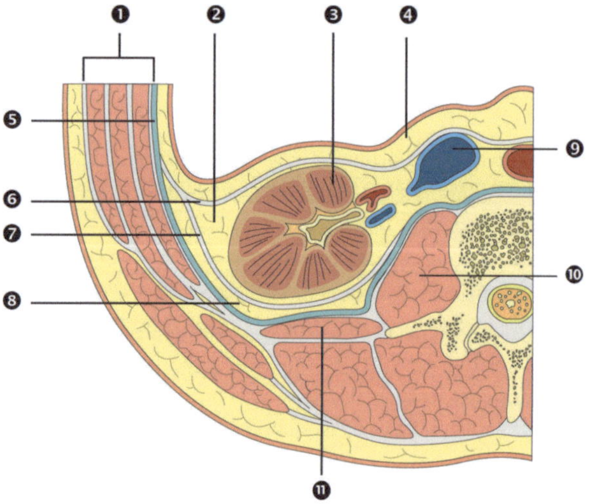

Fig. 9.1 Schematic representation of the retroperitoneum, showing the anatomical relationships of Gerota's fascia. (1) Anterolateral wall abdominal muscle, (2) perirenal fat, (3) kidney, (4) peritoneum, (5) transversalis fascia, (6) anterior leaflet, (7) anterior leaflet, (8) pararenal fat, (9) inferior vena cava, (10) psoas major muscle, (11) lumbar square muscle

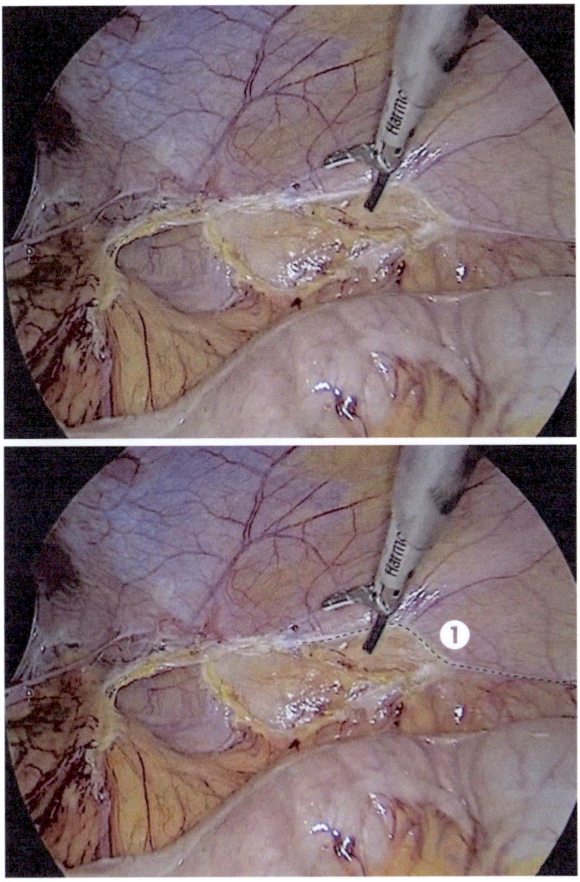

Fig. 9.2 Location of Toldt's line opening in the parietocolic drip (dashed line). (1) Toldt's line

The leaflets also do not fuse in their lower portion, creating a potential open space to the pelvis. The ureter descends into the pelvis in this virtual space between the two leaflets of Gerota's fascia. The Gerota is thinner inferiorly and is easily undone when the periureteral fat and the ureter itself, which rest on the psoas muscle, are dissected. Once the abdominal ureter is identified, its concomitant cranial and lateral tractions help in the exposure of the renal pelvis and the renal hilum. The pararenal fat (external to the Gerota) complements the composition of the retroperitoneum and helps support the kidneys (Fig. 9.5).

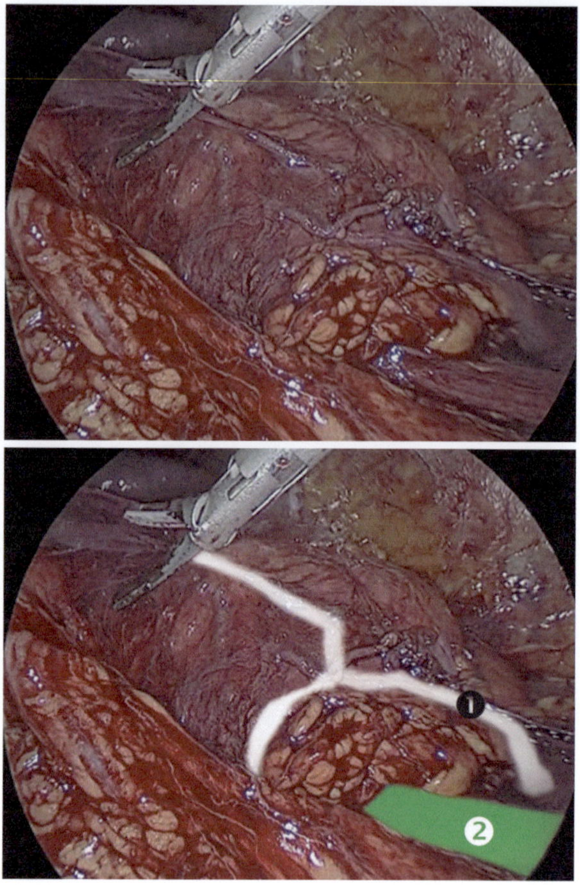

Fig. 9.3 Collapsed colon, ureter, and Gerota's fascia. (1) Gerota's fascia, (2) ureter

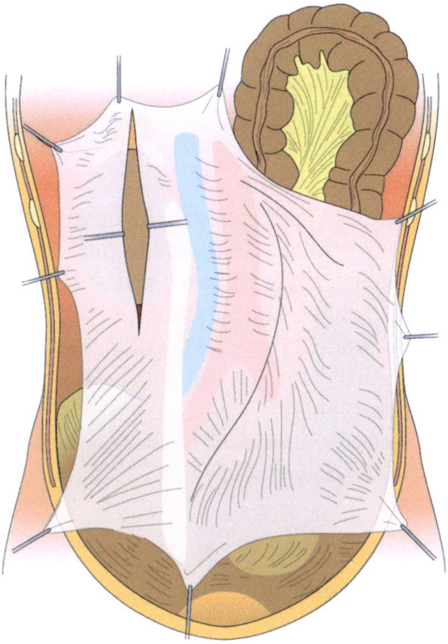

Fig. 9.4 Schematic representation of the medially folded colon and the exposed Gerota over kidney and ureter

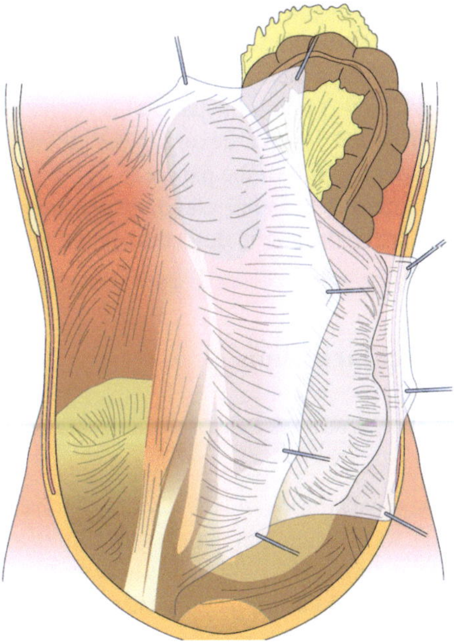

Fig. 9.5 Schematic representation of the posterior leaflet of Gerota's fascia encompassing kidney, perirenal fat, and ureter

Topographic Anatomy

Right Kidney

Limits

Posterior: Upper pole with diaphragm muscle and 12th rib; lower pole with psoas muscle (medial) and quadratus lumborum muscle (lateral).

Cranial: Right adrenal gland and posteroinferior aspect of the liver. At this point, the parietal peritoneum forms the hepatorenal ligament.

Inferior: Hepatic flexure of the colon and loops of the small intestine.

Medial: Close contact with the descending portion of the duodenum; elements of the renal hilum.

Anterior: Border of the liver and adrenal gland (upper pole); hepatic flexure of the colon (lower pole).

Left Kidney

Limits

Posterior: Upper pole with diaphragm muscle and 12th rib; lower pole with psoas muscle (medial) and quadratus lumborum muscle (lateral).

Cranial: Splenic vessels of the left adrenal gland (medial); spleen (laterosuperior). At this point, the parietal peritoneum forms the splenorenal ligament.

Inferior: Splenic flexure of the colon.

Medial: Tail of the pancreas and elements of the renal hilum.

Anterior: Adrenal gland, spleen and tail of the pancreas (upper pole); splenic flexure of the colon, descending colon and jejunum (lower pole).

Vascularization

Arterial

The renal arteries, classically unique on each side, are direct branches of the abdominal aorta, originating just below the superior mesenteric artery at the second vertebral column. The right renal artery exits the aorta laterally and runs anteroposteriorly to the renal hilum, passing behind the inferior vena cava (Fig. 9.6). The left renal artery also runs in a posteroinferior direction (due to the 30° anterior angulation of the renal hilum) and goes directly to the medial surface of the kidney. Both arteries issue branches to the adrenals, the renal pelvis, and the ureters before reaching the hilorenal. These branches may exit either the renal artery or one of its direct segmental branches (Figs. 9.7 and 9.8).

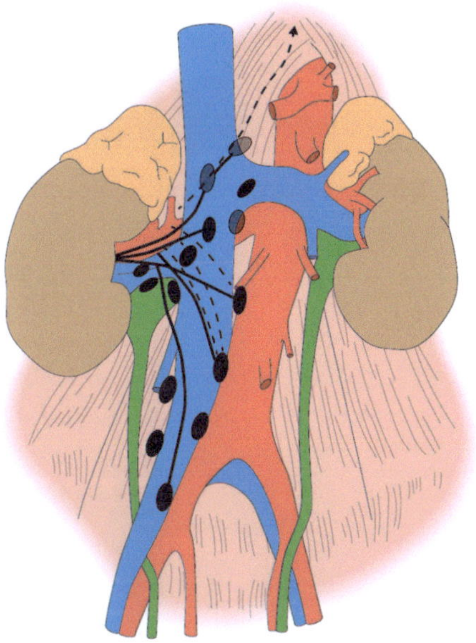

Fig. 9.6 Right renal artery and its anatomical relationships and lymphatic drainage of the left kidney

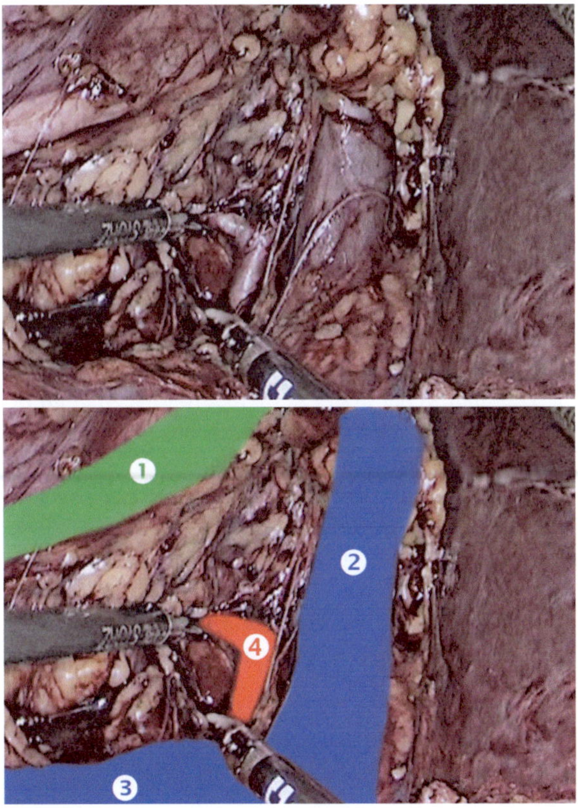

Fig. 9.7 Right kidney and ureter, retracted laterosuperiorly, exposing the renal vein and the bifurcated renal artery. The inferior vena cava is also visible. (1) Ureter, (2) renal vein, (3) inferior vena cava, (4) bifurcated renal artery

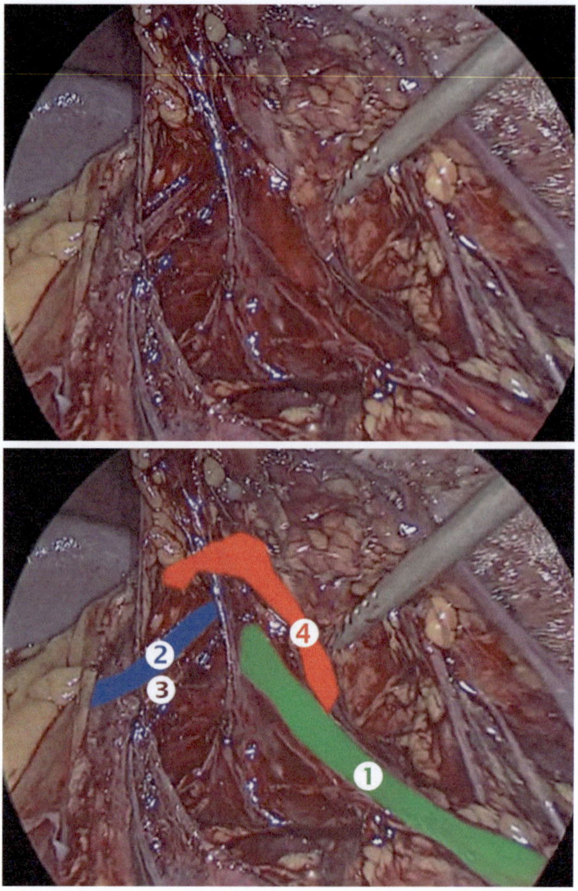

Fig. 9.8 Left kidney folded laterocranially, showing left renal vein, left renal artery, renal pelvis, and ureter. (1) Ureter, (2) renal vein, (3) renal pelvis, (4) renal artery

The renal arteries reach the renal hilum, where they will be in close contact with the ipsilateral renal vein and renal pelvis. All these structures in the renal hilum are surrounded and protected by the renal sinus fat (part of the perirenal fat).

The main renal artery is divided into segmental branches. They are called segmental because each of these branches irrigates a specific segment of the kidney, with no collateral circulation or communication between them. Occlusion of one of these branches, therefore, will cause segmental renal infarction. Already within the renal parenchyma, these segmental arteries subdivide, sequentially forming the lobar, interlobar, arcuate, and interlobular arteries, until reaching the afferent arteries.

Classically, the first segmental branch emitted is the posterior branch, and this occurs even before the renal artery enters the kidney. The anterior branches may appear before or after entering the kidney; they are typically divided into apical, superior, medial, and inferior. As it is the first to issue, the posterior branch usually follows posterior to the renal pelvis before entering the renal parenchyma.

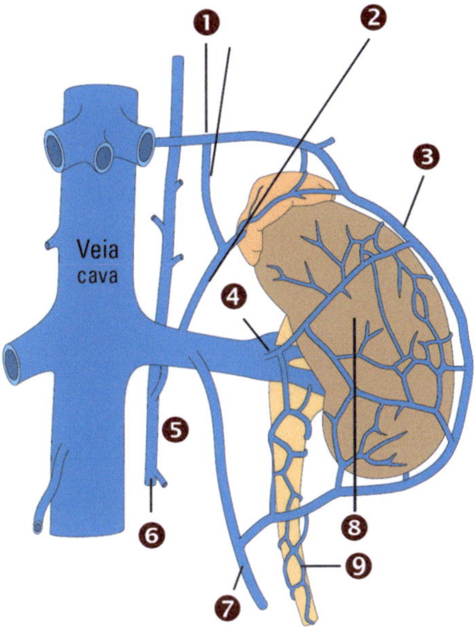

Fig. 9.9 Schematic representation of renal venous drainage showing the extensive communication between the different venous plexuses. (1) Inferior phrenic, (2) adrenal, (3) capsular, (4) renal, (5) lumbar, (6) lumbar vein, (7) gonadal, (8) capsular plexus, (9) urethral plexus

Variations in renal vascular anatomy are not uncommon, affecting 25–40% of individuals. The most frequent variation is the supernumerary renal arteries, with up to five renal arteries in a same side. Supernumerary veins are less frequent. In case of variation in renal positioning (e.g., pelvic kidneys), supernumerary arteries are even more likely.

Venous

Renal venous drainage is closely matched to the arterial supply. The interlobular veins successively form the arcuate, interlobar, lobar, and segmental veins, all following parallel to the corresponding arteries. Unlike the segmental arteries, the segmental veins join together to form a true venous network between them. Therefore, the eventual occlusion of one of these veins has no repercussion for the venous drainage of the kidney (Fig. 9.9).

The right renal vein is usually 2–4 cm long and enters directly into the posterolateral aspect of the inferior vena cava (Figs. 9.6 and 9.9). The left renal vein is longer (between 6 and 10 cm) and, before reaching the lateral aspect of the vena cava, crosses posteriorly the superior mesenteric artery and anteriorly the aorta. Because it is longer, the left renal vein generally receives as affluents the adrenal vein, the inferior lumbar vein, and the left gonadal vein (which flows at an angle of 90° with the renal vein). The right renal vein does not usually receive branches in its path.

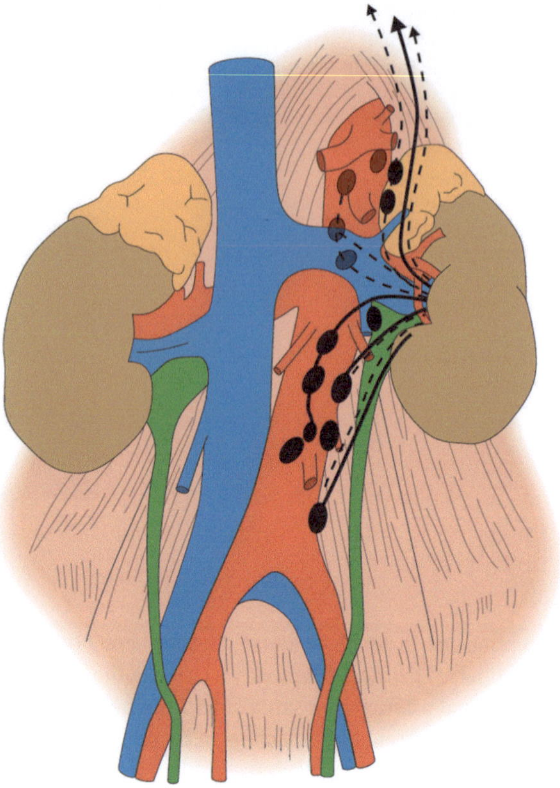

Fig. 9.10 Lymphatic drainage of the right kidney

Lymphatics

The renal lymphatic vessels, with lymphatic inflows from the ureter, renal capsule, and perirenal tissue, drain locally to the hilar lymph nodes; from there, distinct drains follow between the sides: right: right paracaval and interaortocaval lymph nodes (Fig. 9.10), and left: left para-aortic lymph nodes (Fig. 9.6). Eventually, both sides may present drainage to retrocrural lymph nodes. The left side, in turn, may drain directly into the thoracic duct.

Renal Innervation

Sympathetic

These are preganglionic nerves that originate from the thoracolumbar segments and proceed to the celiac and aortorenal ganglia. From there, postganglionic fibers reach the kidney via the autonomic plexus that follows the arterial supply.

- Function: Vasoconstriction

Parasympathetic

Involves fibers of the vagus nerve that go to the kidney through the autonomic plexus, along the renal artery.

- Function: Vasodilation

Bladder

Anatomy

The bladder is a musculomembranous organ, located between the ureters and urethra, and has the function of storing urine. It measures 6 × 5 cm and, when full of urine, it can double in size, with a physiological filling capacity of 500 mL, when it assumes an ovoid shape, coming out of the true pelvis. The empty bladder has a tetrahedral shape with an upper face, from where the urachus exits, which is covered by the visceral peritoneum, and laterally the peritoneum makes a groove called the paravesical fossa; two inferolateral surfaces, covered by perivesical fat and by umbilical-prevesical fascia; and a posteroinferior surface, or base surface, with the bladder neck at the lowest part, which is located between 3 and 4 cm from the symphysis pubis.

The urachus is composed of smooth muscle tissue, 2 mm in diameter and 12 cm long, and connects the bladder to the abdominal wall; near the umbilical scar, it has a more fibrous structure and fuses with one of the obliterated umbilical arteries and is covered by the umbilical-prevesical fascia.

Topographic Anatomy

The base of the bladder and urethra rest on the anterior vaginal wall and uterus and are tightly connected laterally to the levator ani muscle. The contraction of the pelvic diaphragm raises the bladder neck in an anterior direction. In women with urge urinary incontinence, the bladder neck lies below the symphysis pubis. In infancy, the bladder neck is at the height of the upper edge of the symphysis pubis. In puberty, the bladder migrates to the true pelvis. The portion of the bladder fundus that lies above the trigone is located in the supravaginal region of the cervix, forming the vesicouterine septum. The portion just behind the trigone lies in the anterior vaginal wall, forming the vesicovaginal septum.

Bladder Ligaments

- Median umbilical: remnant of the urachus (Fig. 9.11).
- Anterior vesical: from the bladder neck to the symphysis pubis, contains the clitoral vein (Fig. 9.12).

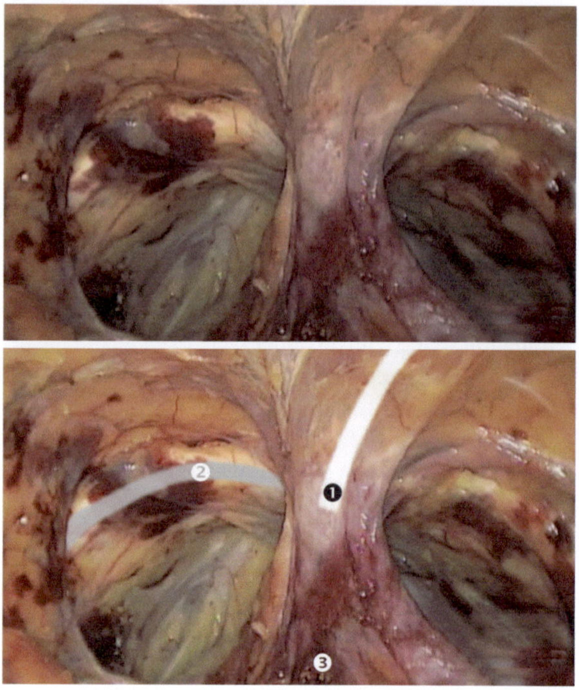

Fig. 9.11 Retzius space dissected. (1) Median umbilical ligament, (2) Cooper's ligament, (3) bladder

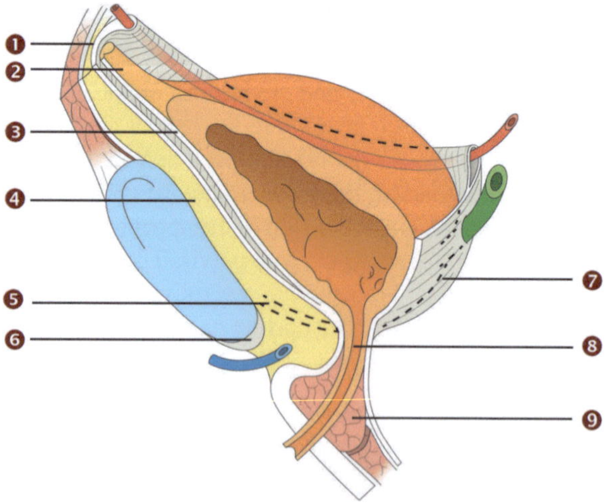

Fig. 9.12 Bladder ligaments. (1) Umbilical-prevesical fascia, (2) median umbilical ligament, (3) vesical fascia, (4) retropubic space, (5) pubovesical ligament, (6) inferior pubic ligament, (7) retrovesical fascia, (8) urethra, and (9) sphincter of the urethra

- Lateral vesical: from the underside of the bladder to the paracervix, contains the superior vesical artery.
- Vesicouterine: from the vesical fundus to the uterine neck, just above the vagina (anterior vesical pillar).

Bladder Structure

The bladder wall is 8–15 mm thick when empty and 2–5 mm when full.

- External tunica: composed of the tunica adventitia, or vesical fascia, and serosa. The tunica adventitia is rich in small autonomous ganglia.
- Muscular tunica or detrusor muscle: composed of muscle tissue and connective tissue (57%); it has a muscular arrangement of complex mesh, without forming distinct layers, which allows the detrusor muscle to happen in a harmonious way, compressing the urine towards the proximal urethra during urination.
- Internal tunica: constituted of a polymorphic epithelium, called urothelium, which rests on the lamina propria.

The inner surface of the bladder is covered by an epithelium that appears to be smooth when the bladder is full, but contracts when the bladder is empty. The urothelium is made up of six layers of cells that rest on the basement membrane. Deeper down, the lamina propria forms a relatively thick layer of fibroelastic connective tissue that allows bladder distension; this layer is traversed by numerous blood vessels and contains a few smooth muscle fibers forming the muscular layer of the mucosa (Fig. 9.13). Below this layer is the smooth muscle of the bladder wall, which consists of large interwoven muscle fibers. This aspect of the detrusor muscle allows the emptying of the spherical organ.

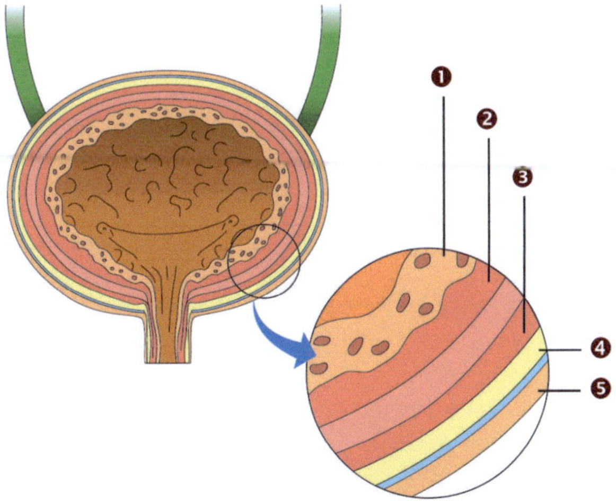

Fig. 9.13 Bladder wall, showing urothelium, lamina propria, muscle layer, perivesical fat, and peritoneum. (1) Urothelial layer, (2) lamina propria, (3) muscle, (4) perivesical fat, (5) peritoneum

Bladder Trigone

As the ureter approaches the bladder, its smooth muscle layer, with a spiral, follows a longitudinal orientation. Then, 2 or 3 cm from the bladder, a fibromuscular layer (Waldeyer's) extends longitudinally over the ureter and follows into the trigone. The ureter enters the bladder longitudinally, crossing 1.5–2 cm, and ends at the ureteral ostium. As it passes through the detrusor muscle hiatus (intramural ureter), considerable compression and narrowing occur, and it is a common site of ureteral stone impaction. The bladder trigone is a region between the two ureteral ostia (with a distance between them of 2.5 cm) and the urethral meatus (with a distance of 2–3 cm), composed of smooth-looking urothelium (Fig. 9.14). In this region, the detrusor muscle fibers do not have an irregular arrangement and in all directions, as in the rest of the bladder, being composed of three layers:

- Superficial: originating from the longitudinal layer of the ureter.
- Deep: continuous with the Waldeyer's fibromuscular layer, which inserts into the bladder neck.
- Detrusor pp. dicta: formed by external longitudinal and internal circular fibers.

This fact is important because when there is contraction of the trigone, the ureteral ostia are pulled caudally, towards the bladder neck, increasing the ureterovesical resistance and preventing ureteral reflux during bladder filling.

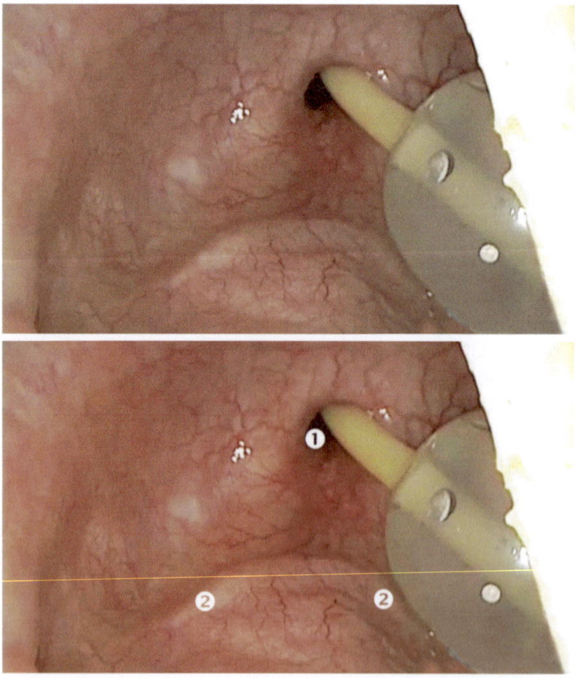

Fig. 9.14 Laparoscopic view after bladder opening. (1) Urethral ostium, (2) ureteral meatus

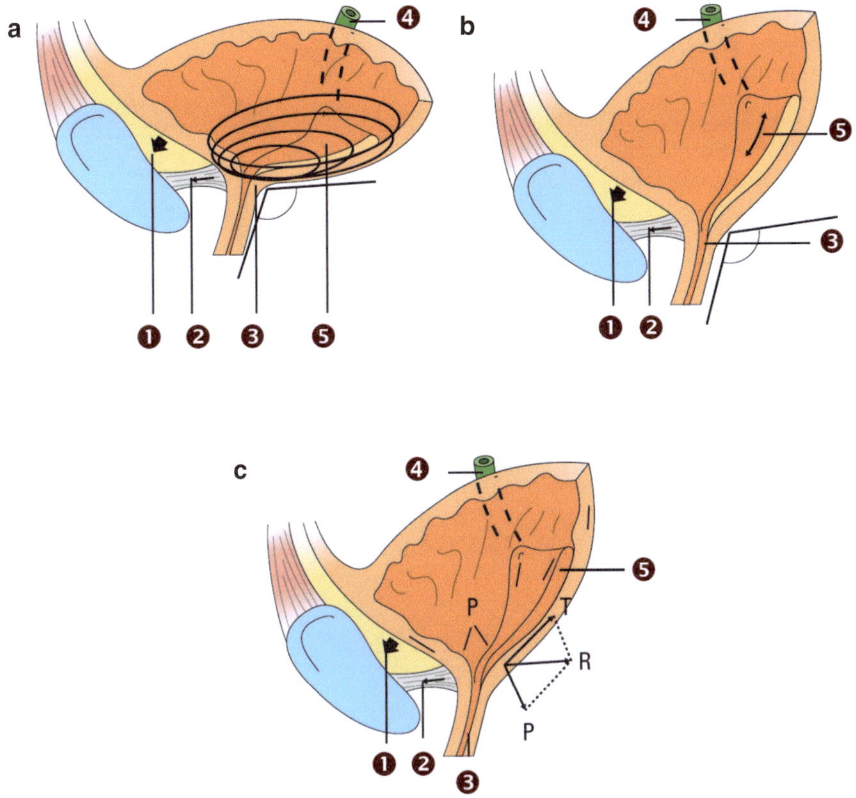

Fig. 9.15 Anatomy of urination: (**a**) detrusor muscle contraction; (**b**) formation of the trigone funnel; (**c**) opening of the bladder neck. (1) Connective tissue of the retropubic space; (2) pubovesical ligament; (3) bladder neck; (4) ureter, and (5) bladder trigone. P = intravesical pressure; T = parietal pressure

In addition, with contraction of the trigone, there is decreased resistance of the bladder neck, which facilitates urination (Fig. 9.15).

The intravesical portion of the ureter is located well below the urothelium; in its posterior part, it presents a firm and thick layer of detrusor muscle. With bladder filling and increasing bladder pressure, there is a passive closing of the ureter, just like a valve (Fig. 9.16).

Bladder Neck

It represents the transition site between the bladder and the urethra. It has muscle fibers of the tunica externa, which constrict the neck, forming a cervical loop.

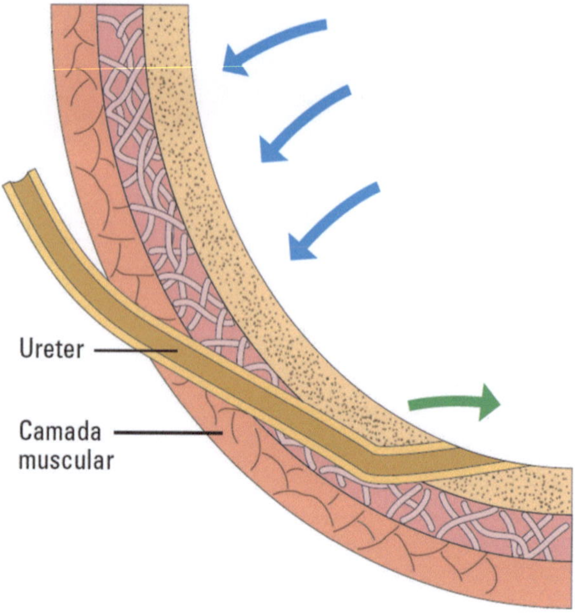

Fig. 9.16 Contraction of the trigone, pulling the ureter caudally (green arrow). Ureteral compression from increased bladder pressure by filling the bladder (blue arrows)

Vascularization

The bladder is irrigated by branches of the internal iliac artery.

- Superior vesical artery: responsible for the major arterial support of the bladder; it originates from the umbilical artery, containing one to four branches (Figs. 9.17 and 9.18).
- Vaginal artery: it irrigates the bladder and is formed by branches that join the uterine artery or the rectus medius artery (Fig. 9.19).
- Branches of the uterine artery, the pudendal artery, and the obturator artery.

The venous drainage from the bladder follows to the bladder plexus and is done to the internal iliac vein. Whereas the lymphatic drainage goes to (Fig. 9.19):

- Medial external iliac lymph nodes
- Obturator lymph nodes
- Internal iliac lymph nodes
- Interiliac lymph nodes

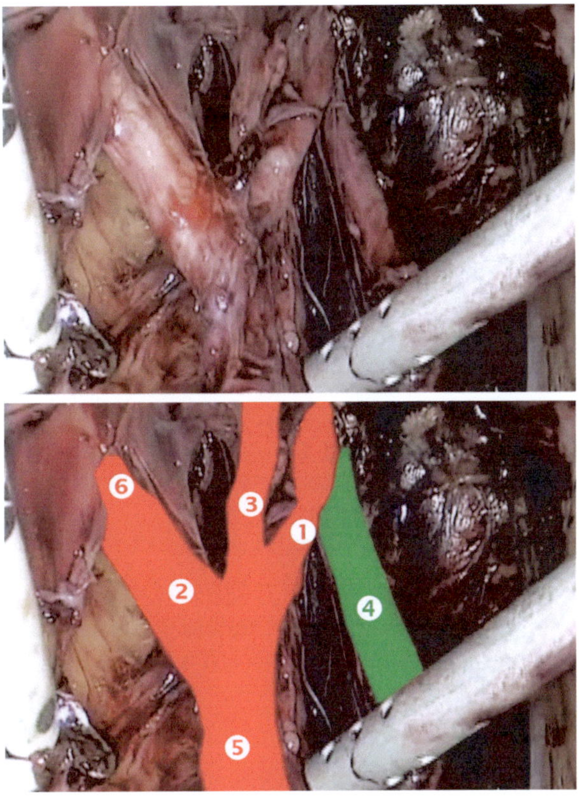

Fig. 9.17 Superior vesical artery originating from the umbilical artery. (1) Uterine artery, (2) umbilical artery, (3) superior vesical arteries, (4) ureter, (5) hypogastric artery, (6) obliterated umbilical artery

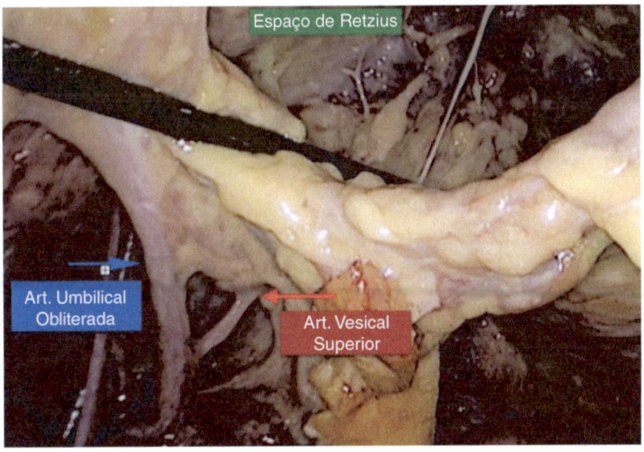

Fig. 9.18 Superior vesical artery (red arrow), obliterated umbilical artery (blue arrow), and dissected Retzius space (green)

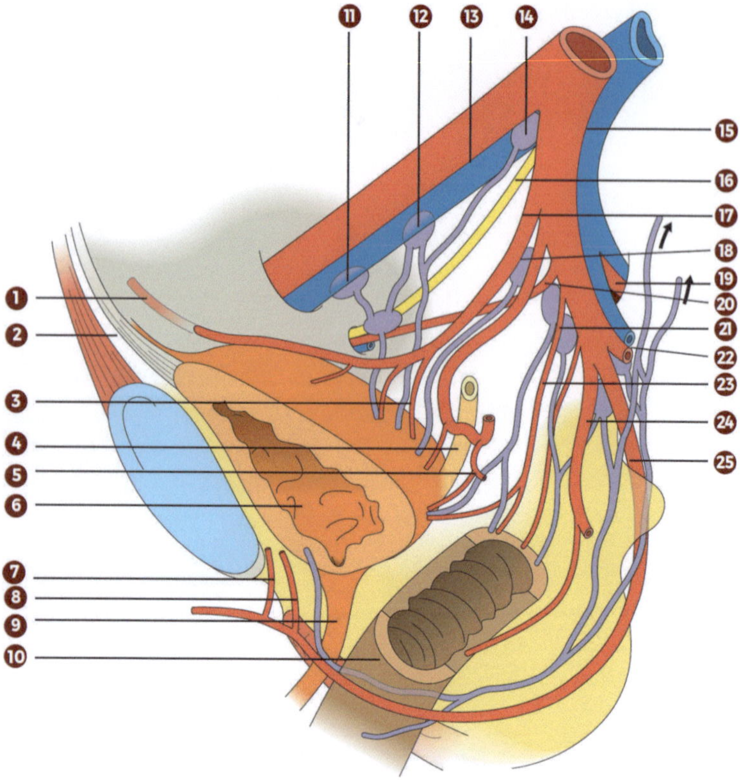

Fig. 9.19 Irrigation and drainage (lymphatic and venous) of the bladder: (1) medial umbilical ligament, (2) median umbilical ligament, (3) superior vesical arteries, (4) ureter, (5) vesicovaginal artery, (6) bladder, (7) retrosymphyseal artery, (8) anterior vesical artery, (9) urethra, (10) vagina, (11) obturator lymph node, (12) medial external iliac lymph node, (13) external iliac artery and vein, (14) interiliac lymph node, (15) internal iliac artery and vein, (16) obturator nerve, (17) umbilical artery, (18) internal iliac lymph nodes, (19) superior gluteal artery and vein, (20) obturator artery, (21) uterine artery, (22) inferior gluteal artery and vein, (23) vaginal arteries, (24) middle rectal artery, (25) internal pudendal artery

Innervation

The innervation of the bladder originates in the inferior hypogastric plexus, containing both sympathetic and parasympathetic fibers (Fig. 9.20). The hypogastric nerve is responsible for proprioception, bladder filling, and contraction of the internal sphincter of the urethra. It originates in the superior hypogastric plexus, derived from the sympathetic trunk, of thoracic origin.

The hypogastric nerve lesion can cause loss of proprioception and stress urinary incontinence.

The splanchnic nerves are parasympathetic, originating in S2 and S4, and with the hypogastric nerve form the inferior hypogastric plexus. They are responsible for

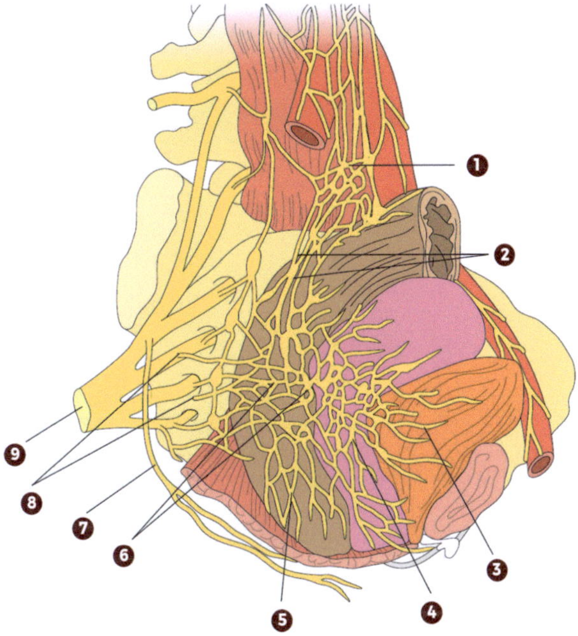

Fig. 9.20 Bladder innervation, highlighting lower hypogastric plexus, hypogastric nerve, and splanchnic nerves: sacral plexus, splanchnic nerves, pudendal nerve, lower hypogastric plexus, rectal fibers, vaginal fibers, bladder fibers, hypogastric nerve, and upper hypogastric plexus: (1) upper hypogastric plexus, (2) hypogastric nerve, (3) bladder fibers (IHP), (4) vaginal fibers (IHP), (5) rectal fibers (IHP), (6) lower hypogastric plexus, (7) pudendal nerve, (8) splanchnic nerves S2–S4, (9) sacral roots

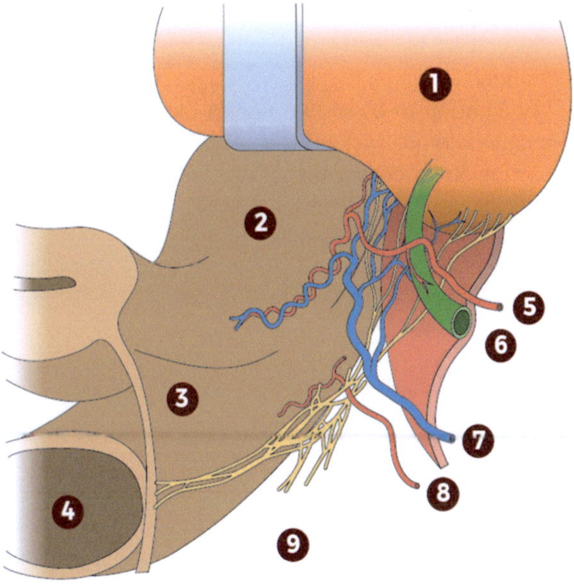

Fig. 9.21 Lower hypogastric plexus one level below the middle rectal artery and the deep uterine vein: (1) bladder, (2) uterine cervix, (3) uterosacral ligament, (4) rectum, (5) uterine artery, (6) ureter, (7) deep uterine vein, (8) middle rectal artery, (9) anterior hypogastric plexus

the contraction of the detrusor muscle, inhibiting signals to the internal sphincter, and for nociception (pain) (Fig. 9.9).

In pelvic surgery, it is possible to identify them by dissecting one level below the middle rectal artery or the deep uterine vein (Fig. 9.21).

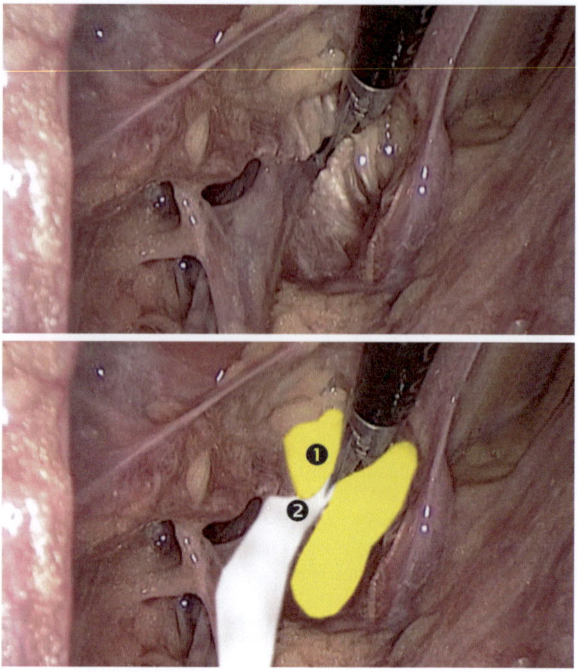

Fig. 9.22 Pudendal nerve evidenced after sectioning the sacrospinal ligament. (1) Pudendal nerve, (2) sacrospinal ligament

Lesion of the pelvic splanchnic nerves can cause bladder atony and urinary retention.

In addition to these two nerves mentioned above, there is the pudendal nerve (somatic nervous system) (Fig. 9.22), which allows conscious control of urination by acting on the contraction of the striated sphincter of the urethra and anus; it determines the urethral and perineal sensitivity. Bladder filling is detected by the urethra and the trigone of the bladder.

Lesion of the pudendal nerve can cause perineal pain, especially in the vagina and clitoris.

Ureters

Knowledge of the anatomy of the ureters is very important, especially when it comes to surgical dissection in the treatment of pelvic diseases. Inadvertent injury to the ureters can cause harm to the patient, and, legally, the literature shows that the physician has no backing in this regard, even when dealing with deep disease and distorted anatomy (Jha S, 2015).

The ureters are bilateral tubular tubes or organs that are located retroperitoneally in the pelvis (Fig. 9.14). Both measure approximately 22–30 cm in length and 5–12 mm in diameter and have the function of carrying urine from the renal pelvis

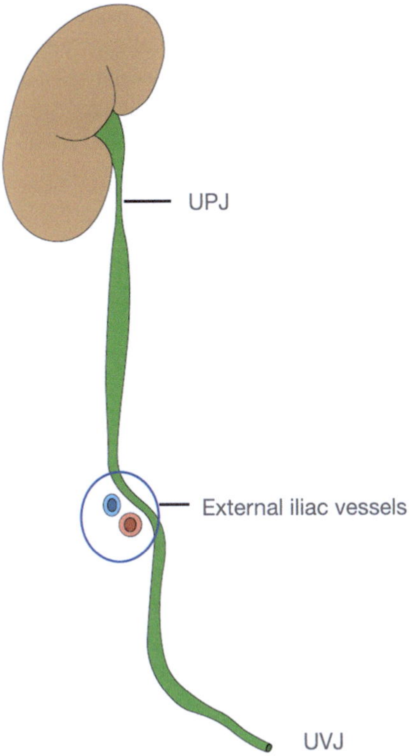

Fig. 9.23 Narrowing of the ureter: (1) ureteropelvic junction (UPJ), (2) iliac vessels, and (3) ureterovesical junction (UVJ)

to the bladder. They have minimal absorption, with dynamics and movement. As for their diameter, points of decreased caliber are observed in both ureters, known as regions of narrowing, located at the ureteropelvic junction, at the crossing of the ilia, and at the ureterovesical junction (Fig. 9.23).

- At the ureteropelvic junction (UPJ), the first narrowing site, the renal pelvis tapers into the proximal ureter, inferior to this junction. The ureters have a descending and retroperitoneal path in the medial region of the psoas muscle. In this narrowing, there is no evidence of obstruction even on radiographic or endoscopic investigation.
- The second region of narrowing occurs when the ureter crosses the iliac vessels. This occurs by a combination of extrinsic compression of the ureter by the iliac vessels and the necessary anterior angulation of the ureter when it crosses the iliac vessels to enter the pelvis. There is also no intrinsic change in ureteral caliber at this site.
- The third site of narrowing seen in a normal ureter is at the ureterovesical junction (UVJ). There is a true physical restriction of the ureter, as the intramural passage is through the bladder wall to the ureteral orifice.

These three sites of ureteral narrowing are clinically significant as they are common sites during the passage of urinary calculi. In addition, the angulation of the ureter, first anteriorly as it passes through the iliac vessels and then posteromedially as it enters the pelvis and runs behind the bladder, may restrict proper passage of rigid endoscopes. An appreciation of this normal angulation and the three-dimensional course of the ureter is critical to safe and successful ureteral endoscopy (Fig. 9.23).

Histology of the Ureters

Histologically, the ureters have three layers: mucosa, muscular, and adventitia (Figs. 9.24 and 9.25).

- The mucosal layer (innermost) has its own lamina and epithelium and is formed by four to five layers of epithelial cells; the most superficial cells present a thickening in the apical region, besides being larger and flatter. In the mucosal layer, a transitional epithelium is noted, that is, several layers of cells with different formats. Its epithelial cells are supported by a basal membrane, and, just below it, there is a layer of connective tissue called the lamina propria or chorion [2, 3].
- The muscle layer (Figs. 9.15 and 9.16), an intermediate layer, has smooth muscle fibers and is divided into an inner and outer longitudinal layer with circular fibers.
- The outermost layer, which covers the ureter, is called adventitia; it is located near the mesoureter and has internally vessels, nerves, and fatty tissue (Fig. 9.24).

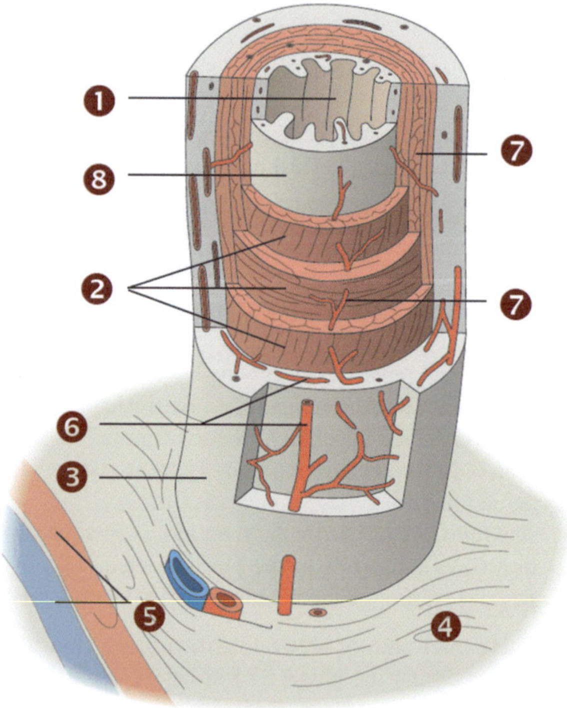

Fig. 9.24 Ureteral histology. (1) Mucosa, (2) muscular, (3) adventitia, (4) mesoureter, (5) artery and vein, (6) vascular plexus, (7) perforating arteries, (8) mucosa vascular plexus

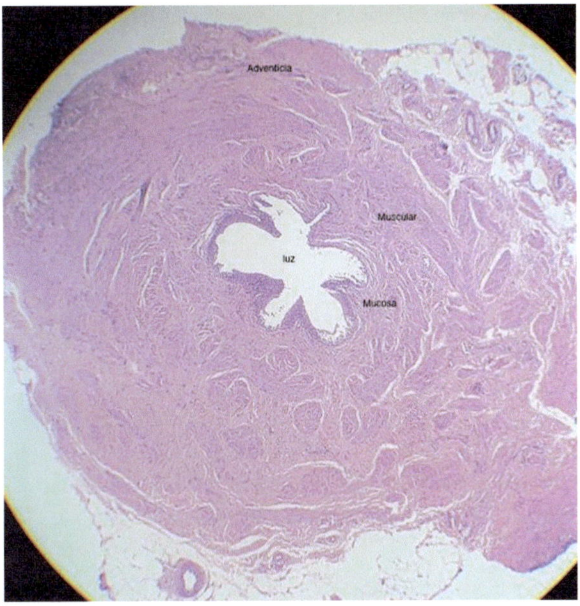

Fig. 9.25 Hematoxylin-eosin-stained ureter; original magnification (AO) 40 times. The three histological layers of the ureter (adventitia, muscular, and mucosa)

Tips and Tricks 1
In ureterolysis, it is important to know that when dissecting the outer (adventitia) layer of the ureter, there is no risk of ureteral fistula, but if it is necessary to advance to the intermediate (muscular) layer, fistula may occur. In deeper ureteral lesions, therefore, it is suggested to place a double-J catheter in the intraoperative stage, allowing the ureter to recover in its integrity.

Vascularization

The ureter has no vessel of its own. It receives blood supply from multiple arterial branches along its path until it penetrates the urinary bladder. The arterial branches of the abdominal ureter are located medially to the pelvis; in the pelvic ureter, the vascularization is lateral. This information is useful mainly when the ureters are dissected in a surgical procedure, thus being able to preserve their vascularization or avoid unnecessary bleeding.

In the abdominal ureter, the branches originate from the renal artery, the gonadal artery, the abdominal aorta, and the common iliac artery.

As for the pelvic ureter, the branches come from the internal iliac artery and the bladder and uterine arteries (Figs. 9.26, 9.27, and 9.28); some authors also place the middle vaginal and the middle rectal arteries among the branches (Fig. 9.29). After reaching the ureter, the arterial vessels run longitudinally through the periureteral

Fig. 9.26 Surgical image of the relationship of the vessels to the left pelvic ureter: (1) uterine artery, (2) superior vesical artery, (3) internal iliac artery, (4) ureter

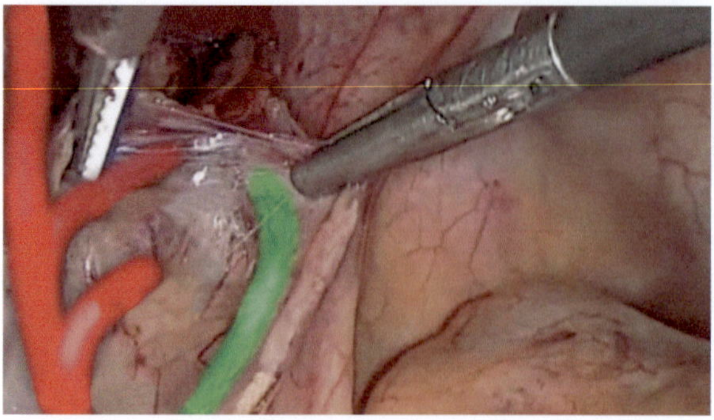

Fig. 9.27 Ureter and its relationship to the pelvic infundibulum and the left hypogastric artery. (1) Left ureter, (2) obliterated umbilical artery, (3) pelvic infundibulum, (4) left uterine artery, (5) ureter vascularization

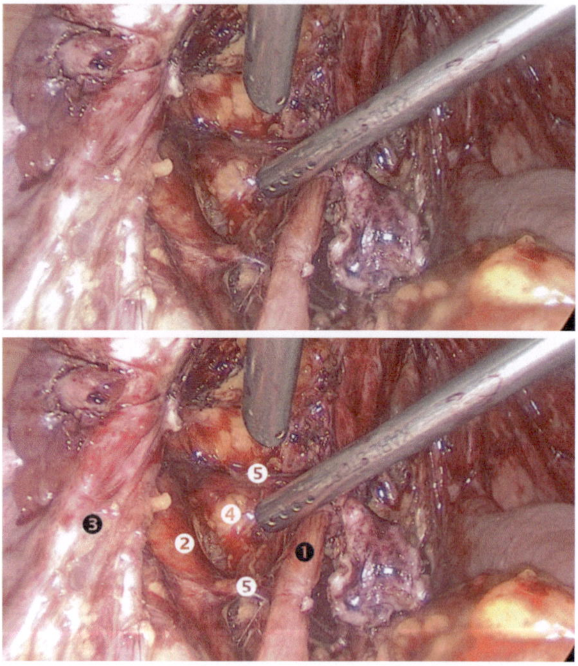

Fig. 9.28 Relationship of the ureter to the uterine artery: (1) ureter, (2) uterine artery

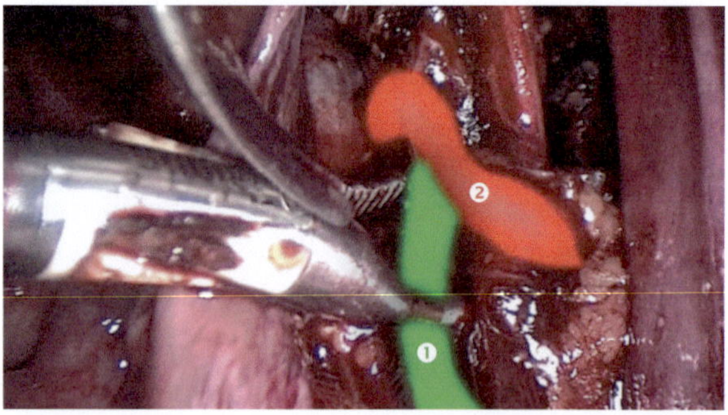

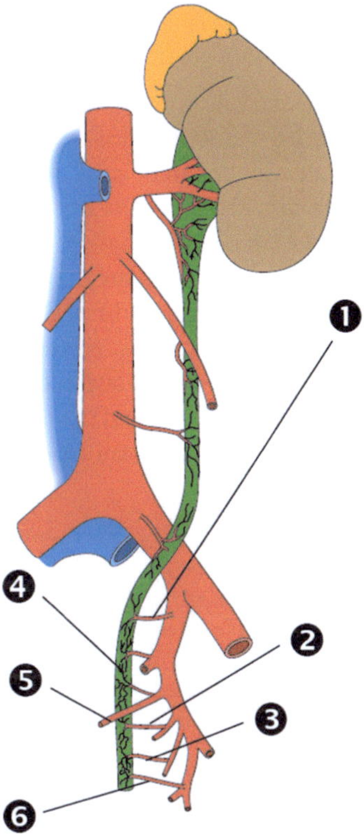

Fig. 9.29 Vascularization of the ureter: (1) common Iliac, (2) rectal middle, (3) vaginal, (4) superior vesical, (5) uterine, (6) inferior vesical

adventitia, which allows safe mobilization of the ureter by the surrounding retroperitoneal tissues, without compromising the vascular supply, provided that the periureteral adventitia is not removed. The venous and lymphatic drainage of the ureter is parallel to the arterial supply.

The lymphatic drainage of the ureters follows a similar path as the arterial supply and varies according to the point where the ureter is located. In the pelvis, drainage comes from the internal, external, and common iliac vessels. In the abdomen, the left para-aortic lymph nodes are the main drainage site for the left ureter, while the abdominal portion of the right ureter is drained primarily to the right paracaval and interaortocaval lymph nodes. The lymphatic drainage of the abdominal ureter and renal pelvis tends to join the renal lymphatics. The middle portion of the ureters drains to lymph nodes associated with common iliac vessels; the lower portion of the home ureter drains to lymph nodes associated with internal and external iliac vessels.

Tips and Tricks 2

When performing ureterolysis, it is important to know that the vascularization of the abdominal ureter—and therefore with a higher risk of bleeding—is concentrated medially, and that of the pelvic ureter, laterally. Thus, in the dissection of the abdominal region, the strategy is lateral, and in the pelvic, medial.

Innervation

The innervation of the ureter is not completely known. Its peristalsis has no direct external nervous intervention, being propagated by the intrinsic smooth muscle, located in the minor calyces of the renal collecting system (when the kidney is filled with urine, the ureters initiate their contractility). The autonomic nervous system exerts some effect on modulation during this process, receiving preganglionic sympathetic fibers from the thoracic T10 to the lumbar spinal segments. Postganglionic fibers arise from various ganglia in the hypogastric, upper and lower autonomic plexuses. The most important nerve preservation of the ureter is concentrated in its distal portion, more specifically in the nerve branches originating from the lower hypogastric plexus and the bladder plexus (Fig. 9.30), because a lesion in this region results in bladder dysfunction (Figs. 9.30, 9.31, and 9.32).

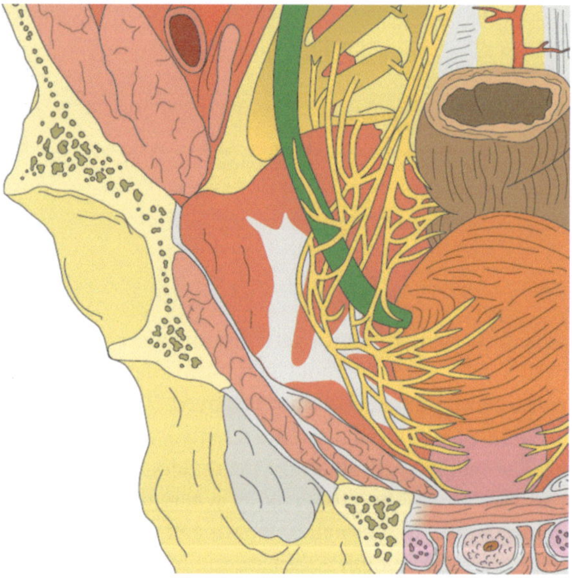

Fig. 9.30 Distal ureter innervation. Ureter in green and inferior hypogastric plexus in yellow

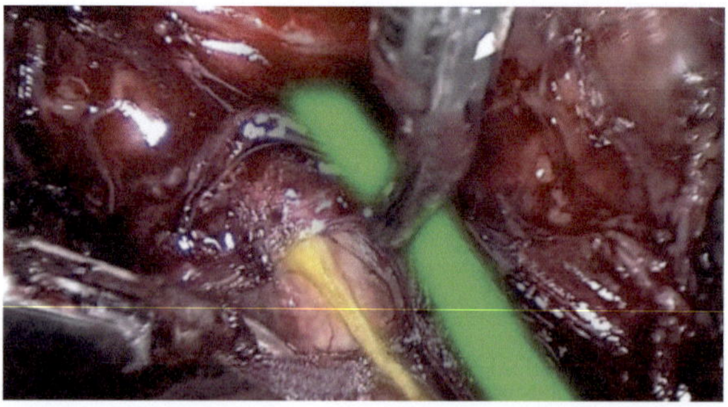

Fig. 9.31 Surgical image of the ureter and its relationship to the hypogastric nerve. Ureter (in green) and hypogastric nerve (in yellow)

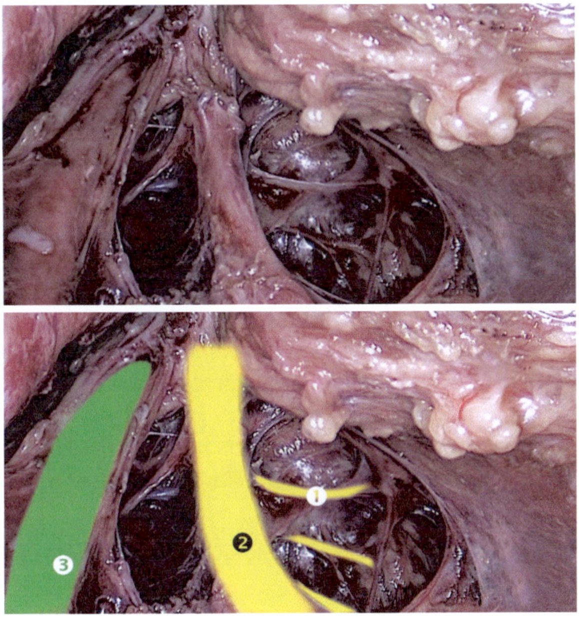

Fig. 9.32 Anatomical relations of the ureter with parasympathetic innervation: (1) splanchnic nerves, (2) inferior hypogastric plexus, (3) left ureter

An obstructive or inflammatory process in the ureter generates a clinical picture according to its location. In the abdominal and pelvic ureters, the referring dermatomes are from T8 to Tl2, generating pain that can vary from the infrascapular region to the region of the labia majora.

Tips and Tricks 3
In the case of the distal ureter, a wide dissection should be avoided, because the lower hypogastric plexus is observed anterior and posterior to the ureter, more specifically in the bladder branch; thus, if there is a lesion, this may cause bladder dysfunction.

Tips and Tricks 4
Unnecessary dissections of the periureteral connective tissue can significantly reduce ureteral compliance and, consequently, renal function.

Topographic Anatomy

Didactically, the ureter's pathway can be divided into abdominal and pelvic; this division takes place at the height of the superior stricture. During its course, the ureter is located in the retroperitoneal loose connective tissue, which ensures the freedom of its movements.

Abdominal Part of the Ureter

It is located in the retroperitoneal space and has two segments: lumbar ureter and iliac ureter.

Lumbar Ureter

- **Posteriorly**: The ureter projects at the top of the transverse processes of the lumbar vertebrae from L2 to L5, resting on and under the psoas major muscle in the iliac fascia; the genitofemoral nerve runs downward and laterally to the posterior superior iliac spine.
- **Anteriorly**: The ureter projects into the abdominal wall, along a line joining the pelvic-renal point and the pubic spine, passing through the upper and middle ureteric points.
  - The renal pelvis point is located in the transpyloric plane, 5 cm from the midline.
  - The superior ureteral point is located on the lateral border of the rectoabdominal muscle, at the height of the umbilical plane (i.e., 4 cm from the umbilicus).
  - The middle ureteral point is the outer third of the line joining the two anterosuperior iliac spines (iliac interspinous line).

The right ureter meets the descending segment of the duodenum and then the ascending mesocolon. It is crossed by the right gonadal (ovarian) vessels at the height of the L3 lumbar vertebra and the right colic and right ileocolic vessels. The left ureter meets the descending mesocolon. It is crossed by the left gonadal vessels at L3 lumbar vertebrae and the left colonic vessels (Figs. 9.33, 9.34, 9.35 and 9.36).

- **Laterally**: After leaving the ureteropelvic junction, the right ureter meets the ascending colon, and the left one, the descending colon.
- **Medially**: The inferior vena cava and the laterocaval lymph nodes are situated medially to the right ureter. The abdominal aorta and lateroaortic lymph nodes lie medially to the left ureter.

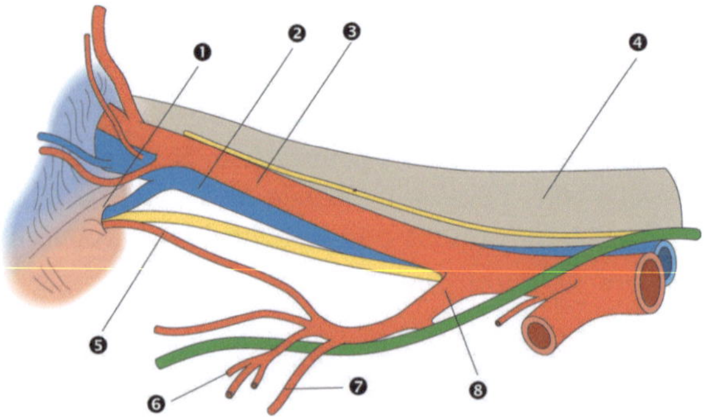

Fig. 9.33 Relationship of the hypogastric nerve to the ureter: (1) obturator fossa, (2) iliac vein, (3) iliac artery, (4) psoas muscle, (5) obturator nerve, (6) inferior vesical artery, (7) upper vesical artery, (8) hypogastric artery

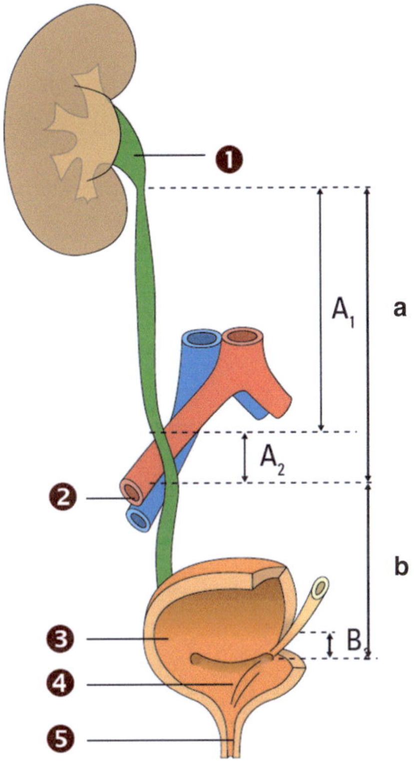

Fig. 9.34 (**a**) Composition of the ureter: (A1) lumbar ureter, (A2) iliac ureter, (**b**) pelvic portion of the ureter, (B1) bladder segment. (1) Renal pelvis, (2) iliac vessels, (3) open bladder, (4) bladder trigone, (5) urethra

Tips and Tricks 5

The transparietal repair of the mesocolon helps contain the loops of the small intestine and improves access to the para-aortic and paracaval spaces. The right ureter is the lateral limit for paracaval lymphadenectomy; the left ureter is the lateral limit for para-aortic lymphadenectomy (Fig. 9.37).

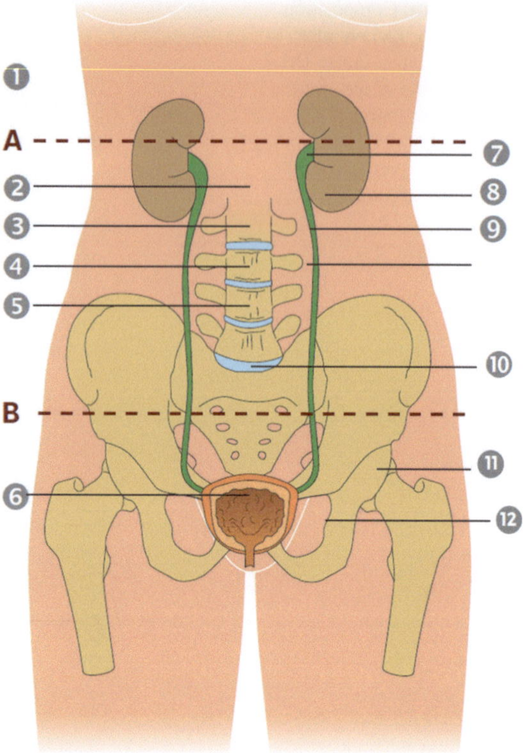

Fig. 9.35 (**a**) Transpyloric plane; (**b**) interspinous iliac plane: (1) right 11th rib, (2) right renal pelvis, (3) right kidney, (4) right ureter, (5) psoas major muscle, (6) bladder, (7) left renal pelvis, (8) left kidney, (9) left ureter, (10) umbilicus, (11) iliac spine, and (12) pubic spine

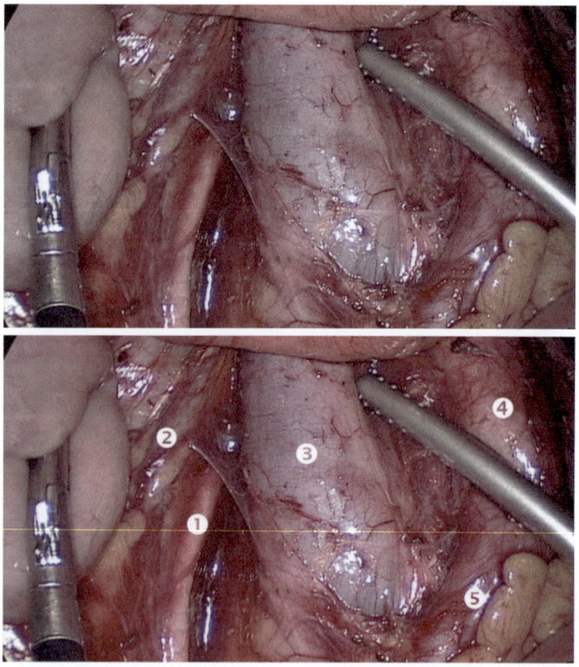

Fig. 9.36 Anatomical relations of the ureter with the aorta, vena cava, and gonadal vessels. (1) ureter (2) gonadal vein (3) vena cava (4) aorta artery (5) common iliac artery

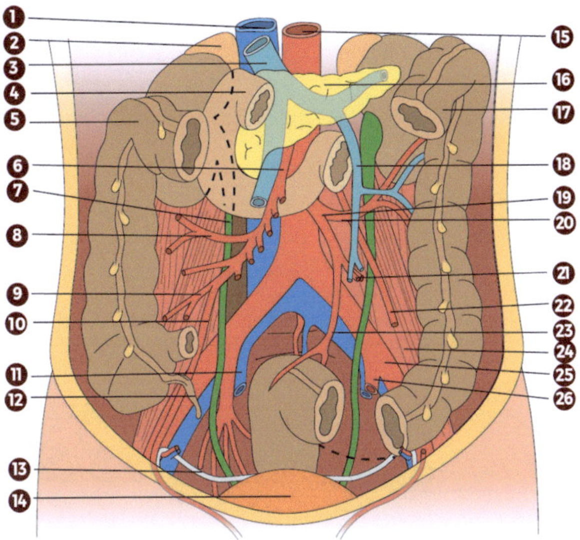

Fig. 9.37 Relationships of the ureters: (1) inferior vena cava, (2) right suprarenal vein, (3) portal vein, (4) duodenum, (5) right colic angle, (6) superior mesenteric artery and vein, (7) right ureter, (8) right colic artery, (9) iliac artery, (10) gonadal artery, (11) right internal iliac artery and vein, (12) appendix, (13) ductus deferens, (14) bladder, (15) abdominal aorta, (16) pancreas, (17) transverse colon, (18) inferior mesenteric vein, (19) inferior mesenteric artery, (20) left colic artery, (21) sigmoid artery, (22) ovarian artery, (23) superior rectal artery, (24) psoas muscle, (25) sigmoid root, (26) left internal iliac artery and vein

Iliac Ureter

- **Posteriorly**: The iliac ureter projects into the posterior superior iliac spine. The right ureter then passes over the external iliac vessels, about 1.5 cm from the origin of the external iliac artery, while the left ureter passes over the termination of the common iliac vessels.
- **Anteriorly**: The right ureter is crossed by the root of the mesenteric and ileocolic vessels, whereas the left ureter is crossed by the sigmoid mesocolon and the sigmoid vessels (Fig. 9.38).

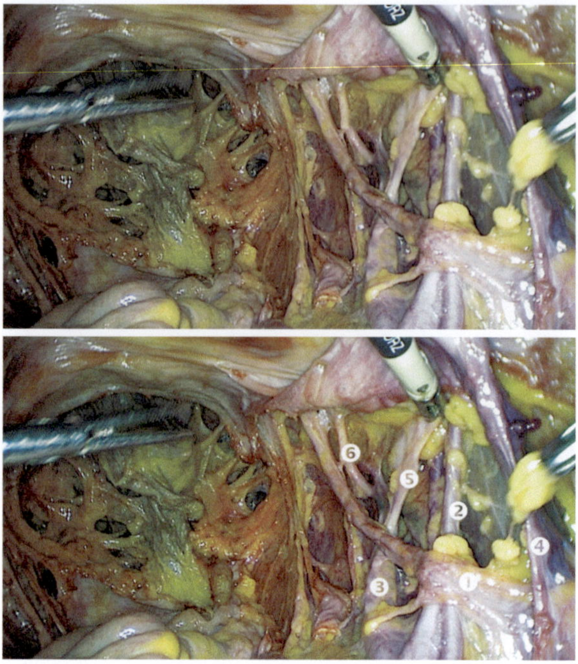

Fig. 9.38 Anatomical relationships of the iliac ureter. (1) Right ureter, (2) right external iliac artery, (3) right internal iliac artery, (4) right pelvic infundibulum, (5) right umbilical artery, (6) right uterine artery

Pelvic Part of the Ureter

It is located in the pelvic retroperitoneal space and has five segments: parietal, retroligamentary, intraligamentary, retrovesical, and vesical.

Parietal Segment

It rests on the lateral pelvic wall, at the anterior margin of the ischial incisure; near the ischial spine, it curves anteriorly. It runs anteromedial to the internal iliac artery, covered by the pelvic peritoneoparietal peritoneum and bordered by the posterior edge of the ovarian fossa (Fig. 9.39).

Tips and Tricks 6
This segment of the ureter is closely related to the pelvic infundibulum. It is therefore a vulnerable anatomical structure when there is hemostasis of this ligament during an oophorectomy.

The right ureter is usually located anterior to the internal iliac artery, while the left ureter is posterior to it. Both, however, can also be medial to this artery.

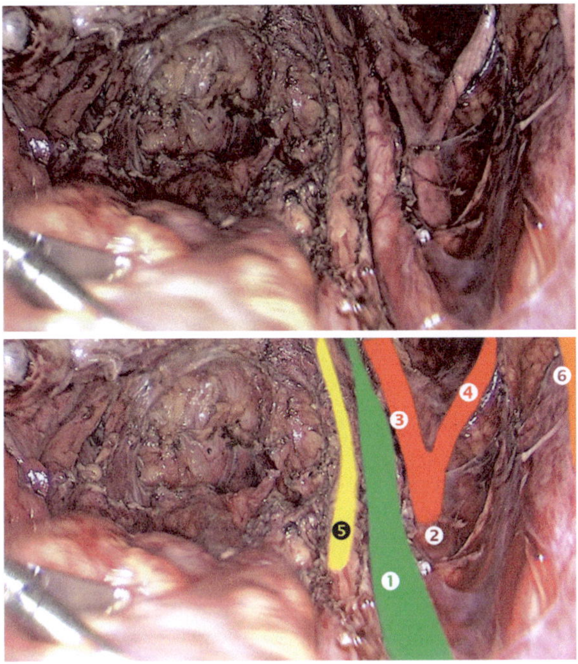

Fig. 9.39 Anatomical relations of the pelvic ureter. (1) Right ureter, (2) internal iliac artery, (3) uterine artery, (4) umbilical artery, (5) right hypogastric nerve, (6) right pelvic infundibulum

- **Laterally**: The segment is related to the internal iliac vein, the obturator nerve, the obturator nerve vessels, and the umbilical, uterine, and vaginal vessels.
- **Medially**: The segment adheres to the deep aspect of the pelvic floor and lies next to the rectum; it separates the pararectal fossa into medial and lateral. It then runs along the posterior border of the ovarian fossa and thus posterior to the ovary and uterine tube.

Retroligamentary Segment

At about 15 mm from the ischial spine, the segment moves anteromedially, passing along the posteromedial border of the uterine artery, and approaches the origin of the uterosacral ligament (Fig. 9.40).

Tips and Tricks 7
The course of this segment may be modified in case of retraction due to endometriosis, sequelae of pelvic inflammatory disease, previous surgery, and presence of intraligamentary myoma. It may then come into contact with the ovary or the uterosacral ligament, and its identification is indispensable before proceeding with surgery.

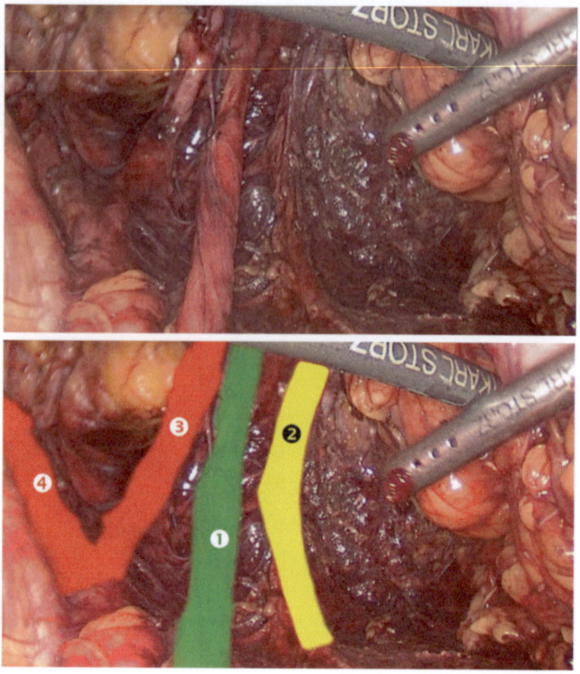

Fig. 9.40 Retroligamentary ureter. (1) Left ureter, (2) left hypogastric nerve, (3) left uterine artery, (4) left umbilical artery

Intraligamentary Segment

This segment of the ureter penetrates under the adventitia of the parametrium, always surrounded by its sheath to preserve its mobility, and crosses posteriorly the uterine artery, moving anteromedially along the posteromedial border of the uterine artery, a little below the uterine isthmus. In the lateral uterine region, it passes between the parametrium and the paracervix. The uterine artery then crosses the ureter 20 mm (23 ± 8) from the isthmus and 15 mm from the lateral fornix of the vagina. It then passes rapidly through the vesicovaginal space, under the vesicouterine ligament, before entering the bladder (Figs. 9.41 and 9.42).

Tips and Tricks 8

Ureteral injuries occur most frequently in this segment during total laparoscopic hysterectomy. To avoid ureteral injury at this site, the uterus should be tractioned cranially and a vaginal delineator used, which will displace the ureter lateral to the ligation of the uterine vessels (Fig. 9.43).

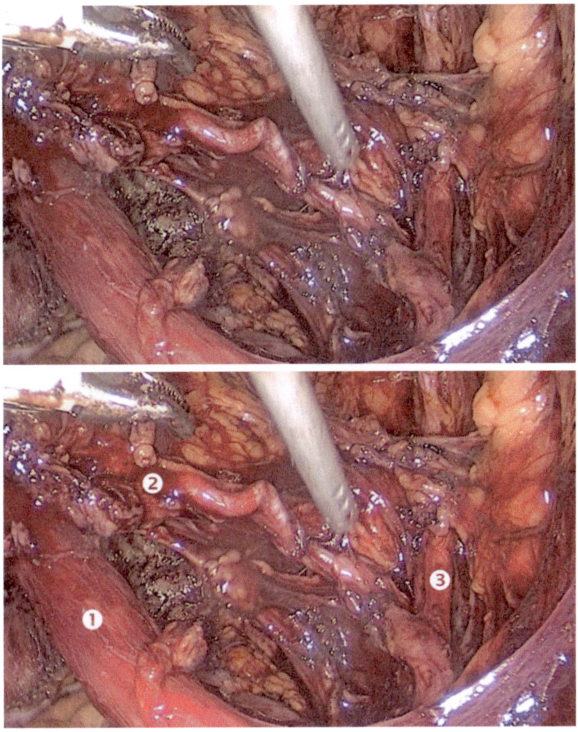

Fig. 9.41 Intraligamentary ureter. (1) Right ureter, (2) right uterine artery, (3) right umbilical artery

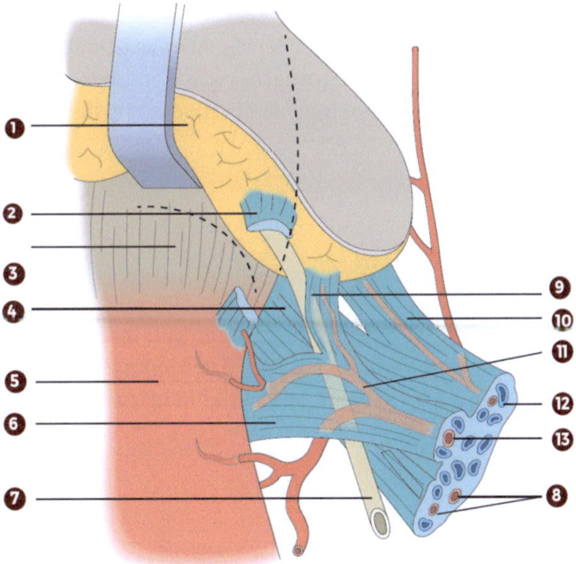

Fig. 9.42 Relationships of the bladder, ureter, and ligaments. (1) Bladder dissected, (2) vesicouterine ligament sectioned, (3) vaginal fornix, (4) paracervix, (5) uterine isthmus, (6) parametrium, (7) right ureter, (8) vaginal arteries, (9) anterior parametrium, (10) lateral bladder ligament, (11) vesicovaginal artery, (12) umbilical artery, and (13) uterine artery

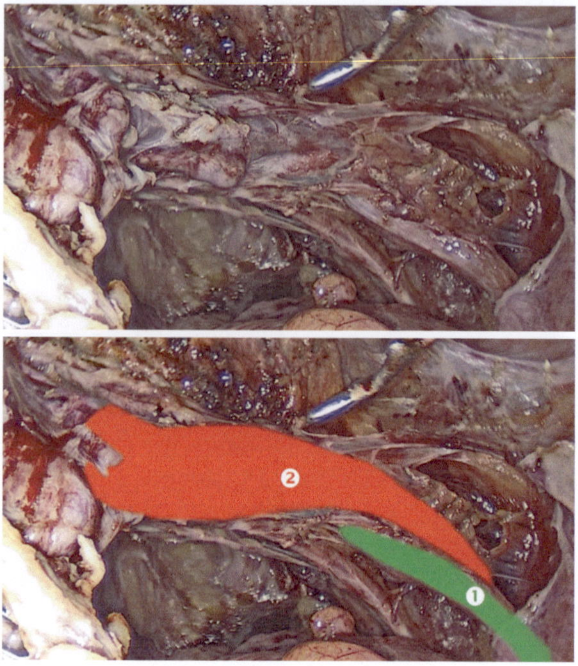

Fig. 9.43 Risk area for ureteral injury in pelvic surgery. (1) Right ureter, (2) right uterine vessels

Retrovesical Segment

This segment of the ureter represents the lateral limit of the Yabuki space. It runs briefly through the vesicovaginal space before entering the bladder. This segment is approximately 10 mm long and is covered by the vesicouterine ligament (Figs. 9.44 and 9.45).

Bladder Segment

It runs obliquely through the bladder wall for 1–2.5 cm. The points of penetration of the ureters are about 4 cm apart. Their openings, at the lateral angles of the bladder trigone, are 2.5 cm apart, and each bladder ostium is elliptical (Fig. 9.45).

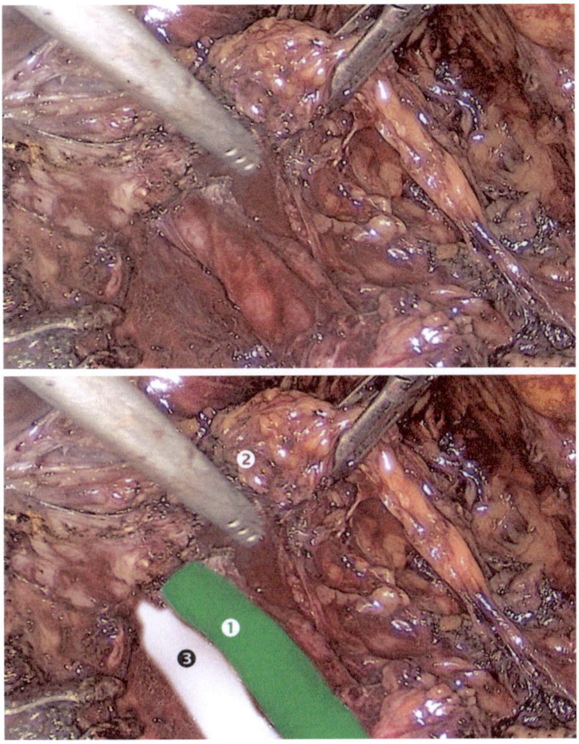

Fig. 9.44 Retrovesical ureter. (1) Right ureter, (2) bladder, (3) Yabuki space

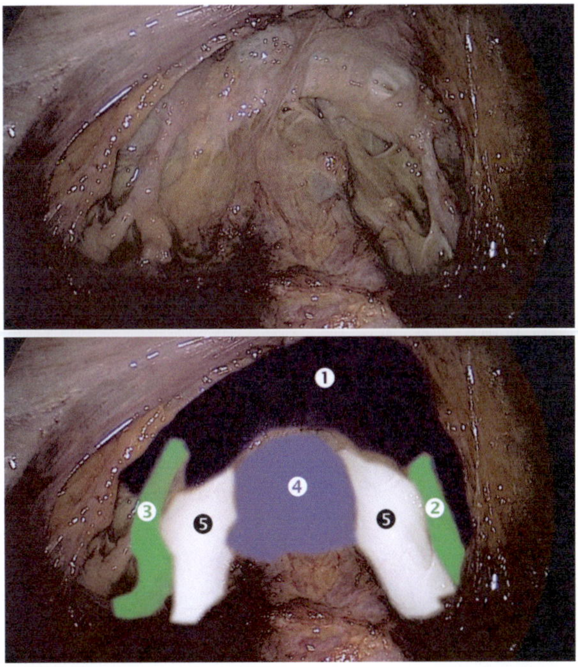

Fig. 9.45 Vesical segment of the ureter. (1) Bladder, (2) right ureter, (3) left ureter, (4) vagina, (5) right and left Yabuki spaces

Bibliography

1. Campbell-Walsh. Urology. 10th Edition. Elsevier Publisher; Herbert S. e Cols.
2. Di Fiore MSH, editor. Atlas de histologia. 7th ed. Rio de Janeiro: Guanabara Koogan; 2005. p. 150.
3. Junqueira LC, Carneiro J, editors. Histologia básica. 8th ed. Rio de Janeiro: Guanabara Koogan; 1981. p. 313–30.
4. Kamina P, Gouazé A. Anatomie clinique: organes urinaires et genitaux, pelvis, coupes du tronc. 2nd ed. Educa Books; 2014. Tome 4.
5. Kraima CA, Derks M, Smit NN, van de Velde CJ, Kenter GG, DeRuiter MC. Careful dissection of the distal ureter is highly important in nerve-sparing radical pelvic surgery: a 3D reconstruction and immunohistochemical characterization of vesical plexus. Int J Gynecol Cancer. 2016;26(5):959–66.
6. Jha S. Ureteric injury: always a guilty verdict? BJOG. 2015;122(4):499.
7. Yabuki Y, Asamoto A, Hoshiba T, Nishimoto H, Nishikawa Y, Nakajima T. Radical hysterectomy: an anatomic evaluation of parametrial dissection. Gynecol Oncol. 2000;77(1):155–63.

Index

H. Salomão Ayroza, P. Ayroza Ribeiro (eds.), *Atlas of Laparoscopic Gynecological Anatomy*, https://doi.org/10.1007/978-3-031-63520-5

Y

MIX
Papier aus verantwortungsvollen Quellen
Paper from responsible sources
FSC® C105338

If you have any concerns about our products,
you can contact us on
ProductSafety@springernature.com

In case Publisher is established outside the EU,
the EU authorized representative is:
Springer Nature Customer Service Center GmbH
Europaplatz 3, 69115 Heidelberg, Germany

Printed by Libri Plureos GmbH
in Hamburg, Germany